Tai Chi Chuan

CLASSICAL YANG STYLE

DR. YANG, JWING-MING

Tai Chi Chuan

CLASSICAL YANG STYLE

THE COMPLETE LONG FORM AND QIGONG

YMAA Publication Center
Wolfeboro, N.H., USA

YMAA Publication Center
  Main Office: PO Box 480
  Wolfeboro, NH 03894
  1-800-669-8892 • www.ymaa.com • info@ymaa.com

ISBN-13: 978-1-59439-200-9
ISBN-10: 1-59439-200-5

10 9 8 7 6 5

Publisher's Cataloging in Publication

Yang, Jwing-Ming, 1946-

  Tai chi chuan, classical Yang style : the complete long form and qigong / Yang, Jwing-Ming. --
2nd ed. -- Wolfeboro, N.H. : YMAA Publication Center, c2010.

    p. ; cm.

    ISBN: 978-1-59439-200-9
    1st ed. issued in 1999 under title: Taijiquan-classical Yang style.
    Includes bibliographical references and index.

    1. Tai chi. 2. Qi (Chinese philosophy) 3. Qi gong. I. Title.
  II. Title: Taijiquan-classical Yang style.

  GV504 .Y373 2010   2010930953
  613.7/148--dc22   1006

Printed in Canada.

Dedication
To a Great Taiji Spiritual Teacher and Father—Jou, Tsung Hwa

Deeply inside, I am experiencing unlimited and uncontrollable sorrow.

Master Jou, such a great taiji teacher, passed away so suddenly from an accident. Although it is so sad to look back now to those happy days when I received your teaching and caring, and I know you would be so disappointed that you cannot fulfill your dream to demonstrate your will and capability of living 150 years, still I can remember how everyone saw you grow younger and younger, your spirit becoming stronger each year. All of us, your students and spiritual children of the Taiji Farm, were convinced that through practicing and understanding taijiquan, we could live for a long time with a healthy body and happy mind, just like you.

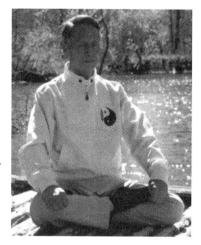

Countless taiji practitioners came each year to your creation, the Taiji Farm, to share your spirit and admire your will power and living force. Like a modern day roundtable of taiji, the Taiji Farm taught us to put aside our differences and petty jealousies and absorb from you your life experience and profound wisdom. Together we learned how to take care of our bodies through practicing taijiquan and qigong, and most importantly of all, we learned that the true journey of our art is the reevaluation of the meaning of our life and an appreciation of the energies that taiji makes visible to our senses. This was your gift to us, to the taiji society, and to the human race.

I feel such a sudden sense of loss, which I know I share with so many. I have appreciated every second we spent together, and I quietly listened to your life philosophy and taiji experience at every opportunity. It is hard for me to accept that you will not be there for further discussions and good-natured arguments about life's different viewpoints. I will miss you whenever the word of taiji appears in my mind. I will never stop talking about the legacy of your life and existence. As I have promised you, I will continue in the promotion of taijiquan, although I know that without you, the burden will be so much greater. I acknowledge my obligation to you, and I promise that as long as I live, I will continue to share what I know without hesitation. Your spirit is my spirit, and the goal of your life is my goal. I only wish the life I can offer, the example I can provide, could be as rich and meaningful as the one that you provided to all of us. I cannot express with words how much I will miss you. But I know that your spirit will live forever and that your name and your story will continue to inspire taiji practitioners far into the future.

Dr. Yang, Jwing-Ming
August 4, 1998

Editorial Notes

Using the book and DVD together. Throughout this book, you will see this icon on certain pages. The DVD icon tells you that companion material is found on the DVD. The larger words indicate the type content (eg. lecture, follow along, etc.), the smaller words indicate the precise menu selection you should choose in the DVD.

Romanization of Chinese Words. This book primarily uses the Pinyin romanization system of Chinese to English. Pinyin is standard in the People's Republic of China, and in several world organizations, including the United Nations. Pinyin, which was introduced in China in the 1950's, replaces the Wade-Giles and Yale systems. In some cases, the more popular spelling of a word may be used for clarity.

Some common conversions:

Pinyin	Also Spelled As	Pronunciation
Qi	Chi	chē
Qigong	Chi Kung	chē gŏng
Qin Na	Chin Na	chĭn nă
Jin	Jing	jĭn
Gongfu	Kung Fu	gŏng foo
Taijiquan	Tai Chi Chuan	tī jē chüén

For more information, please refer to *The People's Republic of China: Administrative Atlas, The Reform of the Chinese Written Language,* or a contemporary manual of style.

The author and publisher have taken the liberty of not italicizing words of foreign origin in this text. This decision was made to make the text easier to read. Please see the comprehensive glossary for definitions of Chinese words.

Contents

Dedication	v
Editorial Notes	vi
Foreword	ix
Preface	xi
Acknowledgments	xv

Chapter 1. General Introduction

1-1. Introduction	1
1-2. Common Knowledge of Chinese Martial Arts	2
A Brief History of Chinese Martial Arts—East and West	3
Northern Styles and Southern Styles	13
Internal Styles and External Styles	15
Martial Power—Jin	18
Hard Styles, Soft-Hard Styles, and Soft Styles	18
Four Categories of Fighting Skills	20
The Dao of Chinese Martial Arts	21
The Real Meaning of Taijiquan	29
1-3. General History of Taijiquan	30
1-4. History of Yang Style Taijiquan	32
1-5. Taijiquan and Health	36
1-6. What is Taijiquan?	38
1-7. Contents of Yang Style Taijiquan Practice	41
1-8. How Do You Learn Taijiquan?	43
1-9. Becoming a Proficient Taijiquan Artist	49

Chapter 2. Qi, Qigong, and Taijiquan

2-1. Introduction	53
2-2. Qi, Qigong, and Man	54
2-3. Categories of Qigong	74
External and Internal Elixirs	76
Schools of Qigong Practice	77

2-4. Qigong Training Theory   84

2-5. Qigong and Taijiquan   98

Chapter 3. Taijiquan Thirteen Postures (Eight Doors and Five Steppings)

3-1. Introduction   107

3-2. Eight Doors (八門)   110

3-3. Five Steppings (五步)   127

Chapter 4. Traditional Yang Style Taijiquan

4-1. Introduction   133

4-2. How to Practice the Taijiquan Sequence   135

4-3. Postures and Taijiquan   136

4-4. Fundamental Eight Stances (*Ji Ben Ba Shi,* 基本八勢)   140

4-5. Taiji Qigong (太極氣功)   145

　　Still Sitting Meditation (Yin)   146
　　Still Standing Meditation (Yang)   147
　　Moving (Yang)   150
　　Stationary (Yin)   160

4-6. Traditional Yang Style Taijiquan   187

Chapter 5. Conclusion   367

Appendix A. Names of Traditional Yang Style Taijiquan Movements   345

Appendix B. Translation and Glossary of Chinese Terms   349

Appendix C. Taijiquan Classical Yang Style DVD   363

Index   365

About the Author   373

Foreword
Grandmaster Jou, Tsung Hwa

In 1985, I wrote a foreword for Dr. Yang when the first edition of his book, *Advanced Yang Style Tai Chi Chuan,* vol. 1, was published. Time flies like an arrow, and already fourteen years have passed. During this period, Dr. Yang has published many more books and videos related to Chinese martial arts and qigong. In addition, he has been offering wushu and qigong seminars and workshops every year in America, Europe, Africa, South America, and the Middle East.

It is said in Chinese society that "Even separated for three days, we should see each other differently." This is really true. Dr. Yang, after more than ten years of further study and in-depth research, together with his abundant teaching experience, has written this new book, *Tai Chi Chuan, Classical Yang Style.* He asked me to write a foreword for him again.

Taijiquan has spread throughout the entire world. Millions of people now practice it. Unfortunately, I believe that almost all the essence of taijiquan has also been gradually lost. Take a look at Wang, Zong-yue's *Taijiquan Classics*, where it is said: "There are many martial art styles. Although the postures are distinguishable from one another, after all, it is nothing more than the strong beating the weak, the slow yielding to the fast. The one with power beats the one without power; the slow hands yield to the fast hands. All this is natural born ability. It is not related to the power that has to be learned." If we look at most of today's taijiquan tournaments, haven't they entered the side door, that is, the wrong path? Again, let us read the following sentence from Wang, Zong-yue, where it is said: "Consider the saying: 'Four ounces repels one thousand pounds.'" It is apparent that this cannot be accomplished by strength. Look, if an eighty- or ninety-year-old man can still defend himself against multiple opponents, it cannot be a matter of speed. Therefore, if we truly wish to learn the real taijiquan, we must free ourselves from the prisons of muscular power (*li*) and speed. Externally, we must learn to use the body movements to replace the hand movements. Internally, we must pursue and cultivate the real contents of essence (*jing*, 精), energy (*qi*, 氣), and spirit (*shen*, 神). To reach this goal and to improve your taijiquan, you are well advised to study Dr. Yang's books, such as *Tai Chi Theory and Power* and this book, *Tai Chi Chuan, Classical Yang Style.*

Jou, Tsung Hwa (1917–1998)
Taiji Farm, Warwick, New York
June 30, 1998

Preface

It has been almost forty years since Master Cheng, Man-ching (鄭曼清) introduced the taijiquan art to the West. Later, when Bruce Lee's (李小龍) motion pictures became popular, they stimulated an interest in studying Chinese culture, especially Chinese martial arts. In addition, President Nixon's visit to the Chinese mainland in the early 1970s led to more intense cultural exchange. The internal healing arts, such as acupuncture and qigong have since become an important part of Western alternative or complementary medicine for illness treatment and prevention.

Qigong is a training system which helps to generate a strong flow of qi (internal energy or known as bioelectricity) inside the body and then circulate it through the entire body. Many martial and non-martial styles of qigong training have been created in the last four thousand years. The most famous martial styles are Taijiquan (太極拳), Baguazhang (八卦掌), Xingyiquan (形意拳), and Liu He Ba Fa (六合八法). These are considered "internal" styles (*nei gong*, 內功 or *nei jia*, 內家), as opposed to "external" styles (*wai jia*, 外家) like Shaolin Gongfu, because they emphasize heavily the development of qi internally. The best known non-martial styles, which emphasize the enhancement of qi circulation to improve health, are Five Animal Sport (*Wu Qin Xi*, 五禽戲), Eight Pieces of Brocade (*Ba Duan Jin*, 八段錦), Da Mo's *Muscle Change Classic (Yi Jin Jing*, 易筋經), and Twelve Postures (*Shi Er Qhuang*, 十二庄).

Taijiquan, which is said to have been created by Zhang, San-feng (張三豐) in the twelfth century, is now the most popular martial qigong style in the world, even though it was shrouded in secrecy until the beginning of 20th century. At present it is widely practiced not only in China and the East, but in the Western world as well.

There are several reasons for the rapid spread of this art. The most important, perhaps, is that the practice of taijiquan can help to calm the mind and relax the body, which are becoming survival skills in today's hectic and stress-filled world. Secondly, since guns are so effective and easy to acquire, taijiquan has been considered less vital for personal self-defense than it used to be. For this reason, more taijiquan masters are willing to share their knowledge with the public. Thirdly, ever since taijiquan was created, it has been proven not only effective for defense, but also useful for improving health and curing a number of illnesses.

Unfortunately, because of this healthful aspect, the deeper theory and practice of taijiquan, especially the martial applications, is being widely ignored. Therefore, the essence of the art has been distorted. Most people today think that taijiquan is not practical for self-defense. To approach the deeper aspects requires much time and patience, and there are very few people willing to make the necessary sacrifices. In addition, a few taijiquan experts are still withholding the secrets of the deeper aspects of the training and not passing down the complete art.

Anyone who practices this art correctly for a number of years will soon realize that taijiquan is not just an exercise for calmness and relaxation. It is a complex and highly developed art. It is one of the most effective methods to understand the way of the Dao and our lives. Through slow meditative movement, taijiquan gives the practitioner a deep inner feeling of enjoyment and satisfaction, which goes beyond that of any other art. This is because taijiquan is smooth, refined, and elegant internally as well as externally. The practitioner can sense the qi (energy or bioelectricity) circulating within his body and can achieve the peaceful mind of meditation. Qi circulation can bring good health and may even help you to reach enlightenment. Furthermore, when a taijiquan practitioner has achieved a high level of qi cultivation and development, he can use this qi in self-defense situations. The principles that taijiquan uses for fighting are quite different from most other martial styles, many of which rely on muscular force. Taijiquan uses the soft to defend against the hard, and weakness to defeat strength. The more you practice, the better you will become, and this defensive capability will grow with age instead of weaken. However, because the martial theory of taijiquan is much deeper and more profound than most other systems, it is much harder to learn and takes a longer time to approach a high level of martial capability. In order to reach an understanding of the deep essence of taijiquan, either spiritually (mentally) or physically, a knowledgeable instructor is very important. Correct guidance from an experienced master can save many years of wandering and useless practice.

Today, more and more taijiquan practitioners are researching and practicing the deeper aspects of taijiquan with the help of the very few qualified experts and/or the limited number of in-depth publications. Many questions have arisen: Which is a good style of taijiquan? How can I tell who is a qualified taijiquan instructor? What is the historical background of the different styles? Which styles can best be applied to my health or to my martial arts training? How is taijiquan different from other qigong practice? How do I generate qi? How do I coordinate my breathing with the qi circulation? How do I use qi in self-defense? What is power (*jin*) and is there more than one kind? How do I train my jin correctly? How does the fighting strategy of taijiquan differ from other styles? All these questions puzzle people even in China today.

I wrote the taijiquan book, *Yang Style Tai Chi Chuan*, published by Unique Publications in 1982. When I wrote this book, it was based on my understanding of taijiquan after twenty years of taijiquan practice. Since then, many years have passed. In these years, my experience and my knowledge have also grown through pondering, studying, practicing, and teaching. In fact, in order to contribute all of my efforts to studying Chinese qigong and internal arts, I resigned from my engineering job in 1984. I then started to write and teach extensively around the world, and my goal through this effort, is that Chinese culture can be introduced to the West more rapidly and correctly. From 1984 until the present, I have written 30 more books and published 60 videotapes and DVDs.

I have gained much knowledge and experience from reading the ancient documents, understanding them, compiling them, and organizing them logically according to my scientific background. I experienced the theories and techniques myself and then published them into books or videotapes. I deeply believe that the ancient secrets must be revealed to the public in order to encourage wide-scale study, research, and development of the Chinese inner arts.

Now, after more than forty-five years of study, I realize that taijiquan is actually a profound training for spiritual enlightenment. Taijiquan was developed in Daoist monasteries nearly one thousand years ago. The final goal of its practice is enlightenment, which all Daoists at all times are pursuing. I realize that the method to reach this goal is understanding the essence of the art through comprehending theory and practice correctly.

Among my writings since 1984, those that relate to taijiquan are:
1. *Tai Chi Theory and Martial Power*, 1986
2. *Tai Chi Chuan Martial Applications*, 1986
3. *The Essence of Taiji Qigong*, 1990
4. *Taiji Chin Na*, 1995
5. *Taiji Sword Classical Yang Style*, 1999
6. *Taijiquan Theory of Dr. Yang, Jwing-Ming*, 2003
7. *Tai Chi Chuan Classical Yang Style* (Revised), 2010
8. *Tai Chi Ball Qigong*, 2010

Over the coming years, I will continue to write more books about taijiquan:
1. *Taiji Saber and Its Applications*
2. *Taiji Fighting Set*
3. *Taiji Pushing Hands*
4. *Taiji Staff and Spear*
5. *Taiji Sparring*

These new books will be based on my personal understanding of taijiquan and my martial arts background. The purpose of these books is to offer you some reference material. You should not treat them as authoritative. Once you do so, you have blocked yourself from further pondering and studying. As we should always remember, the art is alive. As long as it is alive, it should and must grow. Otherwise, it is a dead art and not worth preserving.

In the first chapter of this book, a general discussion will be given, which will provide basic concepts for taijiquan beginners. Next, since taijiquan is considered a branch of qigong training, the relationship between taijiquan and qigong training will be summarized in the second chapter. After you have built a firm understanding in taijiquan theory from the first two chapters, the most important foundation of taijquan practice—the thirteen postures—will be discussed in the third chapter. Finally, the traditional Yang Style Taijiquan form will be introduced in the fourth chapter. If you wish to understand more deeply both theory and martial applications, you should refer to the books previously listed.

Acknowledgments

Thanks to Mei-Ling Yang, and Ramel Rones for general help with the work. Thanks to the editor (first edition), James O'Leary, and special thanks to Erik Elsemans, Chris Hartgrove, and Chris Fazzio for proofing the manuscript and contributing many valuable suggestions and discussions. Thanks to Dolores Sparrow for proof reading and for the editorial style guidance of this revised edition, and thanks to Axie Breen for the cover design and interior layout model. Thanks also to Tim Comrie for typesetting.

CHAPTER 1

General Introduction

概論

1-1. Introduction

Even though Chinese martial arts were imported into Western society more than fifty years ago, many questions still remain. The most common and confusing questions today are the following: Where does the style I am learning come from? What are its theoretical roots and foundation? How good are the styles which I am practicing? What are the differences between the internal styles and the external styles? What are the differences between the southern styles and northern styles? How do we define hard, soft-hard, and soft styles? How is Japanese karate different from Korean taekwondo, and how are these styles different from Chinese martial arts? How do these styles relate to each other? What is martial arts qigong? How different is this qigong from other schools of qigong, such as medical qigong, scholar qigong, and religious qigong?

In order to answer these questions, you must first study and understand the history of Chinese martial arts. Furthermore, you should search and comprehend its theoretical roots and cultural background. Knowledge of its past history and an understanding of its roots will enable you to appreciate the consequences that exist today.

Taijiquan, its theoretical roots and the concept of yin and yang itself, can be traced back four thousand years. From this root, the essence of taijiquan originated. Specifically, the style was created in the Daoist monastery of Wudang Mountain (武當山), Hubei province (湖北). The original motivation behind taijiquan creation was twofold: self-defense and spiritual cultivation.

Taijiquan is a slow and relaxed moving meditation. Through practicing taijiquan, you are able to calm your mind, locate your spiritual center, and consequently find your entire being. Moreover, from the relaxed moving exercises, you can bring your physical body to an ultimate level of relaxation and natural ease. This can result in smooth qi (inner energy or bioelectricity) and smooth blood circulation. This is the key to maintaining health and recovering from sickness.

Since taijiquan's revelation to the Chinese public in 1926 by Yang, Chen-fu (楊澄甫) in Nanking Central Guoshu Institute (南京中央國術館), it has been widely welcomed and has gradually become one of the most effective ways of self-healing exercises or qigong (氣功) in China. Unfortunately, it was also due to its popularity and emphasis on health promotion that the martial essence of taijiquan has been gradually lost. The forms have been changed and the quality has been worsened. The essence of every movement is no longer of importance to the general public.

When Taijiquan was introduced into Western society during the 1960s by Cheng, Man-ching (鄭曼清), it was already popular in China. Before long, it had become a very popular exercise in the West. Today, it is commonly recognized that practicing taijiquan is able to help with many problems such as hypertension, high blood pressure, balance and stability, heart problems, lung-related illness, stomach problems, and many others. It is understood that through these relaxed movements, you can reach a state of self-relaxation and healing. The benefits of practicing taijiquan are reported again and again. In fact, many healthcare providers started encouraging their clients to practice taijiquan, and beginning in the 1990s, some insurance companies even began to contribute to the expense of learning in order to further the health and vitality of their members.

Since 1973 when President Nixon visited mainland China and opened the gate of China, many taijiquan masters have immigrated to the United States. Now, the Western taijiquan practitioners are starting to realize there are many styles of taijiquan that have originated from the same theoretical root. Unfortunately, two major parts of taijiquan essence are still missing. These two are the martial root of taijiquan and its relationship with qigong. The motivation for writing this book is to provide modern taijiquan practitioners with an understanding of the relationship between taijiquan and qigong. After studying this material, if you are interested in knowing more about the taiji qigong and martial applications of taijiquan, you may refer to these books: *The Essence of Taiji Qigong, Tai Chi Theory and Martial Power*, and *Tai Chi Chuan Martial Applications*, published by YMAA.

In the first chapter of this book, common martial arts knowledge will be introduced followed by a brief history of taijiquan. The meaning of taijiquan and its training guidelines, particularly that of Yang style, will then be discussed. After you are familiar with these general concepts, the most important essence of taijiquan will be introduced: the relationship between qi and taijiquan. This relationship will be explored in Chapter 2 through the means of taiji qigong. The third chapter will cover the external manifestations of the theory, as well as the external root of basic taijiquan movement, the thirteen postures. Finally, the traditional Yang Style Long Form of Taijiquan will be introduced in Chapter 4.

I believe that through effort and by coordinating both theory and the practice of qigong and external training, you can glimpse and begin to appreciate the profound essence of taijiquan, instead of just learning how to copy the forms.

1-2. Common Knowledge of Chinese Martial Arts

Since taijiquan is an internal martial art, in order to understand its origin and historical background, it would be wise for us first to learn some of the common knowledge behind Chinese martial arts.

In this section, we will explain some essential points, such as the general definition of Chinese martial arts, martial arts history, and comparisons of the different styles. Hopefully, through study of this section, you will gain a better understanding of Chinese martial arts.

This section will first survey Chinese martial arts history and its cultural relationship with neighboring countries in the past. From this survey, you will obtain a general concept of how this art developed. Then, we will trace how this art was developed and how it became popular today in the West. From this, you can analyze the style you are learning.

Next, we will summarize some of the important concepts in Chinese martial society, such as the differences between internal styles and external styles, how the southern styles developed differently from the northern styles, the definition of the hard, soft-hard, and soft styles, the four fighting categories of Chinese martial arts, and the Dao of Chinese martial arts.

General Definition of Chinese Martial Arts. The word for martial in Chinese is *wu* (武). This word is constructed from two Chinese words *zhi* (止) and *ge* (戈). *Zhi* means to stop, to cease, or to end and *ge* means spear, lance, or javelin, and implies "general weapons." From this you can see that the original meaning of martial arts in China is "to stop or to end the usage of weapons" (止戈為武).

The name of Chinese martial arts has been changed from period to period. However, the most commonly-recognized name is *wuyi* (武藝). Wuyi means "martial arts" and includes all categories of martial arts which are related to battle, such as archery, horse riding, dart throwing, the design and manufacture of weapons, armor, or even the study of battlefield tactics.

In actual combat, individual fighting techniques are called *wushu* (武術), which means "martial techniques." This implies the techniques that can be used to stop a fight. This means that Chinese martial arts were created to stop fighting instead of starting it. It is defensive instead of offensive. This concept was very different from that which was obtained by Western society in the 1960s. At that time, Chinese martial arts were commonly lumped together under the term "kung fu" (功夫) and were considered solely as fighting skills. In fact, the Chinese meaning of kung fu (*gong*, 功) means energy and (*fu*, 夫) means time. If you are learning or doing something that takes a great deal of time and effort to accomplish, then it is called kung fu (*gongfu*). This can be learning how to play the piano, to paint, to learn martial arts, or complete any difficult task that takes time and patience.

A Brief History of Chinese Martial Arts—East and West
It is impossible to survey the history of all the existing Chinese martial arts in a single book. There are two reasons for this:
1. Since ancient times, there have probably been more than five thousand martial styles created in China. After long periods of testing and experimenting in martial arts society or in battle, the arts of quality continued to survive, while those that were ineffective slowly became disregarded and died out. According to recent reports out of China, there could be more than one

thousand martial styles which still exist and are practiced there, each with its own several hundreds or even thousands of years of history. It is not possible to collect all of this history for every style.

2. Since most martial artists in ancient times were illiterate, the history of each style was often passed down orally. After a few generations, the history would become like a story. In fact, there are only a few existing famous styles, such as Taijiquan, Shaolin Quan, and some military martial styles, in which the history was documented in writing. Moreover, the documentation for these styles was extremely scarce and its accuracy often questioned.

Therefore, in this sub-section, I would first like to briefly summarize a portion of the known history of the East. Then, based on my personal observations of the evolution of Chinese martial arts in the West for the past 35 years, I will offer my observations and conclusions on Chinese martial arts in Western society.

Historical Survey of Chinese Martial Arts. Chinese martial arts probably started long before history was recorded. Martial techniques were discovered or created during the long epoch of continuous conflict between humans and animals or between different tribes of humans themselves. From these battles, experiences were accumulated and techniques discovered that were passed down from generation to generation.

Later, with the invention of weapons—whether sticks, stones, or animal bones—different types and shapes of weapons were invented, until eventually metal was discovered. At the beginning, metal weapons were made from copper, tin, or bronze, and after thousands of years of metallurgical development, the weapons became stronger and sharper. Following the advancement of weapon fabrication, new fighting techniques were created. Different schools and styles originated and tested one another.

Many of these schools or styles created their forms by imitating different types of fighting techniques from animals (e.g., tiger, panther, monkey, bear, or snake), birds (e.g., eagle, crane, or chicken), or insects (e.g., praying mantis). The reason for imitating the fighting techniques of animals came from the belief that animals possessed natural talents and skills for fighting in order to survive in the harsh natural environment. The best way to learn effective fighting techniques was by studying and imitating these animals. For example, the sharp spirit of the eagle was adopted, the pouncing, fighting of the tiger and the eagle's strong claws were imitated, and the attacking motions of the crane's beak and wings were copied.

Since the martial techniques first developed in very ancient times, they gradually became part of Chinese culture. The philosophy of these fighting arts and culture has in turn been influenced by other elements of Chinese culture. Therefore, the yin and yang taiji theory was merged into techniques, and the bagua eight trigrams concept was blended into fighting strategy and skills.

Chinese culture initially developed along the banks of the Yellow River (黃河) (Figure 1-1). After many thousands of years, this culture spread so widely that it eventually reached every corner of Asia. China is called Central Kingdom (*Zhong Guo,* 中國) by its neighboring countries. The reason for this was because China possessed a much longer history in artistic, spiritual, religious, and scholastic fields, as well as many others; Chinese history stretches back more than seven thousand years. To the neighboring countries, China was an advanced cultural center from which they could learn and absorb cultural forms. Over thousands of years, the Chinese people themselves have immigrated to every corner of Asia, carrying with them their arts and customs. From this prolonged exchange, Chinese culture became the cultural foundation of many other Asian countries. Naturally, Chinese martial arts, which were considered a means of defense and fighting in battle, have also significantly influenced other Asian societies.

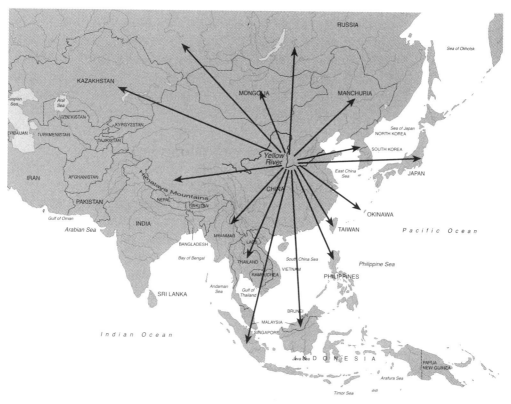

Figure 1-1. China and Her Neighboring Countries

However, since the martial arts techniques and the methods of training could decide victory or defeat in battle, almost all Chinese martial arts were considered highly secret between countries, and even between different stylists. In ancient times, it was so important to protect the secret of a style that usually a master would kill a student who had betrayed him. It is no different from a modern government protecting its technology for purposes of national security. For this reason, the number of Chinese martial techniques that were revealed to outside countries was limited. Often, when an outlander came to China to learn martial arts, he first had to obtain the trust of a master. Normally, this would take more than ten years of testing from the teacher in order to achieve mutual understanding. Moreover, the techniques exported were still limited to the surface level. The deeper essence of the arts, especially the internal cultivation of qi and how to apply it to the martial techniques, normally remained a deep secret.

For example, it is well known in China that in order to compete and survive in a battle against other martial styles, each martial style must contain four basic categories of fighting techniques. They are kicking (*ti*, 踢), hand striking (*da*, 打), wrestling (*shuai*, 摔), and joint locking or seizing and controlling techniques (*qin na* or *chin na*) (*na*, 拿). When these techniques were exported to Japan, they splintered over time to become many styles. For example, punching and kicking became karate, wrestling became judo, and qin na became jujitsu. Actually, the essence and secret of Chinese martial arts developed in Buddhist and Daoist monasteries were not completely revealed to Chinese lay society until the Qing dynasty (清, A.D. 1644-1912). This secret has been revealed to Western countries only in the last three decades.

There was an extreme scarcity of documentation before A.D. 500 with regard to martial arts organization and techniques. The most complete documents that exist today concern the Shaolin Temple (少林寺). However, since Shaolin martial arts significantly influence the overwhelming majority of Chinese martial arts society today (and this includes taijiquan), we should be able to obtain a fairly accurate concept from studying Shaolin history. The following is a brief summary of Shaolin history according to recent publications by the Shaolin Temple itself.

The Shaolin Temple. Buddhism traveled to China from India during the Eastern Han Ming emperor period (東漢明帝) (A.D. 58-76). Chinese emperors were given special names upon their coronation; it was customary to address them by this name, followed by the title "emperor." Several hundred years later, as several emperors became sincere Buddhists, Buddhism became very respected and popular in China. It is estimated that by A.D. 500, there probably existed more than ten thousand Buddhist temples. In order to absorb more Buddhist philosophy during these five hundred years, some monks were sent to India to study Buddhism and bring back Buddhist classics. Naturally, some Indian monks were also invited to China to preach.

According to one of the oldest books *Deng Feng County Recording* (*Deng Feng Xian Zhi*, 登封縣志), a Buddhist monk named Batuo (跋陀) came to China to preach Buddhism in A.D. 464 Deng Feng is the county in Henan Province where the Shaolin Temple was eventually located.[1]

Thirty-one years later, A.D. 495, the Shaolin Temple was built by the order of Wei Xiao Wen emperor (魏孝文帝) (A.D. 471-500) for Batuo's preaching. Therefore, Batuo can be considered the first chief monk of the Shaolin Temple. However, there is no record regarding how and what Batuo passed down by way of religious qigong practice. There is also no record of how or when Batuo died.

However, the most influential person in this area was the Indian monk Da Mo (達摩). Da Mo, whose last name was Sardili (刹地利) and who was also known as Bodhidarma, was once the prince of a small tribe in southern India. He was of the Mahayana school of Buddhism and was considered by many to have been a *bodhisattva*, that is, an enlightened being who had renounced nirvana in order to save others. From the fragments of historical records, it is believed that he was born about A.D. 483.

Da Mo was invited to China to preach by the Liang Wu emperor (梁武帝). He arrived in Canton, China in A.D. 527 during the third year of the reign of the Wei Xiao Ming emperor Xiao Chang (魏孝明帝孝昌) (A.D. 516-528) or the Liang Wu emperor (梁武帝) (A.D. 502-557). When the emperor decided he did not like Da Mo's Buddhist theory, the monk withdrew to the Shaolin Temple. When Da Mo arrived, he saw that the priests were weak and sickly, so he shut himself away to ponder the problem. When he emerged after nine years of seclusion, he wrote two classics: the *Muscle/Tendon Changing Classic (Yi Jin Jing*, 易筋經) and the *Marrow/Brain Washing Classic (Xi Sui Jing*, 洗髓經).

The *Yi Jin Jing* taught the priests how to build their qi to an abundant level and use it to improve health and change their physical bodies from weak to strong. After the priests practiced the *Yi Jin Jing* exercises, they found that not only did they improve their health, they also greatly increased their strength. When this training was integrated into the martial arts forms, it increased the effectiveness of their martial techniques. This change marked one more step in the growth of the Chinese martial arts: martial arts qigong.

The *Xi Sui Jing* taught the priests how to use qi to clean their bone marrow and strengthen their immune systems, as well as how to nourish and energize the brain, helping them to attain Buddhahood. Because the *Xi Sui Jing* was hard to understand and practice, the training methods were passed down secretly to only a very few disciples in each generation. Da Mo died in the Shaolin Temple in A.D. 536, and was buried on Xiong Er Mountain (熊耳山). If you are interested in knowing more about *Yi Jin Jing* and *Xi Sui Jing*, please refer to my book, *Qigong The Secret of Youth, Da Mo's Muscle/Tendon Changing and Marrow/Brain Washing Classics* published by YMAA.

During the revolutionary period between the Sui dynasty (隋) and the Tang dynasty (唐), in the fourth year of Tang Gao Zu Wu De (唐高祖武德四年), A.D. 621, Qin king Li, Shi-ming (秦王李世民) had a serious battle with Zheng king Wang, Shi-chong (鄭帝王世充). When the situation was urgent for the Qin king, thirteen Shaolin monks assisted him against the Zheng. Later, Li, Shi-ming became the first emperor of the Tang dynasty (A.D. 618-907), and he rewarded the Shaolin Temple with 40 *qing* (about 600 acres) of land. He also permitted the Temple to own and train its own soldiers. At that time, in order to protect the wealthy property of the Shaolin Temple from bandits, martial arts training was a necessity for the monks. The priest martial artists in the temple were called "monk soldiers" (*seng bing*, 僧兵). Their responsibility, other than studying Buddhism, was training in the martial arts to protect the property of the Shaolin Temple. For nearly three hundred years, the Shaolin Temple legally owned its own martial arts training organization.

During the Song dynasty (A.D. 960-1278) the monks of the Shaolin Temple continued to gather more martial skills from outside sources. They blended these arts into the Shaolin training. During this period, one of the most famous Shaolin martial monks, Jueyuan, (覺遠) traveled around the country in order to learn and absorb high levels of martial skill into Shaolin training. He went to Lan Zhou (蘭州) to meet one of the most famous martial artists, Li Sou (李叟). From Li Sou, he met Li Sou's friend, Bai, Yu-feng (白玉峰) and his son. Later, all four returned to the Shaolin Temple and studied together. After ten years of mutual study and research, Li Sou left Shaolin; Bai, Yu-feng and his son decided to stay and became monks. Bai, Yu-feng's monk's name was Qiu Yue Chan Shi (秋月禪師) who was known for his bare hand fighting and narrow blade sword techniques. According to the book *Shaolin Temple Record* (少林寺志), he developed the existing eighteen Buddha hands techniques into one hundred and seventy-three techniques. Moreover, he compiled the existing techniques contained within Shaolin and wrote the book, *The Essence of the Five Fists* (五拳精要). This book included and discussed the practice methods and applications of the five fist animal patterns. The five animals included dragon, tiger, snake, panther, and crane. This record confirms that the five animal patterns martial skills already existed for some time in the Shaolin Temple.

From the same source, it is recorded that in the Yuan dynasty (元代), in the year A.D. 1312, the monk Da Zhi (大智和尚) came to the Shaolin Temple from Japan. After he studied Shaolin martial arts (bare hands and staff) for nearly thirteen years A.D., in1324, he returned to Japan and spread Shaolin gongfu to the Japanese martial arts society. Later, in A.D. 1335, another Buddhist monk named Shao Yuan (邵元和尚) came to Shaolin from Japan. He mastered calligraphy, painting, chan theory (i.e., *Zen*, 忍) and Shaolin gongfu during his stay. He returned to Japan in A.D. 1347 and was considered and regarded as "country spirit" (*guohuen*, 國魂) by the Japanese people. This helps to confirm that Shaolin martial techniques were imported into Japan for at least seven hundred years.

Later, when the Manchus took over China and established the Qing dynasty, in order to prevent the Han race (pre-Manchurian Chinese) from rebelling against the government, martial arts training was forbidden from (A.D. 1644 to 1911). In order to preserve the arts, Shaolin martial techniques spread to laymen society. All martial arts training in the Shaolin Temple was carried out secretly during this time. Moreover, the Shaolin monk soldiers decreased in number from thousands to only a few hundred. According to *Shaolin Historical Records*, the Shaolin Temple was burned three times from the time it was built until the end of the Qing dynasty A.D. 1911. Because the Shaolin Temple owned such a large amount of land and had such a long history, it became one of the richest temples in China. It was also because of this that Shaolin had been attacked many times by bandits. In ancient China, bandit groups could number more than ten thousand; robbing and killing in Chinese history was very common.

During Qing's ruling period, the most significant influence on the Chinese people occurred during A.D. 1839-1840, (Qing Dao Guang's twentieth year, 清道光二十年). This was the year that the Opium War between Britain and China broke out. After losing this war, China started to realize that traditional fighting methods, i.e., using traditional weapons and bare hands, could not defeat an opponent armed with guns. The values of the traditional Chinese culture were questioned. The traditional dignity and pride of the Chinese people started to waver, and doubt that China was the center of the world began to arise. Their confidence and trust in self-cultivation weakened, and this situation continued to worsen. In A.D. 1900 (in Qing Guangxu's twentieth year, 清光緒二十年), when the joint forces of the eight powerful countries of Britain, France, the United States, Japan, Germany, Austria, Italy, and Russia occupied Beijing in the wake of the Boxer Rebellion, Chinese dignity was degraded to its lowest point. Many Chinese started to despise their own culture, which had been built and developed on principles of spiritual cultivation and humanistic morality. They believed that these traditional cultural foundations could not save their country. Instead, they needed to learn from the West. Chinese minds started to open and guns and cannons became more popular.

After 1911, the Qing dynasty fell in a revolution led by Dr. Sun, Yat-sen (孫中山). Due to the mind-expanding influence of their earlier occupation, the value of traditional Chinese martial arts was reevaluated, and their secrets were gradually revealed to the public. From the 1920s to the 1930s, many martial arts books were published. However, this was also the Chinese Civil War period, during which Chiang, Kai-shek (蔣介石) tried to unify the country. Unfortunately, in 1928, there was a battle in the area of the Shaolin Temple, and the temple was burned for the last time by warlord Shi, You-san's (石友三) military. The fire lasted for more than forty days, and all the major buildings were destroyed. The most priceless books and records on martial arts were also burned and lost.

It was also during this period that, in order to preserve Chinese martial arts, President Chiang, Kai-shek ordered the establishment of the Nanking Central Guoshu Institute (南京中央國術館) at Nanking in 1926. For this institute, many famous masters and practitioners were recruited. The traditional name for martial techniques (*wushu*, 武術) was renamed Chinese martial techniques (*zhong guo wushu*, 中國武術) or simply country techniques (*guoshu*, 國術). This was the first time in Chinese history that under the government's power, all the practitioners of the different styles of Chinese martial arts sat down and shared their knowledge. Unfortunately, after only three generations (that is, the time it takes to train a group of students from novice to advanced), World War II started in 1937 and all training was discontinued.

In 1945, after the Second World War, mainland China was taken over by communists. Under communist rule, all religions were forbidden. Naturally, all Shaolin training was also prohibited. Later, under the communist party, wushu training was established by the Chinese Athletic Committee (中國國家体委). In this organization, the communist party purposely deleted portions of the martial training and their applications in order to discourage possible unification of martial artists against the government. From Chinese history, it is well known that almost all revolutions that succeeded did so due to the unification of Chinese martial artists. Unfortunately, only the aesthetic and acrobatic parts of the arts were preserved and developed. Eventually, it became known that the athletes trained during this period did not know how to fight or defend themselves. Performance was the goal of this preservation. This situation was not changed until the late 1980s. After the communist government realized that the essence of the arts—martial training and applications—started to die out following the death of many traditional masters, the traditional training was once again encouraged. Regrettably, many masters had already been killed during the so-called "Cultural Revolution," and many others had lost their trust of the communist party and were not willing to share their knowledge.

In order to bring Chinese wushu into Olympic competition, China expended a great deal of effort to promote it. With this motivation, the Shaolin Temple again received attention from the government. New buildings were constructed and a grand hotel was built. The Shaolin Temple became an important tourist attraction. In addition, many training activities and programs were created for interested martial artists around the world. Moreover, in order to preserve the dying martial arts, a group called the Martial Arts Investigation Team (武術挖掘小組) was organized by the government. The mission of this team was to search for surviving old, traditional masters and to put their knowledge in books or videos.

This situation was very different in Taiwan. When Chiang, Kai-shek retreated from mainland China to Taiwan, he brought with him many well-known masters, who passed down the Chinese martial arts there. Traditional methods of training were maintained and the arts were preserved in the traditional way. Unfortunately, due to modern lifestyles, not many youngsters were willing to dedicate the necessary time and patience for the training. Therefore, the level of the arts reached the lowest level in Chinese martial history. Many secrets of the arts, which were the accumulation of thousand years of human experience, rapidly died out. In order to preserve the arts, the remaining secrets began to be revealed to the general public and even to Western society. It is good that books and videotapes have been widely used both in mainland China and Taiwan to preserve the arts.

Many of the Chinese martial arts were also preserved in Hong Kong, Indo-China, Malaysia, the Philippines, Indonesia, Japan, and Korea. It is now widely recognized that in order to preserve the arts, all interested Chinese martial artists should be united and share their knowledge openly.

If we look back at the martial arts history in China, we can see that in the early 1900s, the Chinese martial arts still carried on the traditional ways of training. The level of the arts remained high. But from then until World War II, the level of arts degenerated very rapidly. From the war until now, in my opinion, the arts have not reached even one-half of their traditional levels.

All of us should understand that today's martial arts training is no longer useful for war. The chances for using it in self-defense have also been reduced to a minimum compared to that of ancient times. This is an art whose knowledge has taken the Chinese thousands of years to accumulate. What remains for us to learn is the spirit of the arts. From learning these arts, we can discipline ourselves and promote our understanding of life to a higher spiritual level. From learning the arts, we can maintain healthy conditions in our physical and mental bodies.

A History of Chinese Martial Arts in the West. If we trace back the history of Chinese martial arts in Western society, we can see that even before the 1960s, karate and judo had already been imported into Western society and had been popular for nearly twenty years (Figure 1-2). Yet most Chinese culture was still isolated and conservatively hidden in communist China. Later, when Bruce Lee's (李小龍) motion pictures were introduced to the public, they presented a general concept of Chinese kung fu (*gongfu*), which stimulated and excited Western oriental martial arts society

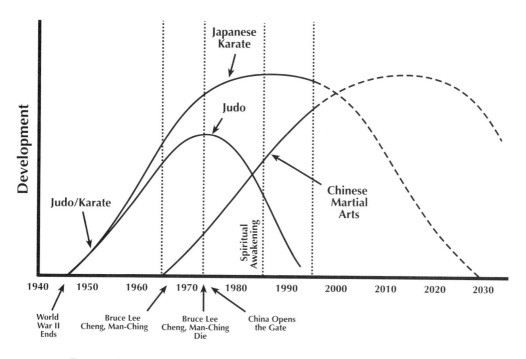

Figure 1-2. History of Oriental Martial Arts Developed in Western Society.

to a great level. This significantly influenced the young baby-boomer generation in America. During the period of unrest in America during the war in Vietnam, these films provided both a heroic figure for young Americans to admire, as well as a positive Asian personality with whom they could easily relate. Many troubled youngsters started to abuse drugs during this time, perhaps as an attempt either to escape from the reality of a capricious world or to prove to themselves that they had courage and bravery. Under these conditions, Bruce Lee's movies brought to the young generation both excitement and challenge. Since then, Chinese kung fu has become popular in Western society.

At that time the term "kung fu" was widely misinterpreted to mean "fighting," and very few people actually knew that its meaning is "hard work," an endeavor which normally requires a person to take a great deal of time and energy to accomplish. It was even more amazing that after the young generation saw these movies, they started to mix the concepts from what they had learned from the movies with the background they had learned from karate, judo, aikido, and their own imagination. Since then, a new generation of American styles of Chinese kung fu originated, and hundreds of new kung fu styles have been created. These practitioners did not know that the movies they had watched were a modified version of Chinese martial arts derived from Bruce Lee's Chinese martial art, Wing Chun (*Yongchun*) Style. For cinematic purposes, it had been mixed with the concepts of karate, Western boxing, and some kicking techniques developed by Bruce Lee himself. At that time, there were only a very few traditional Chinese martial arts instructors residing in the West, and even fewer were teaching.

During this period Cheng, Man-ching (鄭曼清) brought the concept of one of the

Chinese internal martial arts, taijiquan, to the West. Through his teaching and publications, a limited portion of the public finally grasped the correct concepts of a small branch of Chinese martial arts. This again brought to Western society a new paradigm for pursuing Chinese martial arts. Taijiquan gradually became popular. However, the American style of Chinese kung fu still occupied the major market of the Chinese martial arts society in America.

When President Nixon levered open the tightly closed gate to mainland China in the early 1970s, the Western public finally had a better chance to understand Chinese culture. From the more frequent communications, acupuncture techniques for medical purposes, used in China for more than four thousand years, were exported to the West. In addition, Chinese martial arts also slowly migrated westward. The period from the 1970s to the early 1980s can be regarded as an educational time for this cultural exchange. While the Americans' highly developed material sciences entered China, Chinese traditional medical and spiritual sciences, qigong, started to influence American society.

During this period, many Western doctors went to China to study traditional Chinese medicine, while many Chinese students and professors came to America to study material sciences. In addition to this, many American Chinese martial artists started to awaken and reevaluate the art they had learned during the 1960s. Many of the younger generation went to China to explore and learn directly from Chinese martial arts masters. It was a new and exciting period in the late 1970s and early 1980s. Because of the large market and new demand, many Chinese martial artists poured into America from China, Taiwan, Hong Kong, and Indo-China. However, this generated a great force that opposed the American styles of Chinese kung fu created during the 1960s. The Chinese martial arts society was then divided more or less against each other. Moreover, martial artists who came from different areas of Asia also grouped themselves into camps against each other. Coordination and mutual support in Chinese martial arts for tournaments or demonstration was almost nonexistent.

In the late 1980s, many American Chinese martial artists trained in China became aware of some important facts. They discovered that what they had learned emphasized only the beauty of the arts, and that martial purposes, the essence and root of the arts, were missing. They started to realize that what they had learned were arts that had been modified by the Chinese communist party in the 1950s. All of the actual combative Chinese martial arts were still hidden from lay society and were passed down conservatively in traditional ways. Many of these artists were disappointed and started to modify what they had learned, transforming their techniques into more martial forms, while many others started to learn from martial artists from Taiwan, Hong Kong, and Indo-China.

When mainland China finally realized this in the late 1980s, they decided to bring the martial purpose once again into the martial arts. Unfortunately, the roots of the beautiful martial arts that had been developed for nearly forty years were already firm and very hard to change. As mentioned earlier, the situation was especially unacceptable when it was realized that many of the older generation of martial artists had been either killed by the Red Guard during the "Cultural Revolution" or had died of old age. Those who controlled the martial and political power and could change the wrong path into the correct one had already built successful lives in the "beauty arts." The government therefore established the Martial Arts Investigating Team (武術挖掘小組) to find those surviving members of the old generation in order to preserve the arts through videotapes or books while still possible. They also started to bring sparring into national tournaments in hopes that through this effort, the real essence of the martial arts could be rediscovered. Sparring (*san shou* or *san da*, 散手、散打) was brought back to the tournament circuit in the early 1990s. In san shou training, certain effective fighting techniques were chosen for their special training, and each successfully delivered technique was allocated a point value. It was much like many other sports. However, the strange fact is that many wushu athletes in China today do not know how to fight, and many san shou fighters do not train wushu at all. In my opinion, wushu is san shou and san shou is wushu. They cannot and should not be separated.

In Europe, Bruce Lee's movies also started a fashion of learning kung fu. People there were only one step behind America. Unfortunately, from 1960 to 1980, there were very few traditional Chinese martial artists immigrating to Europe. The few traditional masters there dominated the entire market. Later, in the early 1980s, many European martial artists went to mainland China, Taiwan, and Hong Kong to train for short periods of time to learn kung fu. Unfortunately, after years of training, they realized that it was very difficult to comprehend the deep essence of an art simply by studying a few months here and there. The situation was especially difficult for martial artists who went to mainland China at that time. At the beginning of the 1990s, China significantly changed its training from gymnastic wushu to more traditional styles. The worst outcome was that after many years of effort to bring wushu into the Olympic games, China failed in its bid to host the summer games. China has since paid less attention to the development of wushu. Even the young generation in China now treats wushu as an old fashioned pursuit and pays more attention to Western material satisfaction and political reform. The spirit of training has been reduced significantly.

In America, since 1985, Mr. Jeffery A. Bolt and many other Chinese martial arts practitioners, such as Nick Gracenin, Pat Rice, Sam Masich, and more have tried to unify the Chinese martial arts community, hoping to bring together the great martial artists from China, Taiwan, Hong Kong, and Indo-China through tournaments and friendship demonstrations. Their ultimate goal is that these masters would become friends and finally promote Chinese martial arts to a higher quality. After ten years of effort, the organization, the United States of America Wushu-Kung Fu Federation (USAWKF) was established. Although there are still many opposing forces and obstacles to this unification, I believe that the future is bright, and I can foresee the continued success of this enterprise in the future.

Northern Styles and Southern Styles

Chinese martial arts can be categorized into northern styles and southern styles. The geographic line making this distinction is the Yangtze River (*Chang Jiang*, 長江), which means Long River (Figure 1-3). The Yangtze River runs across southern China from the west to the east.

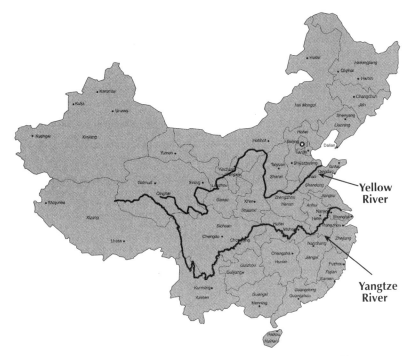

Figure 1-3. The Yangtze and Yellow Rivers in China

Generally speaking, the northern region of the Yangtze River is bordered by large fields, highlands, and desert. For this reason, horse riding was common, like Texas in the United States. People in the north are more open-minded compared to those of the south. The common foods are wheat, soybeans, barley, and sorghum that can be grown in the dry highlands.

In the southern region, there are more plains, mountains, and rivers. Rain is common in the south. Population density is much higher than that in the north. The common food is rice. Other than horses, the most common means of transportation is by boat. There is a common saying: "southern boats and northern horses" (南船北馬). This implies that the southern people use boats for travel and communication, while the northern people use horses.

Because of a long history of development shaped by these distinctions, the northern Chinese are generally taller than southern Chinese. It is believed that this is from the difference in diet. Moreover, northern Chinese are used to living in a wide-open environment. After thousands of years of martial arts development, northern people perfected long-range fighting, and therefore they preferred to use their legs more. This is not the case in southern China, which is more crowded and where the people, generally speaking, are shorter than those of the north. Moreover, because boats are so common, many martial techniques were actually developed to fight on boats. Since a fighter must be steady on a boat, the techniques developed emphasized hands with a firm root. High kicks were limited.

From these factors, we can conclude:

1. Northern Chinese are generally taller, and therefore prefer long- or middle-range fighting, while southern Chinese are shorter, so middle- and short-range fighting are emphasized.

2. Northern styles emphasize more kicking techniques for long-range fighting, while southern stylists specialize in more hand techniques and a limited number of low kicks. This is why it is commonly said in Chinese martial arts society: "southern fist and northern leg" (南拳北腿).

3. Southern stylists focus on training a firm root, while northern stylists like to move and jump around. Moreover, northern martial stylists have more expertise in horse riding and martial techniques from horseback, while southern martial styles specialize more in fighting on boats and on the ground.

4. Because southern styles generally emphasize more hand techniques, grabbing techniques such as qin na were developed.

Many styles were created near the Yellow River, which carried within them the characteristics of both northern and southern styles. For example, the Shaolin Temple is located in Henan Province (河南省), just to the south of the Yellow River. The Shaolin Temple has trained both northern and southern styles for most of its history. In fact, there were a few branches of the Shaolin Temple in existence at different locations throughout its history. These include the Quan Zhou Shaolin Temple (泉州少林寺) in Fujian (福建) established during the Chinese year of Tang Qian Fu (唐乾符年) (A.D. 874-878), and five others established by the head monk Fuyu (福裕) during the first year of the Chinese Huang Qing of Yuan dynasty (皇慶元年), A.D. 1312. These five were located at Jixian of Hebei (河北、薊縣), He Lin of Wai Meng (外蒙、和林), Changan of Shanxi (陝西、長安), Taiyuan of Shanxi (山西、太原), and Lo Yang of Henan (河南、洛陽). Among these branches, two were located in the south of China.[2]

Internal Styles and External Styles

Before we go into the differences between internal and external styles, you should first recognize one important point: all Chinese styles, both internal and external, come from the same root. If a style does not share this root, then it is not a Chinese martial style. This root is the Chinese culture. Throughout the world, various civilizations have created many different arts, each one of them based on that civilization's cultural background. Therefore, it does not matter which style you are discussing; as long as it was created in China, it must contain the essence of Chinese art, the spirit of traditional Chinese virtues, and the knowledge of traditional fighting techniques that have been passed down for thousands of years.

Martial artists of old looked at their experiences and realized that in a fight there are three factors which generally decide victory: speed, power, and techniques. Among these, speed is the most important. This is because if you are fast, you can get to the opponent's vital areas more easily and get out again before he can get to you. Even if your power is weak and you know only a limited number of techniques, you still have a good chance of inflicting a serious injury on the opponent. The reason for this is because there are many vital areas, such as the eyes, groin, and throat, where you do not need too much power to make an attack effective.

If you already have speed, then what you need is power. Even if you have good speed and techniques, if you don't have power, your attacks and defense will not be as effective as possible. You may have met people with great muscular strength but no martial arts training; yet they were able to defeat skilled martial artists whose power was weak. Finally, once you have good speed and power, if you can develop good techniques and a sound strategy, then there will be no doubt that victory will be yours. Therefore, in Chinese martial arts, increasing speed, improving power, and studying the techniques are the most important subjects. In fact, speed and power training are considered the foundation of effectiveness in all Chinese martial arts styles.

It does not matter what techniques a style creates; they all must follow certain basic principles and rules. For example, all offensive and defensive techniques must effectively protect vital areas such as the eyes, throat, and groin. Whenever you attack, you must be able to access your opponent's vital areas, without exposing your own.

The same applies to speed and power training. Although each style has tried to keep its methods secret, each follows the same general rules. For example, developing muscle power should not be detrimental to your speed, and developing speed should not decrease your muscular power. Both must be of equal concern. Finally, the training methods you use or develop should be appropriate to the techniques that characterize your style. For example, in eagle and crane styles, the speed and power of grabbing are extremely important and should be emphasized.

In Chinese martial arts society, it is also said: "First, bravery; second, power; and third, gongfu."[3] The word "gongfu" here means the martial skills that a person has achieved through long, arduous training. When the situation occurs, among the factors necessary for winning, the first and most crucial is how brave you are. If you are afraid and nervous, then even if you have fast speed, strong power, and good techniques, you will not be able to put all of these into action. From this proverb, you can see that compared to all other winning factors bravery is the most important.

It is generally understood in Chinese martial arts society that before the Liang dynasty (梁) (A.D. 502-557), martial artists did not study the use of qi to increase speed and power. As explained earlier, after the Liang dynasty, martial artists performing *Muscle/Tendon Changing Qigong* from Da Mo realized the value of qi training in developing speed and power. This type of training quickly became a major component of almost all styles. Because of this two-part historical development, the examination of this topic will cover two distinct eras. The dividing point will be the Liang dynasty, when Da Mo came to China (A.D. 527-536).

It is generally believed that before Da Mo, although qi theory and principles had been studied and widely applied in Chinese medicine, they were not used in the martial arts. Speed and power, on the other hand, were normally developed through continued training. Even though this training emphasized a concentrated mind, it did not provide the next step and link this to developing qi. Instead, these martial artists concentrated solely on muscular power. This is why styles originating from this period are classified as external styles.

Da Mo passed down two classics: the *Muscle/Tendon Changing Classic (Yi Jin Jing)* and the *Marrow/Brain Washing Classic (Xi Sui Jing)*. The *Yi Jin Jing* was not originally intended to be used for fighting. Nevertheless, the martial qigong based on it was able to significantly increase power, and it became a mandatory course of training in the Shaolin Temple. This had a revolutionary effect on Chinese martial arts, leading to the establishment of an internal foundation based on qi training.

As time passed, several martial styles were created which emphasized a soft body instead of the stiff muscular body developed by the Shaolin priests. These newer styles were based on the belief that since internal energy (qi) is the root and foundation of physical strength, a martial artist should first build up this internal root. This theory holds that when qi is abundant and full, it can energize the physical body to a higher level so that power can be manifested more effectively and efficiently. In order to build up qi and circulate it smoothly, the body must be relaxed and the mind must be concentrated. We can recognize at least two internal styles, post-heaven techniques (*hou tian fa*, 後天法) and small nine heavens (*xiao jiu tian*, 小九天), as having been created during this time (A.D. 550-600). Both later became popular during the Tang dynasty (唐朝) (A.D. 618-907). According to some documents, these two styles were the original sources of Taijiquan, the creation of which is credited to Zhang, San-feng of the late Song dynasty ca. A.D. 1200.[4]

In summary: The various martial arts are divided into external and internal styles. While the external styles emphasize training techniques and building up the physical body through some martial qigong training, the internal styles emphasize the building up of qi in the body. In fact, all styles, both internal and external, have martial qigong training. The external styles train the physical body and hard qigong first and gradually become soft and train soft qigong, while the internal styles train soft qigong first and later apply the built-up qi to the physical techniques. It is said: "Externally, train tendons, bones, and skin; and internally, train one mouthful of qi."[5] This means that it does not matter whether you are studying an external or an internal style; if you want to manifest the maximum amount of power, you have to train both externally and internally. Externally means the physical body, and internally means the qi circulation and level of qi storage in the body that is related to the breathing.

It is said: "The external styles are from hard to soft and the internal styles are from soft to hard; the ways are different but the final goal is the same."[6] It is also said: "External styles are from external to internal, while internal styles are from internal to external. Although the approaches are different, the final goal is the same."[7] Again, it is said: "External styles are first muscular strength (*li*) and then qi, while internal styles are first qi and later li."[8] The preceding discussion should give you a general idea of how to distinguish external and internal styles. Frequently, internal and external styles are also judged by how the jin is manifested. Jin is defined as "li and qi," (力氣). Li means muscular strength. It is how the muscles are energized by the qi and how this manifests externally as power. It is said: "The internal styles are as soft as a whip, the soft-hard styles (half external and half internal) are like rattan, and the external styles are like a staff." The concept of jin will be discussed next.

Martial Power—Jin

Jin training is a very important part of the Chinese martial arts, but there is very little written on the subject in English. Theoretically, jin can be defined as "using the concentrated mind to lead the qi to energize the muscles and thus manifest the power to its maximum level." From this, you can see that jin is related to the training of the mind and qi. That means qigong.

Traditionally, many masters have viewed the higher levels of jin as a secret that should be passed down only to a few trusted students. Almost all Asian martial styles train jin. The differences lie in the depth to which jin is understood, in the different kinds of jin trained, and in the range and characteristics of the emphasized jins. For example, Tiger Claw Style emphasizes hard and strong jin, imitating the tiger's muscular strength; muscles predominate in most of the techniques. White Crane, Dragon, and Snake are softer styles, and the muscles are used relatively less. In Taijiquan and Liu He Ba Fa, the softest styles, soft jin is especially emphasized and muscle usage is cut down to a minimum.

The application of jin brings us to a major difference between the Oriental martial arts and those of the West. Oriental martial arts traditionally emphasize the training of jin, whereas this concept and training approach is relatively unknown in other parts of the world. In China, martial styles and martial artists are judged by their jin. How deeply is jin understood and how well is it applied? How strong and effective is it, and how is it coordinated with martial technique? When a martial artist performs his art without jin it is called "flower fist and brocade leg" (花拳繡腿). This is to scoff at the martial artist without jin who is weak like a flower and soft like brocade. Like dancing, his art is beautiful but not useful. It is also said: "Train *quan* and not *gong*, when you get old, all emptiness."[9] This means that if a martial artist emphasizes only the beauty and smoothness of his forms and doesn't train his gong, then when he gets old, he will have nothing. The "gong" here means "qigong" (氣功) and refers to the cultivation of qi and its coordination with jin to develop the latter to its maximum and to make the techniques effective and alive. Therefore, if a martial artist learns his art without training his "qigong" and "jin gong" (勁功), once he gets old the techniques he has learned will be useless because he will have lost his muscular strength.

Often jin has been considered a secret transmission in Chinese martial arts society. This is so not only because it was not revealed to most students, but also because it cannot be passed down with words alone. Jin must be experienced. It is said that the master "passes down jin." Once you feel jin done by your master, you know what is meant and can work on it by yourself. Without an experienced master it is more difficult, but not impossible, to learn about jin. There are general principles and training methods which an experienced martial artist can use to grasp the keys of this practice. If you are interested in this rather substantial subject, please refer to my book: *Tai Chi Theory and Martial Power*, published by YMAA.

Hard Styles, Soft-Hard Styles, and Soft Styles

Chinese martial styles can also be distinguished from the ways they manifest jin (martial power); they can thus be categorized into hard, soft-hard, and soft styles.

Generally speaking, the hard styles use more muscular power. In these styles, the qi is led to the muscles or generated in the local area; then the muscles are tensed up to trap the qi there in order to energize muscular power to its maximum efficiency. In order to reach this goal, once the qi is led to the muscles, commonly the breath is held temporarily to trap the qi in the muscles. Then this muscular power is used for attack or defense. This kind of jin manifestation is like using a staff to strike. It is easy for a beginner to manifest hard jin. When this power is used upon an opponent's body, external injury can be inflicted immediately. A typical hard style is Tiger Claw (虎爪), which imitates the tiger's use of strong muscular power for fighting. With hard jin, because the muscles and tendons are more tensed in order to protect the ligaments of the joints, few injuries are caused from power manifestation. Generally speaking, external styles are more likely to be hard styles.

The second category is soft-hard styles. In these styles, the muscles and tendons remain relaxed, and the movements are soft to allow the qi to move freely from the lower dan tian to the limbs. Just before the attack reaches the opponent's body, suddenly the muscles and tendons are tensed. This kind of power is first soft and then hard. According to my own experience, this kind of power is like the strike of rattan. When this soft-hard power is applied to the opponent's body, both external and internal injuries can be inflicted. The reason for softness at the beginning is to allow the qi to move freely from the lower dan tian to the limbs, and the reason for the hardening through tensing the muscles and tendons is to protect against pulling and damaging the ligaments in the joints. It also offers the attacker strong physical support for the power, which can be bounced back from the opponent's body when the techniques are applied with enough speed and precision. Typical soft-hard styles are White Crane (白鶴) and Snake (蛇).

Finally, the third category is soft styles. In these styles, the muscles and tendons are relaxed as much as possible to allow the qi to circulate from the lower dan tian to the limbs for striking. However, right before contact with the opponent's body, the physical body remains relaxed. In order to protect the ligaments in the elbows and shoulders from being pulled and injured, right before the limbs reach their maximum extension they are immediately pulled back. From this pulling action, the muscles and tendons are tensed instantly to protect the ligaments, and then immediately relaxed again. This action is just like the whipping of a whip. Although the physical body is relaxed, the power generated is the most harmful and penetrating possible and can reach to the deep places of the body. Therefore, internal injury or organ damage can occur. Naturally, this kind of jin manifestation is dangerous for beginners. The reason for the penetration of the power is the whipping motion. Theoretically speaking, when you propel a whip forward with a speed (v), and then pull back with another speed (v), at the turning point between forward and backward, the speed at which the whip contacts the target is $2v$ (Figure 1-4). From here, you can see that speed

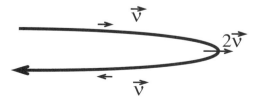

Figure 1-4. Whipping Speed

in whipping is the key to power penetration. This is like a surgical technology from the 1970s in which water from a high-pressure nozzle was used for cutting. Typical soft styles are Taijiquan (太極拳) and Liu He Ba Fa (六合八法).

At this point, we can superficially perceive the internal styles or soft styles and the external styles or hard styles. Consider Figure 1-5. The left line represents the amount of muscular power manifested, and the right line represents the qi which is built up. From this figure, you can see that those styles which emphasize mostly muscular power or that use local qi to energize the muscles are toward the left, while those styles which

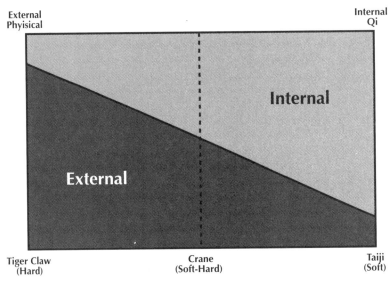

Figure 1-5. Hard Styles, Soft-Hard Styles, and Soft Styles

use less muscular power are toward the right. Naturally, the more a style is toward the right, the softer and more relaxed the physical body should be, and greater concentration is needed to build up qi and lead it to the limbs.

Four Categories of Fighting Skills

After many thousands of years of knowledge accumulation and fighting experience, martial techniques can be divided into four major categories: kicking (*ti*, 踢), hand striking (*da*, 打), wrestling (*shuai*i, 摔), and joint locking (*qin na* or *chin na*) (*na*, 拿).

Kicking is using the legs to kick the opponent's vital areas, sweep the opponent's legs, or block the opponent's kick. Hand striking is using the hands, forearms, elbows, or shoulders to block an attack or to strike the opponent. Wrestling is using grabs, trips, sweeps, bumps, etc., to make the opponent lose his balance, and then to take him down. Finally, qin na itself has four categories of techniques, including sealing the veins and arteries, sealing the breath, cavity press, and joint locking.

Technically speaking, wrestling techniques are designed against kicking and striking; qin na techniques are to be used in countering wrestling; and kicking and hand striking are used to conquer the techniques of qin na joint locking. From this, you can see that all have special purposes and mutually support and can conquer each other.

In order to make the techniques effective, all four categories of fighting techniques are required in any Chinese martial style.

Therefore, in order to become a proficient martial artist, you must learn northern styles and southern styles, allowing you to cover all ranges of fighting skills. You should also understand both internal and external styles. Although the basic theory of qi cultivation for both styles is the same, the training methods are often quite different. Learning both internal and external styles will offer you various angles for viewing the same thing. Most importantly, in order to make your martial arts training complete, you should learn all four categories of fighting techniques. These four categories should be included in any Chinese martial arts style.

The Dao of Chinese Martial Arts

As mentioned earlier, the word "martial" (武) is constructed by two Chinese words "stop" (止) and "weapons" (戈), and when combined means "to cease the battle." This concept is very important, especially in ancient times when there was even more violence and fighting between different races and nations than there is today. In order to protect yourself and your country, you needed to learn the martial arts. From this perspective, you can see that martial arts are defensive and are a way of using fighting skills to stop actual fighting. If you examine Chinese history, you will see that even after China had become a huge country and its culture had reached one of the highest levels in the world, it never thought of invading or conquering other countries. On the contrary, throughout its history, China has tried to prevent invasion by the Mongols from the north, the Manchus from the northeast, and many small incursions from Korea and the tribes to its west. Even though China invented gunpowder before the Song dynasty, it did not develop as a purely military power. If China had possessed the intention of conquering the world at that time, its military technologies were probably up to the task.

China's most basic human philosophies originated with Confucianism and Daoism. These philosophies emphasize peace, harmony, and the love of the human race. War is necessary only when it is needed for self-protection. From this fundamental philosophy and cultural development, we can understand that almost all the Chinese martial arts techniques were developed under the motivation for self-defense, and not for offense. However, there is one style called Shape-Mind Fist (*Xingyiquan*, 形意拳) that was created by Marshal Yue Fei (岳飛) during the Chinese Southern Song dynasty (南宋) (A.D. 1127-1280), which emphasizes attack. If we consider the background of the creation of this style, we can appreciate why this style was created for offense. At that time, the Mongols had taken over the northern half of China and captured the Song emperor. For survival purposes, a new emperor was established and the empire moved to the south of China. At all times, the Chinese were preparing against an invasion by the Mongols. Martial arts training was one of the most important aspects of the country's affairs in order to survive. Xingyiquan was created as a military style, with which a person could reach a higher fighting capability in a short time. Xingyiquan trains forward movements instead of backward. Although the basic techniques are simple, they are powerful and effective. If you are interested in more information on Xingyiquan, please refer to the book *Xingyiquan—Theory and Applications*, published by YMAA.

According to Chinese philosophy, in order to achieve harmony and peace with your enemy, when there is a conflict, you must not merely conquer his or her body. True power or capability for fighting is in showing your opponents that they do not have a chance of victory. Therefore, after a physical conflict, there should be spiritual harmony with your enemy. Only then can peace be reached. Killing and conquest can only produce more hate and killing in the future. In China, the highest level of fighting is not fighting. If you can anticipate and avoid a fight, then you have won the war.

For example, there is a tavern near my studio. Occasionally, an inebriated person decides that he wants to come in and challenge the students in my school. Often, this will agitate them, and the younger ones want to fight. One time, a drunken Vietnam veteran walked into the school and challenged them to fight. Again, some students were agitated and angry. I told them I would handle it this time. I politely and carefully approached him, asked his name and if there was anything that I could do to help him. He told me how strong and great he used to be, how brave he was in the war, and how well he was able to fight. I listened and nodded my head to show my acknowledgment of his past glory. After he saw that I was actually listening to his story, his manner became gentler. Then I asked him to sit down and told him I was busy with class right now and that I would fight him after class if it were all the same to him. Next, I went to prepare some hot tea and gave it to him. I told him the tea would help him while he was waiting. Half an hour later, he woke up and sneaked out the door without being noticed. Since then, every time he passes the studio, he will smile and wave to me. Although we do not know each other deeply, at least we have become friends, and he understands that I recognize his honor. Since that night we have never had a problem with him. Another story was told to me by my Grandmother. A long time ago, there was a family that owned a small farm. The father worked very hard to make the farm successful so that he would be able to leave it to his two sons when he died. The elder son, who was married, was named De-xin (德信), while the younger son, who was not married, was named De-yi (德義).

One day, the father became very sick, and he knew that he would soon die. He gathered his sons together and said to them, "I wish to give this farm to both of you. Share it equally, and help each other to make it successful. I hope that it makes you as happy as it has made me." With these words the father quietly passed away.

The sons divided the land equally and set about the task of building their own farms. Even though they had divided the land, they still cooperated, helping each other with the more difficult chores. However, not long after the father died, De-xin's wife decided that she and De-xin had not received enough land. After all, De-yi was single and didn't need as much land as they did. She began urging her husband to request more land from his brother.

Finally, after considerable provocation from his wife, De-xin demanded more land from De-yi. Because De-xin was much bigger and stronger, the only thing De-yi could do was to concede in angry silence and let his brother occupy more land.

However, De-xin's wife was still not satisfied. When she saw how easy it was to get more land from her brother-in-law, she again urged her husband to demand more land. Again, De-yi could only consent to his brother's demands. Still, De-xin's wife was not satisfied, and finally she demanded that De-yi leave all the land to her and her husband.

De-yi requested help from his relatives and friends and begged them to mediate the conflict. No one would help. They knew it was unfair for De-yi to be forced off his land, but they were afraid because they knew of De-xin's violent temper.

Finally, De-yi decided to take a stand for what he knew was right. He decided to stay, even though his brother wanted him to leave. For this defiance, De-xin beat him very, very badly. De-yi was finally forced to leave his home and become a traveling street beggar.

One day, while traveling in the Putian (浦田) region of Fujian Province (福建), he saw several Shaolin priests in town on an expedition to purchase food. He knew that the Shaolin monks were good in gongfu, and he thought that if he could learn gongfu, he could beat De-xin and regain the land that was rightfully his. He decided to follow the monks, and when they reached the temple he would request that they accept him as a student of gongfu.

When he arrived at the temple, he requested to see the Head Priest. The Head Priest welcomed him and asked why he had requested the meeting. De-yi told the Head Priest his sad story and asked to be taught gongfu so that he could regain his land.

The Head Priest looked at him, pondered for a few minutes, and finally said, "De-yi, if you are willing to endure the painfully hard training, then you are accepted as a student here." With deep appreciation, De-yi knelt down and bowed to the Head Priest.

Early the next morning, De-yi was summoned to the backyard of the temple. The Head Priest was standing in front of a young willow tree, holding a calf. He said to De-yi, "Before you learn any gongfu, you must first build up your strength. To do this you must hold this calf in your arms and jump over this willow tree fifty times in the morning and fifty times in the evening. De-yi replied, "Yes, master. This is a simple task and I will do it every day."

From then on, De-yi held the calf in his arms and jumped over the willow tree every morning and every evening. Days passed, weeks passed, months passed, years passed. The calf grew into a cow and the small willow tree grew into a big tree. Still, De-yi held the cow in his arms and jumped over the tree.

One day, he requested to see the Head Priest. He asked, "Dear Master, I have held the cow and jumped over the willow tree for three years already. Do you think I am strong enough to train gongfu?"

The Head Priest looked at him and the cow. He smiled and said: "De-yi, you do not have to learn anymore. You have completed your gongfu training. Your strength is enough to regain your lost land. You should take this cow home with you and use it to cultivate your land."

De-yi looked at the Head Priest with surprise and asked: "If I have not learned any martial arts, what do I do if my brother comes to fight me again for my land?" The Head Priest laughed and said, "Do not worry, De-yi. If your brother comes to fight you again, simply pick up the cow and run towards him. There will be no fight."

De-yi half believed the Head Priest, but he also thought that perhaps the Head

Priest was joking with him. He took the cow and left the Shaolin Temple. When he arrived home, he started to cultivate his land.

De-xin soon discovered his brother's return. He decided to beat up his younger brother again and teach him an unforgettable lesson. After that, De-yi would never dare to return. When De-yi came to the rice field, he saw his brother running towards him, shouting in anger.

When De-yi saw his brother running toward him, he remembered what the Head Priest had said and immediately picked up the cow and ran towards his brother. This surprised and shocked De-xin. He just could not believe that his brother possessed such strength. He turned around and ran away, never to return again.

From this story, I learned two lessons. The first is that you need patience and endurance to succeed. Great success always comes from many little efforts. The second lesson is that the best way to win a fight is without fighting. Often you can win a fight with wisdom, and this is better than beating up someone.

I remember that my White Crane master told me something that affected my perspective of Chinese martial arts completely. He told me that the goal of a martial artist's learning was not fighting. It is neither for showing off nor for proving you are capable of conquering other people. He said the final goal of learning is to discover the meaning of life. Therefore, what I was learning from him was not a martial art, but the way of life. I could not accept this concept when I was young. However, now that I am much older, I can start to understand what he meant at that time.

In the last twenty years, I have had many questions in my mind. Why are we here? What do we expect to accomplish in our lifetime? Do we come to this life as just an animal, without a deep meaning, or do we come to this life to comprehend and to experience the deep meaning of our lives?

In my opinion, there are many ways of understanding the meaning of life. You can learn to play the piano with all of your effort (energy and time). From the learning process, you learn to know yourself and to discipline yourself. Hopefully, you achieve the capability to use your wisdom mind to control your emotional mind and reach a high stage of spiritual understanding of your life. Often, whenever I listen to music composed by Beethoven, Mozart, or another great composer or musician, I am so touched and inspired. I always wonder how these people could create such a spiritually high level of music that has influenced the human race for hundreds of years. I deeply believe that in order for them to reach such a deep level of understanding, they must have gone through the same process of emotional and physical self-conquest. I believe that through music, these composers comprehended the meaning of their lives. Of course, the meaning may well be beyond our understanding; however, their spirit has inspired following generations.

Naturally, you may also learn painting or any art, which can cultivate your spirit to a higher level. It does not matter which way you choose; in order to reach a high level of spiritual growth, you must face your greatest enemy. This enemy is you. The only way to defeat this enemy is through self-discipline and an understanding of life.

Have you ever thought about why the highest levels of Chinese martial arts were always created either in Buddhist or Daoist monasteries? Why has it been monks who developed all these deadly martial arts? One of the main reasons, as explained earlier, was self-defense against bandits. The other reason is that through martial arts training, you learn how to use your wisdom mind to conquer or control your emotional mind. This is one of the most effective ways of reaching a high level of spiritual understanding of life.

I also remember a story told to me by my master about a very famous archer, Yang, You-ji (養由基), who lived during the Chinese Spring and Autumn period (春秋) (722-481 B.C.). When Yang, You-ji was a teenager, he was already well-known for his superior skill in archery. Because of this, he was very proud of himself. One day, he was in his study when he heard the call of an oil peddler just outside his house. Curious, he went out of his house and saw an old man selling cooking oil on the street. He saw the old man place the oil jar, which had a tiny hole the size of a coin, on the ground and then use the ladle to scoop a full measure of oil and pour it from chest height into the jar without losing a single drop or even touching the sides of the hole. Yang, You-ji was amazed at this old man's steady hand and the accuracy with which he was able to pour the oil into the jar. He asked the old man: "Old man, how did you do that?" (To call an aged person old man in China is not impolite, but a sign of respect.) The old man looked at him, the well-known teenaged archer of the village, and said: "Young man, would you like to see more?" Yang, You-ji nodded his head.

The old man then asked him to go into the house and bring out a bench. The old man placed a Chinese coin that had a very tiny hole in the center for threading pur-poses, on the hole in the jar. Then, the old man ladled a full scoop of oil and climbed onto the bench. Standing on the bench, he poured the oil all the way down from such a high place, through the hole in the coin and into the jar. This time, Yang, You-ji kept his eyes wide open and was shocked at the old man's amazing skill. He asked the old man: "How did you do that? I have never seen such an amazing thing before." The old man looked at him and smiled. He said: "There is nothing but practicing."

Suddenly, Yang, You-ji understood that his archery was good because he practiced harder than others. There was nothing of which to be proud. Thereafter, he became very humble and practiced even harder. When he reached his thirties, he was consid-ered the best archer in the entire country and was honored to serve the emperor as a bodyguard. But in his late fifties, he disappeared from the palace, and nobody ever knew where he went.

Twenty years later, one of his friends heard that Yang, You-ji was on Tian Mountain in Xinjiang Province (天山，新疆) and decided to find him. After months of travel-ing, he finally arrived at the mountain and located his friend. He stepped into Yang's house and they recognized each other. However, when Yang saw his friend's bow and arrow on his shoulder, he opened his eyes and said: "What are those funny things you are carrying on your back?" His friend looked at him and with mouth agape and said: "You must be the best archer existing today, since you have already gone through the entire experience of archery."

When I heard this story, I could not understand its actual meaning. Now, I begin to understand. Everything we have experienced before is just one learning process in reaching the spirit of our life. Once this learning is completed, the process of learning is no longer necessary and ceases to exist. It is just like the Buddhists who believe that our physical body is used only to cultivate our spirit; once we have reached a high level of spirit, the physical body is no longer important.

Learning martial arts is the same. You are using the way of learning martial arts to understand the meaning of your life. The higher you have reached, the better you experience the spirit which is beyond other martial artists. One day, you will no longer be able to train or perform martial arts. However, your understanding and spirit will remain, and you will retain your knowledge and spirit.

You should understand that the arts are alive and are creative. To Chinese philosophy, if an art is not creative, then the art is dead. It is also because the art is creative that, after hundreds of years of development and creation, there can be many styles of the same art.

One afternoon, I went to visit my master and asked him why the same movement was applied differently by two of my classmates. He looked at me and asked: "Little Yang? How much is one plus one? Without hesitation, I said: "Two." He smiled and shook his head and said: "No! Little Yang, it is not two." I was confused and thought he was joking. He continued: "Your father and your mother together are two. After their marriage, they have five children. Now, it is not two but seven. You can see one plus one is not two but seven. The arts are alive and creative. If you treat them as dead, it is two. But if you make them alive, they can be many. This is the philosophy of developing Chinese martial arts. Now, I am forty-two; when you reach forty-two, if your understanding about the martial arts is the same as mine today, then I will have failed you, and also you will have failed me."

This also reminds me of a story I heard from Master Liang, Shou-yu a few years ago. He said he knew a story of how Master Zhang, San-feng taught the taiji sword techniques to one of his students. After this student completed his three years of taiji sword learning from Master Zhang, he was so happy and could perform every movement in exactly the same way and feeling as Master Zhang had taught him.

Then Master Zhang asked him to leave and practice for three years and then come to see him. The student left. After three years of hard practice, the student came to see Master Zhang. However, he was sad and ashamed to meet Master Zhang. He bowed his head down and felt so sorry. He said: "Master Zhang, after three years of practice, I am now very sad. The more I have practiced, the more I have lost the feeling I had three years ago. Now, I feel about a third of the forms are different from what you taught me originally."

Master Zhang looked at him and said: "No good! No good! Go home and practice another three years and then come to see me." The student left in sorrow and sadness. He practiced harder and harder for the next three years. Then he came to see Master Zhang again. However, he felt even worse than the first time he came back. He looked at Master Zhang very disappointedly. He said: "Master Zhang! I don't know why. The more I have practiced, the worse it has become. Now, two-thirds of the forms feel different from what you taught me."

Master Zhang again looked at him and said: "No good! No good! Go home again and practice another three years and then come to see me." The student left feeling very, very sad. This time, he practiced even harder than before. He put all his mind into understanding and feeling every movement of the forms he learned. After three years, again he returned to see Master Zhang. This time, his face turned pale and he dared not look at Master Zhang's face directly. He said: "Master Zhang! I am sorry. I am a failure. I have failed you and myself. I feel now not even one form has the same feeling as you taught me."

When Master heard of this, he laughed loudly and very happily. He looked at the student and said: "Great! You have done well. Now, the techniques you have learned are yours and not mine anymore."

From this story, you can see that the mentality of the arts is creative. If the great musician Beethoven, after he learned all the techniques from his teacher, never learned to create, then he would not have become so great. It is the same with the great painter Picasso. If he did not know how to be creative, then after he learned all the painting techniques from his teacher, he would never have become such a genius. Therefore, you can see that arts are alive and not dead. However, if you do not learn enough techniques and have not reached a deep level of understanding, then when you start to create, you will have lost the correct path and the arts will be flawed. It is said in Chinese martial arts society: "Sifu leads you into the door; cultivation depends on oneself."[10]

When you learn any art, you should understand the mentality of learning is to feel and to gain the essence of the art. Only if your heart can learn the essence of the arts, then will you have gained the root. With this root, you can grow and become creative.

My master told me a story. Once upon a time a boy came to see an old man and asked him: "Honorable old man, I have heard that you can change a piece of rock into gold. Is that true?" "Yes, young man. Like others, do you want a piece of gold? Let me change one for you." The boy replied. "Oh no! I do not want a piece of gold. What I would like is to learn the trick you use to change rocks into gold."

What do you think about this short story? When you learn anything, if you do not gain the essence of the learning, you will remain on the surface, just holding the branches and flowers. However, if you can feel the arts deeply, then you can create. Feeling deeply enables you to ponder and finally to understand the situation. Without this deep feeling, what you see and what you are will be only on the surface.

Once there was a wise king in Korea who had a fifteen-year-old son. This son had grown up comfortably in the palace, with all of the servants' attention. This made the king very worried, and he believed that his son would never be a good king whose concern was for his people. Therefore, he summoned a well-known wise old man living in the deep woods.

In response to this call, the old man came to the palace. After he promised to teach the prince to be a wise, good king, he took the prince to the deep woods. After they arrived in the deep woods, the old man taught the young prince how to find food, how to cook, and how to survive in the woods. Then he left the prince alone in the woods. However, he promised that he would come back a year later.

A year later, when the old man came back, he asked the prince what he thought about the woods. The prince replied: "I am sick of them. I need a servant. I hate it here. Take me home." However, the old man merely said: "Very good. That is good progress, but not enough. Please wait here for another year, and I will be back to see you again." Then he left.

A year again passed, and the old man came back to the woods, asking the prince again the same question. This time the prince said: "I see birds, I see trees, I see flowers and animals." His mind had started to accept the surrounding environment, and he recognized his role in the woods. The old man was satisfied and said: "This is great progress. However, it is not enough, and therefore you must stay here for another year." This time, the prince was not even upset and said: "No problem." Once again, the old man left.

Another year passed, and the old man came back again. This time, when the old man asked the prince what he thought, the prince said: "I feel birds, woods, fish, animals, and many things around me here." This time, the old man was very happy and said: "Now I can take you home. If you can feel the things happening around you, then you can concern yourself with the people's feelings, and you will be a good king." Then the old man took him home.

This story is only to tell you that when you do anything, you must put your mind into it, feel it, taste it, and experience it. Only then may you say that you understand it. Without this deep feeling and comprehension, the arts you create will be shallow and lose their essence.

I would like to point out something important. Normally, after more than thirty years of learning, studying, pondering, and practicing, all masters have experienced most of the possible creations of their art, and their understanding of it has reached to a very deep level. It is common that the master will keep this personal secret to himself until he has found someone he can really trust. This is often called the secret of the art.

There is another story which was told to me by Master Liang, Shou-yu. About fifty years ago, there was a very famous clay doll maker in Beijing. Because he was so famous, he had many students. However, it did not matter how, when people purchased a doll, they could always tell which ones were made by the master and which ones were made by the students. It also did not matter how the students tried and pondered, they could not catch the secret of their master. They continued to believe that their master's dolls were better because he had more years of experience.

One day, this master became very sick and was dying. After he realized that he would die soon, he decided to reveal his last secret to his most trustworthy student. He summoned his student to his bed, and said: "You are the student whom I can trust most. You have been loyal to me in the past. Here, I would like to tell you the last of my secrets. But remember, if you keep this secret to yourself, you will always enjoy wealth and glory. However, if you reveal it to everyone else, then you will be as poor as others." Then he asked this student to make a doll in front of him.

Not long after, this student had completed his doll. Although the doll was well made, it looked like a student's doll instead of the master's. Then, the master looked at the student and said: "The difference between your doll and my doll is the expression on the face. The expression of the face must be natural and delightful. This is the final trick for you to remember." Then, he placed his index finger under the chin of the wet clay doll and gently pushed the chin slightly upward. Immediately, the facial expression of the doll changed and became very natural. Now, the doll looked like the master's.

From this, you can see that normally a secret is hidden in the obvious place. A practitioner can realize this secret suddenly when time passes by through continued pondering and practice. It is said in Chinese martial arts society, "The great Dao is no more than two or three sentences. Once spoken, it is worth less than three pennies."[11]

From these stories, you may have understood that the creation of an in-depth art comes from continued learning, pondering, and practice. Only then will the spirit of the art be high and the art created be profound.

Conclusions:

1. Chinese martial arts were created mainly for defense and not for offense.

2. The best fight is "the fight of no fight."

3. The meaning of learning arts is to find and to understand yourself. With this understanding, you can promote the meaning of your life to a higher spiritual level.

4. The arts are creative. It is the same in Chinese martial arts. After you have learned and practiced for a long time, then you should blend what you have learned with your own ideas to make the arts even greater.

5. A deeply touching art is created from deep spiritual feelings. It is not an outward form. Forms are only the manifestation of the internal feeling.

6. The greatest secret is hidden in the most obvious place and can be obtained only from continued pondering and practice.

The Real Meaning of Taijiquan

People practice taijiquan for different reasons. Some practice for health or to cure an illness, and others for defense, relaxation, or solely for fun. However, when you approach the highest level of taijiquan, you will probably feel that the above reasons are not really important anymore. At this time, you must seek the real meaning of the practice; otherwise you will soon become satisfied with your achievement and lose enthusiasm for further research. You must ponder what is really behind this highly meditative art. Many religious Daoists practice taijiquan in their striving to eliminate their baser elements and become immortal. Many non-religious people practice taijiquan to gain a peaceful mind and reinvigorate their lives.

You should understand that taijiquan emphasizes meditation both in movement and in stillness. Through this meditation a taijiquan practitioner, like a Buddhist priest, trains himself to be calm and concentrated. It is possible to achieve a state of peace and centeredness, which allows you to judge things and events in a neutral way, without emotional disturbance. When your mind is truly clear and calm, the spiritual side of things starts to open up. You start to see more deeply into things. Skilled practitioners can sense a person's intentions before they are expressed, and they often develop the ability to look more deeply into people and events in non-martial ways too. Many martial arts masters came to be considered wise men and were consulted for their insight into the meaning of human life, this world, and the universe. They learned to live in this world without confusion or doubt and to find peace and happiness. All of this comes through meditation and continuous pondering.

There is a song passed down since ancient times about the real meaning of taijiquan.

It says:

1. "No shape, no shadow" (無形無象). This means that when you have approached the higher levels of taiji meditation, you find your physical body seems not to exist—you feel that you are a ball of energy, part of the natural world and inseparable from it. Your actions and self are part of the natural order of things, fitting in smoothly and unobtrusively, seeming to have no independent shape of their own, casting no shadow.

2. "Entire body transparent and empty" (全身透空). When you feel you are only a ball of energy, there is nothing in your mind, no desire or intention. Since your mind and ego are not there to interfere, you can see clearly and respond correctly.

3. "Forget your surroundings and be natural" (忘物自然). Once you are transparent you will easily forget your surroundings and your energy flow will be smooth and natural.

4. "Like a stone chime suspended from West Mountain" (西山懸磬). This implies that your mind is wide-open, free, and unrestricted. Like a stone chime suspended from the mountain, all things are clear under you, while your mind is still controlled by you just as the thread suspends the stone chime.

5. "Tigers roaring, monkeys screeching" (虎吼猿鳴). When you move the energy you have cultivated, it can be as strong as a tiger's roar and reach as far as a monkey's screech.

6. "Clear fountain, peaceful water" (泉清水靜). Even when your energy is strong, your mind is clear, still, and peaceful.

7. "Turbulent river, stormy ocean" (翻江鬧海). In taiji, if you have to use your energy it can be strong and continuous like a turbulent river or the stormy ocean.

8. "With your whole being, develop your life" (盡性立命). During all your practice and meditation, you must concentrate your whole attention in order to develop the highest level of the art. This dedication and concentration will carry over to the rest of your life, and the striving for perfection becomes the real inner meaning of taiji.

1-3. General History of Taijiquan

Many people have learned Yang Style Taijiquan, but few really understand the history, background, and variations of the style. Often a person who has learned Yang Style Taijiquan will see forms that claim to be Yang style, but which look different from what he has learned. This sometimes causes consternation and doubt about which form, if any, is the correct 'Yang style.' A knowledge of the history can help to explain this discrepancy.

Historically, the most important aspect of taijiquan is its creation from the theory of yin and yang, including the way yin and yang are derived from *wuji*, defined as "no extremity" (無極).

The concept of yin and yang was first detailed in the *Book of Changes (Yi Jing*, 易經) around 1122 B.C. This means that the theory behind taijiquan actually has historical roots going back more than three thousand years.

The manner in which the concept of yin and yang gave birth to taijiquan is unknown. However, since the theory of yin and yang has been such an all-pervading influence on Chinese culture and thinking since the *Yi Jing*, it is possible to piece together the history of taijiquan's origin from the remnants of historical documentation that still exist.

It is said that Taijiquan was created by Zhang, San-feng in the Song Hui Zong era (宋徽宗) ca. A.D. 1101. It is also said that techniques and forms with the same basic principles as taijiquan were already in existence during the Liang dynasty (梁朝) (A.D. 502-557), and were being taught by Han, Gong-yue (韓拱月), Cheng, Ling-xi (程靈洗), and Cheng, Bi (程鉍). Later, in the Tang dynasty (唐朝) (A.D. 618-907), it was found that Xu, Xuan-oing (許宣平), Li, Dao-zi (李道子), and Yin, Li-peng (殷利亨) were teaching similar martial techniques. They were called thirty-seven postures (*san shi qi shi*, 三十七勢), post-heaven techniques (*hou tian fa*, 後天法), and small nine heaven (*xiao jiu tian*, 小九天) that had seventeen postures. The accuracy of these accounts is somewhat questionable, so it is not really known when and by whom taijiquan was created. Because there is more formal history recorded about Zhang, San-feng, he has received most of the credit.[4]

According to the historical record *Nan Lei Ji Wang Zheng Nan Mu Zhi Ming* (南雷集王征南墓志銘), "Zhang San-feng, in the Song dynasty, was a Wudang Daoist. Hui Zong (a Song Emperor, 宋徽宗) summoned him, but the road was blocked and he couldn't come. At night, (Hui Zong) dreamed Emperor Yuan (the first Jin emperor, 元帝) taught him martial techniques. At dawn, he killed a hundred enemies by himself."[12] Also recorded in the Ming history *Ming Shi Fang Ji Zhuan* (明史方技傳) is the following:

Zhang, San-feng, from Liao Dong Yi county (遼東懿州). Named Quan-yi (全一). Also named Jun-bao (君寶). San-feng was his nickname. Because he did not keep himself neat and clean, Zhang, La-ta (Sloppy Zhang, 張邋遢). He was tall and big, shaped like a turtle, and had a crane's back. Large ears and round eyes. Beard long like a spear tassel. Wears only a priest's robe winter or summer. Will eat a bushel of food, or won't eat for several days or a few months. Can travel a thousand miles. Likes to have fun with people. Behaves as if nobody is around. Used to travel to Wudang (mountain) with his disciples. Built a simple cottage and lived inside. In the 24th year of Hong Wu (洪武), around A.D. 1392, Ming Tai Zu (the first Ming emperor, 明太祖) heard of his name, and sent a messenger to look for him but he couldn't be found.[13]

The following was also recorded in the Ming dynasty in *Ming Lang Ying Qi Xiu Lei Gao* (明郎瑛七修類稿):

Zhang the Immortal, named Jun-bao, also named Quan-yi, nicknamed Xuan-xuan (玄玄), also called Zhang, La-ta. In the third year of Tian Shun (天順) A.D. 1460 he visited Emperor Ming Ying Zong (明英宗). A picture was drawn. The beard and mustache were straight, the back of the head had a tuft. Purple face and big stomach, with a bamboo hat in his hand. On the top of the picture was an inscription from the emperor honoring Zhang as 'Tong Wei Xian Hua Zhen Ren' (通微顯化真人), a genuine Daoist who finely discriminates and clearly understands much. (Figure 1-6).[14]

This record is suspect, because if it were true, Zhang, San-feng would have been at least 500 years old at that time. Other records state that Zhang, San-feng's techniques were learned from the Daoist Feng, Yi-yuan (馮一元). Another story tells that Zhang, San-feng was an ancient hermit meditator. He saw a magpie fighting against a snake, had a sudden understanding, and created taijiquan,

After Zhang, San-feng, there were Wang Zong (王宗) in Shanxi province (陝西), Chen, Tong-zhou (陳同州) in Wen County (溫州), Zhang, Song-xi (張松溪) in Hai Yan (海鹽), Ye, Ji-mei (葉繼美) in Si Ming (四明), Wang, Zong-yue (王宗岳) in Shan You (山右), and Jiang, Fa (蔣發) in Hebei (河北). The taijiquan techniques were passed down and divided into two major styles, southern and northern. Later, Jiang, Fa passed his art to the Chen family at Chen Jia Gou

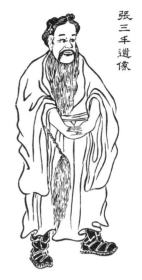

張三丰遺像

Figure 1-6. Zhang, San-Feng

(陳家溝) in Huai Qing County, Henan (河南懷慶府). Taijiquan was then passed down for fourteen generations and divided into old and new styles. The old style was carried on by Chen,

Chang-xing (陳長興) and the new style was created by Chen, You-ben (陳有本).

The old style successor Chen, Chang-xing then passed the art down to his son, Geng-yun (耕云), and his Chen relatives, Chen, Huai-yuan (陳懷遠) and Chen, Hua-mei (陳華梅). He also passed his taijiquan outside of his family to Yang, Lu-chan (楊露禪) and Li, Bo-kui (李伯魁), both of Hebei province (河北). This old style is called thirteen postures old form (*shi san shi lao jia*, 十三勢老架). Later, Yang, Lu-chan passed it down to his two sons, Yang, Ban-hou (楊班侯) and Yang, Jian-hou (楊健侯). Then, Jian-hou passed the art to his two sons, Yang, Shao-hou (楊少侯) and Yang, Cheng-fu (楊澄甫). This branch of taijiquan is popularly called Yang Style. Also, Wu, Quan-you (吳全佑) learned from Yang, Ban-hou and started a well known Wu Style.

Also, Chen, You-ben passed his new style to Chen, Qing-ping (陳清萍) who created Zhao Bao (趙堡) Style Taijiquan. Wuu, Yu-rang (武禹讓) learned the old style from Yang, Lu-chan and new style from Chen, Qing-ping and created Wuu Style Taijiquan. Li, Yi-yu (李亦畬) learned the Wuu Style and created Li Style Taijiquan. Hao, Wei-zhen (郝為楨) obtained his art from Li Style and created Hao Style Taijiquan. Sun, Lu-tang (孫祿堂) learned from Hao Style and created Sun Style.

All the above-mentioned styles are popular in China and Southeast Asia. Among them, Yang Style has become the most popular. In the next section we will discuss the history of the Yang Style.

1-4. History of Yang Style Taijiquan

Yang Style history starts with Yang, Lu-chan (楊露禪) (A.D. 1799-1872), also known as Fu-kuai (福魁) or Lu-chan (祿纏). He was born at Yong Nian Xian, Guang

Ping County, Hebei Province (河北，廣平府永年縣). When he was young he went to Chen Jia Gou in Henan province to learn taijiquan from Chen, Chang-xing. When Chen, Chang-xing stood he was centered and upright with no leaning or tilting, like a wooden signpost, and so people called him Mr. Tablet. At that time, there were very few students outside of the Chen family who learned from Chen, Chang-xing. Because Yang was an outside student, he was treated unfairly, but still he stayed and persevered in his practice.

One night, he was awakened by the sounds of "Hen" (哼) and "Ha" (哈) in the distance. He got up and traced the sound to an old building. Peeking through the broken wall, he saw his master Chen, Chang-xing teaching the techniques of grasp, control, and emitting jin in coordination with the sounds "Hen" and "Ha." He was amazed by the techniques and from that time on, unknown to master Chen, he continued to watch this secret practice session every night. He would then return to his room to ponder and study. Because of this, his martial ability advanced rapidly. One day, Chen ordered him to spar with the other disciples. To his surprise, none of the other students could defeat him. Chen realized that Yang had great potential and after that taught him the secrets sincerely.

After Yang, Lu-chan finished his study, he returned to his hometown and taught taijiquan for a while. People called his style Yang Style (*Yang Quan*, 楊拳), Soft Style (*Mian Quan,* 綿拳), or Neutralizing Style, (*Hua Quan,*化拳) because his motions were soft and able to neutralize the opponent's power. He later went to Beijing and taught a number of Qing officers. He used to carry a spear and a small bag and travel around the country, challenging well-known martial artists. Although he had many fights, he never hurt anybody. Because his art was so high, nobody could defeat him. Therefore, he was called "Yang Wu Di" (楊無敵) which means "Unbeatable Yang." He had three sons, Yang Qi (楊琦), Yang Yu (楊鈺) also called Ban-hou (班侯), and Yang Jian (楊鑒) also called Jian-hou (健侯). Yang Qi died when he was young. Therefore, only the last two sons succeeded their father in the art.

Yang's second son, Yang, Yu (A.D. 1837-1890), was also named Ban-hou. People used to call him "Mr. The Second." He learned taijiquan from his father even as a child. Even though he practiced very hard and continuously, he was still scolded and whipped by his father. He was good at free fighting. One day he was challenged by a strong martial artist. When the challenger grasped his wrist and would not let him escape, Yang, Ban-hou used his jin to bounce the challenger away and defeat him. He was so proud that he went home and told his father. Instead of praise, his father laughed at him because his sleeve was torn. After that, he trained harder and harder, and finally became a superlative taijiquan artist. Unfortunately, and perhaps not surprisingly, he didn't like to teach very much and had few students, so his art did not spread far after he died. One of his students called Wu, Quan-you later taught his son Wu, Jian-quan (吳鑒泉), whose art became the Wu Style Taijiquan. Yang, Ban-hou also had a son, called Zhao-peng (兆鵬), who passed on the art.

The third son of Yang, Lu-chan was Yang Jian (A.D. 1842-1917), also named Jian-hou and nicknamed Jing-hu (鏡湖). People used to call him "Mr. The Third." He also learned taijiquan from his father since he was young. His personality was softer and gentler than his brother's, and he had many followers. He taught three postures—large, medium, and small—although he specialized in the medium posture. He was also expert in using and coordinating both hard and soft power. He used to spar with his disciples who were good at sword and saber, while using only a dust brush. Every time his brush touched the student's wrist, the student could not counter, but would be bounced away. He was also good at using the staff and spear. When his long weapon touched an opponent's weapon, the opponent could not approach him, but instead was bounced away. When he emitted jin, it happened at the instant of laughing the "ha" sound. He could also throw small metal balls called "bullets." With these balls in his hand, he could shoot three or four birds at the same time. The most impressive demonstration he performed was to put a sparrow on his hand. The bird would not be able to fly away because, when a bird takes off, it must push down first and use the reaction force to lift itself. Yang, Jian-hou could sense the bird's power and neutralize this slight push, leaving the bird unable to take off. From this demonstration, one can understand that his listening jin and neutralizing jin must have been superb. He had three sons: Zhao-xiong (兆熊), Zhao-yuan (兆元), and Zhao-qing (兆清). The second son, Zhao-yuan died at an early age.

Yang, Jian-hou's first son, Yang, Zhao-xiong (A.D. 1862-1929), was also named Meng-xiang (夢祥) and later called Shao-hou (少侯). People used to call him "Mr. Oldest." He practiced taijiquan since he was six years old. He had a strong and persevering personality. He was expert in free fighting and very good at using various jins like his uncle Yang, Ban-hou. He reached the highest level of taijiquan gongfu. Specializing in small postures, his movements were fast and sunken. Because of his personality, he didn't have too many followers. He had a son called Yang, Zhen-sheng (振聲).

Yang, Jian-hou's third son was Yang, Zhao-qing (兆清) (A.D. 1883-1935), also named Cheng-fu (澄甫). People called him "Mr. The Third." His personality was mild and gentle. When he was young, he did not care for martial arts. It was not until his teens that he started studying taijiquan with his father. While his father was still alive Yang, Cheng-fu did not really understand the key secrets of taijiquan. It was not until his father died in 1917 that he started to practice hard. His father had helped him to build a good foundation, and after several years of practice and research, he was finally able to approach the level of his father and grandfather. Because of his experiences, he modified his father's taijiquan and specialized in large postures. This emphasis was completely reversed from that of his father and brother. He was the first taijiquan master willing to share the family secrets with the public, and because of his gentle nature he had countless students. When Nanking Central Guoshu Institute (南京中央國術館) was founded in 1928, he was invited to be the head taijiquan teacher, and his name became known throughout the country. He had four sons, Zhen-ming (振銘), Zhen-ji (振基), Zhen-duo (振鐸), and Zhen-guo (振國).

Yang Style Taijiquan can be classified into three major postures: large, medium, and small. It is also divided into three stances: high, medium, and low. Large postures were emphasized by Yang, Cheng-fu. He taught that the stances can be high, medium, or low, but the postures are extended, opened, and relaxed. Large postures are especially suitable for improving health. The medium posture style requires that all the forms be neither too extended nor too restricted and the internal jin neither totally emitted nor too conserved. Therefore, the form and jin are smoother and more continuous than the other two styles. The medium posture style was taught by Yang, Jian-hou. The small posture style—in which the forms are more compact and the movements light, agile, and quick—was passed down by Yang, Shao-hou. This style specializes in the martial application of the art. In conclusion, for martial application the small postures are generally the best, although they are the most difficult, and the large posture style is best for health purposes.

To summarize:

1. Chen Style Taijiquan was derived from Jiang Style . Before Jiang, the history is vague and unclear.

2. Chen Style Taijiquan was divided into two styles: old and new. Chen, Chang-xing learned old style and later passed it down to Yang, Lu-chan. New style was created by Chen, You-ben.

3. Yang Style Taijiquan was derived from Chen Style Taijiquan fourteen generations after the Chen family learned from Jiang.

4. Chen, You-ben passed his art to Chen, Qing-ping who created Zhao Bao Style.

5. Wuu, Yu-rang obtained the new style from Chen, Qing-ping and the old style from Yang, Lu-chan and created Wuu Style Taijiquan.

6. Li, Yi-yu learned Wuu Style Taijiquan and created Li Style Taijiquan.

7. Hao, Wei-zhen obtained his art from Li Style Taijiquan and started Hao Style Taijiquan.

8. Sun, Lu-tang learned from Hao Style Taijiquan and began Sun Style Taijiquan.

9. Wu Style Taijiquan was started by Wu, Quan-you who learned from Yang, Lu-chan's second son Yang, Ban-hou.

10. Yang Style Taijiquan has been famous since its creation by Yang, Lu-chan in the early part of the 20th century.

11. Yang, Cheng-fu's taijiquan is not the same as his father's, uncle's, or brother's. He modified it and emphasized large postures and improving health.

You should now understand why there are so many variations within the art, even within a style such as the Yang Style. After so many years and so many generations, countless students have learned the style and have made many modifications in light of their own experiences and research. It is understandable that a student today might learn taijiquan and find that his or her style is different from another claiming to be from the same source. No one can really tell which one is the original style, or which is more effective than the others. Observations from nature and contemplation of the Dao can help you to determine a style's emphasis—either for healing or self-defense—but it is purely a subjective, human determination whether one is in fact "better" than any other. This is a deeply profound area of the art. Self-defense and good health are indeed closely related concepts, separated only by a philosophical frame of mind.

Ultimately, such comparisons of techniques are meaningless. It is the time, consistency, and quality of your practice that matters. If you can understand this, even as you strive for deeper mastery of your chosen art, then you have already reached a profound understanding of Dao.

1-5. Taijiquan and Health

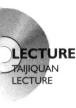

Since ancient times, taijiquan has been recognized as one of the most effective ways of maintaining health. However, this treasure was not revealed to the general Chinese public until the beginning of the 20th century. Since then, taijiquan has become widely accepted as the most popular martial qigong exercise for health. This section will compare taijiquan with other martial qigong, to provide an idea of its relative effectiveness for improving health and preventing disease.

First, you should recognize that taijiquan is a qigong practice, even though it was originally created for self-defense purposes. Second, taijiquan was created based on the theory of yin and yang, the most basic natural concept in the Dao, or "natural way." It is because of this that the balance of the yin and yang remains the most important goal of all practice. It is also because of this that the body's healthy condition, which depends on the balance of yin and yang, can be attained. Third, taijiquan was created in the Daoist monastery, where the final goal of training was spiritual enlightenment. Because of this, the meaning of life was constantly pondered, and a peaceful, harmonious environment was created, both externally and internally. The product of this environment, taijiquan, is a calm and peaceful mind and a relaxed, healthy body. These elements are the critical keys to health both mentally and physically.

Because taijiquan is a qigong training, it was developed following the natural cultivation and training procedures of qigong—also known as the five regulations (*wu tiao*, 五調). Here, we will summarize how this training path can be beneficial for human health.

Regulating the Body (*Tiao Shen*, 調身). The first step in learning taijiquan, other than learning to do the movements accurately, is the emphasis on physical relaxation. In order to obtain a deep level of relaxation, you must first relax your mind. Moreover, you must feel the balance of your body and maintain your physical and mental centers. In order to reach this goal, you must practice until you have strengthened and firmed your legs and torso. This key to maintaining your spiritual center is to first stabilize your mental and physical centers.

Once you have reached the goal of relaxation, you have achieved the most basic condition for your health. If you can relax deeply in your body, the blood and qi circulation can flow smoothly. This will make cell replacement in the body occur without error. Maintaining cell replacement in the body is the key to health and longevity

Regulating the Breathing (*Tiao Xi*, 調息). Once you can relax physically, then you must pay attention to your breathing and come to a full appreciation of how your body absorbs oxygen and expels carbon dioxide smoothly and profoundly. Every cell in the body requires oxygen. If you can take in oxygen smoothly and abundantly, you will provide a crucial ingredient for the creation of new cells in your body. In addition, through deep breathing, you can help to eliminate dead cells from your body through exhalation (carbon dioxide). The carbon in our exhalation originates from two sources: one is from the biochemical combustion of the food we eat, which is primarily composed of carbon, nitrogen, hydrogen, and oxygen. The other source is from our body's own decay and replenishment. Every cell in our body has a lifetime (e.g., a skin cell is 28 days). Amazingly, a trillion (10^{12}) cells die in our body each day.[15] When these cells die, the body must eliminate them and their consituent carbon molecules. Each of our exhalations is a part of this ongoing process.

In order to increase your lung capacity and slow down your breathing, it is necessary to practice either your qigong or taijiquan with an emphasis on the breath. No matter whether you use regular or reverse abdominal breathing, it is necessary to use as much of the lungs' volume as possible without tensing up. Notice that if you inhale to the full capacity of your lungs, you will feel a tightness right under your sternum and possibly into your back and abdomen. You want to avoid this feeling of tightness while still using as much of your lungs' capacity as possible. A good method of practicing is to simply focus on your breathing, filling the lungs from the bottom to the top, and emptying them from the top to the bottom. Remember to avoid tension and to let the breath flow in and out in a controlled, smooth, soft, and uniform manner.

In addition, the breathing helps to prepare you for the next stage of regulating the mind. The breath is a pathway linking the external and the internal universes, and you can use it to guide yourself to this deeper level of existence. The speed, depth, and quality of your breathing will have a direct impact on your taiji, your mental and emotional states, and your physical and energetic bodies. Therefore, in taijiquan practice, you must learn how to breathe deeply and correctly.

Regulating the Mind (*Tiao Xin,* 調心). The mind is the general who directs the body's battle against sickness. If the command post is disordered and the general is confused, naturally the battle will be lost. Remember, in Chinese culture the mind is viewed as having two distinct aspects. The first is the yi, or wisdom mind. The wisdom mind is responsible for the intellect and the higher mental functions, but it is somewhat sterile. The second aspect of the mind is the xin, or emotional mind. The emotional mind encompasses all emotional states and passions. It is the originator of desire and aggression and from it flows all actions and intentions manifested to the physical world. However, it is also selfish and fearful, and if not properly regulated by the wisdom mind, it will lead you to destructive purposes and possibly even self-destruction. Regulating the mind means learning how to calm down your emotional mind and strengthen your wisdom mind. Throughout this process, you must constantly conquer yourself and ponder the meaning of your life. The goal of regulating the mind is to lead you into a deeply profound, peaceful, and harmonious state. Once you are in this state, you can use your whole mind to lead the qi and circulate it through the entire body. From this training, you build clear connections between the mind, body, and qi.

Regulating the Qi (*Tiao Qi,* 調氣). As mentioned previously, if you have a peaceful mind, a relaxed body, and correct breathing, you can lead the qi to anyplace in your body. For a martial artist, the first step is to lead the qi to the limbs to energize the muscles there for defensive purposes. The result of this is the production of strong internal power called jin (勁).

For a person who is training only for health, the mind can be used to circulate the qi in the body through Small Circulation (*Xiao Zhou Tian*, 小周天) and Grand Circulation (*Da Zhou Tian*, 大周天) meditation practice. If you are interested in knowing more about jin and qi circulation, you should refer to additional books and videos published by YMAA.

Regulating the Spirit (*Tiao Shen*, 調神). The final stage of taijiquan practice is regulating the spirit and strengthening the spiritual center. In this training, you use your mind to lead the qi though the thrusting vessel (*chong mai*, 衝脈), that is, the spinal cord to the brain, energizing it and opening the third eye for enlightenment. Since this subject is very profound and of interest only to the most advanced taiji practitioners, it will not be explored further in this work.

From the above, you can appreciate the reasons why taijiquan can reward you with a healthy body, both mentally (yin) and physically (yang). If you practice for only a few minutes every day, you can bring your mind to a peaceful and harmonious level and open your perception to an entire new world of living energy.

1-6. What is Taijiquan?

Let us see what is Taijiquan, as it was written down in the past. First, we must define what we mean by "taiji." It is stated in Wang, Zong-yue's (王宗岳) *Taijiquan Classic*.[4,16]

> *"What is taiji? It is generated from wuji and is a pivotal function of movement and stillness. It is the mother of yin and yang. When it moves, it divides. At rest it reunites."*

太極者，無極而生，動靜之機，陰陽之母也，動之則分，靜之則合。

According to Chinese Daoist scripture, the universe was initially without life. The world had just cooled down from its fiery creation and all was foggy and blurry, without differentiation or separation, with no extremities or ends. This state was called "wuji" (無極) that literally means no extremity, no dividing, or no discrimination. Later, the existing natural energy divided into two extremities, known as yin and yang. This polarity, or tendency to divide, is called taiji, which means grand ultimate or grand extremity, and also means very ultimate or very extreme. It is this initial separation that allows and causes all other separations and changes.

From the above, you can see that taiji, which is derived from wuji, is not yin and yang but is instead the mother of yin and yang. How then do we interpret and define "grand ultimate" as the characters for which taiji is usually translated? And how can we apply this concept to taijiquan practice? Let us turn to the beginning movement of the taijiquan form for an illustration that reveals the answers to these questions.

When you stand still, before you start the sequence, you are in a state of wuji, that is, a state of formlessness. Your mind should be calm, quiet, peaceful, and centered. Your mind, and hence your qi, should focus at your energetic and physical center, i.e., your lower dan tian or center of gravity. Your body is relaxed, with no intention. Your weight is evenly distributed on both legs.

However, once you generate the intention to start the sequence and you begin to move, you are in a state of taiji (i.e., yin and yang start to be differentiated to perception). As the form continues, you shift from side to side, from foot to foot, and each part of your body becomes at times alternately substantial and insubstantial. The taiji in the taijiquan form is thus actually the intention or the motivation generated from the mind that causes the yin and yang to be discriminated. It is this mind that shapes reality. It is this mind that guides us to a deeper and more profound understanding. And it is this living and active mind that continues to achieve further perceptions of yin and yang. From this, you can see why taiji is called "grand ultimate," and why the mind is the Dao in taijiquan practice. Therefore, taijiquan is primarily an art of the mind.

Through the mind's action, the entire art becomes alive. Once you start a motion it is possible to modify or redirect it, but this modification is possible only after the motion has been started. If one change is made, others can be made, and each change opens up other possibilities for variation. Each factor in the situation introduces other factors as possible influences. The initial motion made all other motions possible, and in a sense "created" the other motions. The Chinese express this by saying that taiji is the mother of yin and yang: "Taiji begets two poles, two poles produce four phases, four phases generate eight trigrams (gates), and eight trigrams initiate sixty-four hexagrams" (Figure 1-7).[17]

The yin and yang theory is used to classify everything, whether ideas, spirit, strategy, or force. For example, female is yin and male is yang, night is yin and day is yang, weak is yin and strong is yang. It is from the interaction of all the yin and yang that life was created and grew. Taijiquan is based on this theory and applies it to form, motion, force, and fighting strategy. In the thousands of years since the taiji theory was first stated, many taiji symbols have been designed. The best one for both theory and

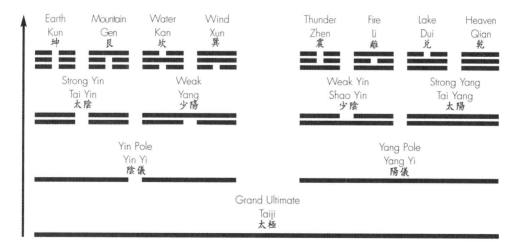

Figure 1-7. The Eight Trigrams are derived from Taiji

application is a circle that contains yin and yang (Figure 1-8). In this figure, the circle and the curved dividing line between yin and yang imply that both yin and yang are generated and contained in roundness. The smooth dividing line between yin and yang means that they interact smoothly and efficiently. Extreme yang weakens and evolves into yin, first weak and then extreme yin. Extreme yin, in turn, evolves into yang. One evolves into the other and back again, continuously and without stopping. The diagram also shows a small dot of yin in the center of the greatest concentration of yang, and a little bit of yang inside the greatest concentration of yin. This means that there is no absolute yin or yang.

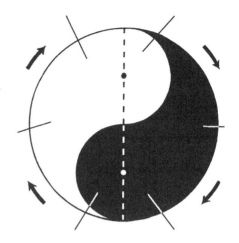

Figure 1-8. The Taiji diagram

Yang always reserves some yin and vice versa. This also implies that there is a seed or source of yin in yang and of yang in yin.

Taijiquan is based on this theory, and therefore it is smooth, continuous, and round. When it is necessary to be soft, the art is soft, and when it is necessary to be hard, the art can be hard enough to defeat any opponent. Yin-yang theory also determines taiji fighting strategy and has led to thirteen concepts which guide practice and fighting. Thus, taijiquan is also called "thirteen postures."

Zhang, San-feng's (張三豐) *Taijiquan Treatise* states:[16]

> *What are the thirteen postures? peng (wardoff), lu (rollback), ji (press or squeeze), an (press down, forward, upward), cai (pluck or grab), lie (split or rend), zhou (elbow), kao (bump), these are the eight trigrams. Jin bu (step forward), tui bu (step backward), zuo gu (beware of the left), you pan (look to the right), zhong ding (central equilibrium), these are the five elements. Wardoff, rollback, press, and push are qian (heaven), kun (earth), kan (water), and li (fire), the four main sides. Pluck, split, elbow, and bump are xun (wind), zhen (thunder), dui (lake), and gen (mountain), the four diagonal corners. Step forward, step backward, beware of the left, look to the right, and central equilibrium are jin (metal), mu (wood), shui (water), huo (fire), and tu (earth). All together they are the thirteen postures.[16]*

> 十三勢者？　　掤、攦、擠、按、採、挒、肘、靠，此八卦也。進步、退步、左顧、右盼、中定，此五行也。掤、攦、擠、按，即乾、坤、坎、離，四正方也。採、挒、肘、靠，即巽、震、兌、艮，四斜角也。進、退、顧、盼、定，即金、木、水、火、土也。合之為十三勢也。

The eight postures are the eight basic fighting jin patterns of the art and can be assigned directions according to where the opponent's force is moved. Peng (wardoff) rebounds the opponent back in the direction he came from. Lu (rollback) leads him further than he intended to go in the direction he was attacking. Lie (split) and kao (bump) lead him forward and deflect him slightly sideward. Cai (pluck) and zhou (elbow) can be done so as to catch the opponent just as he is starting forward, and strike or unbalance him diagonally to his rear. Ji (press or squeeze) and an (press down, forward, and upward) deflect the opponent and attack at right angles to his motion. The five directions refer to stance, footwork, and fighting strategy. They concern the way you move around in response to the opponent's attack, and how you set up your own attacks. We will discuss the thirteen postures in more detail in Chapter 3.

Since ancient times, many taiji masters have tried to explain the deeper aspect of these thirteen postures by using the eight trigrams and the five elements. In order to find a satisfactory explanation, various correspondences between the eight basic techniques and the eight trigrams, and also between the five directions and the five elements have been devised. Unfortunately, none of the explanations are completely reasonable and without discrepancy.[16]

In addition to the thirteen postures, taijiquan is also commonly called soft sequence (*mian quan*, 綿拳). This is because when taiji is practiced, the forms are soft and smooth, the mind is calm, the qi is round, and jin is fluid. Taijiquan is also called Long Sequence (*Chang Quan* or *Changquan,* 長拳). Zhang, San-feng's *Taijiquan Treatise* states:[16]

> *What is Long Fist [i.e., Long Sequence]? [It is] like a long river and a large ocean, rolling ceaselessly.*

長拳者，如長江大海滔滔不絕也 。

Originally, the name "Changquan" came from the Shaolin Temple. Changquan means Long Fist. It can also be translated as Long Range or Long Sequence. Ancient documents suggest that the meaning of Changquan in Taijiquan means the Long Sequence like a long river that acts as a conduit to the open ocean, which also means that when taiji is practiced, the forms flow smoothly and continuously. The qi flow is smooth and continuous, and the jin is unbroken. There is another martial style also called Chang Quan. However, this Shaolin style should be translated as Long Fist because it specializes in long-range fighting.

1-7. Contents of Yang Style Taijiquan Practice

Taijiquan has been evolving for more than seven hundred years, and it is very difficult to state just exactly what makes up the art. The content of the art has varied from one generation to the next. For example, one generation might specialize in the taiji spear and gradually come to ignore other aspects of the art such as the sword or saber. The contents of the system can also vary from one teacher to another. A student might have learned only the sword from his master, and so naturally the sword would be the only weapon he could teach. Some masters will emphasize a particular principle or training method because of their experience, temperament, or research, or perhaps they will create a new training style for a new weapon.

Since the beginning of this century, taiji weapons' practice has been increasingly ignored. Frequently only the bare hand solo sequence is taught. In some cases the solo sequence has been modified to make it simpler and shorter, and therefore more accessible to a greater number of people. Although a number of techniques have been eliminated, the sequence still serves the purpose of improving health. However, a simplified sequence may not be enough if you are interested in deeper research and practice. Additionally, the coordination of breath and qi circulation is often ignored. Most people these days learn taijiquan without ever being exposed to the martial applications of the postures, the concept of jin, bare hand fighting sets, or taijiquan sparring.

Taiji sword and saber sequences, because of their beauty, are practiced in the West, although the applications of the techniques are seldom taught. Qi enhancement and extension training seems almost to have disappeared. Taiji spear, taiji staff, taiji ball qigong, and taiji ruler can hardly be found in this country.

The reason for this is nothing new. The practitioners today are usually looking for a relatively quick and easy way to improve and maintain their health. Very few are willing to sacrifice their time for the long, hard training required to develop the other aspects of the art. Because of this, both in China and the rest of the world, even if a master is qualified to teach the whole art, he may be reluctant to pass it down to an unappreciative, if not actually doubting, generation. It seems very possible that the deeper aspects of Taijiquan will die out in the near future.

The various aspects of taijiquan that are still available are listed below for reference:
1. Barehand
    Taiji solo sequence
    Applications from the solo sequence
    Fast taiji training
    Still meditation
    Qi circulation training
    Jin training
    Pushing hands and its applications
    Taiji fighting set and deeper martial applications
    Taiji free-pushing hands and sparring
2. Taiji Sword
    a. Taiji sword solo sequence
    b. Qi enhancement and extension training
    c. Martial applications
    d. Taiji sword matching forms
    e. Taiji sword sparring
3. Taiji Saber
    a. Taiji saber solo sequence
    b. Martial applications
    c. Taiji saber matching forms
    d. Taiji saber sparring

4. Taiji Spear and Staff
    a. Individual spear and staff martial techniques
    b. Spear and staff sticking-matching practice
    c. Long weapons sparring

5. Taiji Ball
    a. Listening and understanding jin training
    b. Adhere-stick jin training
    c. Qi Enhancement and extension training
    d. Two-person taiji ball training

6. Taiji Ruler
    a. Qi enhancement and extension training for health. Detail unknown.

It can be seen that some of the training areas are already incomplete. For example, there is no longer a complete traditional staff or spear sequence, although a few individual techniques are still taught by some masters. In mainland China, complete sequences are being practiced for a number of weapons, but these sequences have been developed only in the last few years. There are very few masters anywhere who still know and train with the taiji ruler or taiji ball. However, even with the abridged list of taiji activities available today, it would still take about twenty years to learn the art.

1-8. How Do You Learn Taijiquan?

The Attitude of Learning Taijiquan. Whether or not a person learns something depends upon his attitude and seriousness. First he must make a firm decision to learn it, and then he must have a strong will to fulfill his intention. He needs perseverance and patience to last to the end. Even if a person has all these virtues, his achievement might still be different from that of another person's who has the same qualities and personality. The difference is due to his manner of learning. If a person practices and then ponders every new thing he has learned and keeps going back to research and master it, he will naturally be better than the person who never explores what he has learned.

Taijiquan theory is deep and profound. It takes many years of learning, research, pondering, and practice to gradually grasp the key to the art and "enter into the temple." However, the more you learn, the less you are likely to feel you understand. It is just like a bottomless well or a ceaselessly flowing river. There is an ancient list of five mental keys the student of taijiquan needs in order to reach the higher levels of the art.[16] It is said: 1. Study wide and deep (博學); 2. Investigate, ask (審問); 3. Ponder carefully (慎思); 4. Clearly discriminate (明辨); and 5. Work perseveringly (篤行). If you follow this procedure you can learn anything, even how to become a wise and knowledgeable person.

In addition to the above learning attitude, a good master is also an important key to learning the high art of taijiquan. In China, there is a saying: "A disciple inquires and searches for a master for three years, and a master will test the disciple for three years."[18] It also says: "A disciple would rather spend three years looking for a good master than learn three years from an unqualified one." A good master who comprehends the art and teaches it to his students is the key to changing a rock into a piece of gold. It is the teacher who can guide you to the doorway by the shortest path possible and help you avoid wasting your time and energy. It is said: "To enter the door and be led along the way, one needs oral instruction; practice without ceasing, the way is through self-practice."[19] It is also said: "Famous masters create great disciples."[20] On the other hand, a good master will also judge if a disciple is worth his spending the time and energy to teach. A student can be intelligent and practice hard in the beginning, and change his attitude later on. A student who practices, ponders, humbly asks, and researches on his own will naturally be a good successor to the style. Usually a master needs three years to see through a student's personality and know whether he is likely to persevere in his studies and maintain a good moral character.

In the last seventy years since taijiquan has been popularized, many good taijiquan books and documents have been published. A sincere taiji practitioner should collect and read them. Books are the recording of many years of learning, study, and research. If you do not know how to use this literature to your advantage, you will surely waste more time and energy wandering in confusion. However, you should not completely believe what any book says. What is written is only the author's opinions and personal experience. You should read widely, investigate, and then clearly discriminate between the worthwhile and the not so worthwhile. If you do this well you can minimize confusion and avoid straying too far from the right path.

In addition, you should take advantage of seminars, summer camps, and other ways to get in touch with experienced masters. In this way you can catch many key points and gain a feeling for many things which you may have only read about. But remember, you must research on your own in great detail in order to achieve a deeper understanding of the art. Thus it is said: "You don't ever want to give up your throat; question every talented person in heaven and earth. If [you are] asked: how can one attain this great achievement, [the answer is] outside and inside, fine and coarse, nothing must not be touched upon."[21]

Taijiquan Learning Procedures. When you learn an internal art such as qigong or taijiquan, you should always follow the training procedures. In the beginning, you should pay attention to the movements and try to be as accurate as possible. These movements were created and experienced by many wise pioneers of taijiquan. Only after you have mastered these movements skillfully will you be on the right path for learning taijiquan. Moreover, you must also learn how to relax physically to a profound level, keeping yourself centered and rooted both physically and mentally. This process is called regulating the body (*tiao shen*, 調身). Only after you have reached the stage of regulating without regulating, should you proceed to the next stage. While you are training at this level, you will not have to constantly regulate the body consciously, since you will have already made it into a habit and can perform your physical forms naturally. This is what is meant by "regulating without regulating."

The next step is learning how to coordinate your breathing with the movements. With correct breath coordination, you can relax more deeply, which allows you to bring your mind to a more sagacious state. This is the step of regulating the breathing (*tiao xi*, 調息). You should practice until you can regulate without the use of your conscious mind, the aforementioned regulating without regulating. Your breathing must become natural, smooth, deep, slender and calm. Once you have reached this stage, you will have provided a good environment for your wisdom mind to regulate the emotional mind (*tiao xi*, 調心).

If you practice taijiquan simply for relaxation and health when you regulate your mind, then you will learn how to lead the qi to the centers of the palms and the soles of the feet. This is called Four Gate Breathing (*Si Xin Hu Xi*, 四心呼吸). You can also lead the qi to the skin and beyond, to enhance your guardian qi. This will strengthen your immune system and raise your spirit.

However, if you practice taijiquan for martial arts, then you must learn to use your mind to lead the qi to the arms for performing techniques, and to the legs for rooting. In order to manifest power efficiently, you must build a sense of enemy. To do this, you imagine that you are in a combat situation, using each of your performed techniques to defend yourself against an enemy. You must have a sense of controlled urgency because in such a combat situation, you must be alert but not in a state of panic. Only by training all of your techniques with this sense of enemy will you build up your skills to a level that will be useful to you in a real emergency. You must know the martial applications of each movement without having to stop and think. These martial applications are the essence and the root of taijiquan. This leading of the qi is called regulating the qi (*tiao qi*, 調氣).

Finally, your ultimate goal in taijiquan practice is to harmonize your energy with the energy of the natural universe. In order to achieve this goal, you must regulate your spirit (*tiao shen*, 調神) to a firm, strong, peaceful and enlightened state. Only then may you reach the final cultivation of the Dao: the unification of heaven (i.e., universe) and humanity (*tian ren he yi*, 天人合一). When you reach this stage, you will find that even your purpose in studying taijiquan, the very ego that holds the desire to learn and improve, will itself disolve into the patterns of taiji. Taijiquan is only the way or path to understanding life and comprehending the universe. As you near your goal, you will find that your motivation to learn martial arts is sublimated, and the health of your body, mind, and spirit can be unified and maintained without conscious effort.

More information will be given on the five regulating processes of taijiquan practice in Chapter 4. If you would like to know more about the above qigong regulating procedures, please refer to the books, *The Root of Chinese Qigong* and *The Essence of Taiji Qigong*, published by YMAA.

Training Sequence. Every taijiquan master has his own sequence of training, emphasizing his methods and content. In this section, the author lists the general training procedures according to his learning experience with three taijiquan masters and his teaching experience of more than forty years. This section is a guide only to the bare hand training procedures of taijiquan.

The general sequence of taijiquan training is as follows:

1. Understanding the fundamental theory of taijiquan
2. Relaxation, calmness, and concentration practice
3. Breath training
4. Experiencing and generating qi
5. Qi circulation and breathing
6. Still meditation
7. Fundamental stances
8. Breath coordination drills
9. Fundamental moving drills
10. Solo taijiquan
11. Analysis of the martial applications of the sequence
12. Beginning stationary taiji pushing hands
13. Fundamental forms of taiji jin training
14. *Hen* and *ha* sound training
15. Fast taijiquan
16. Advanced taiji pushing hands (both stationary and moving)
17. Advanced taiji jin training
18. Qi expansion and transportation training
19. Martial applications of taiji pushing hands
20. Free-pushing hands (both stationary and moving)
21. Taiji fighting set
22. Taiji free fighting

Before the taijiquan beginner starts training, he should ask himself several questions: Why do I want to learn taijiquan? What benefits do I hope to gain? Am I likely to continue training for a long time?

After you have answered these questions you should then ask: Does this taijiquan style offer what I want? Is this master qualified? Does this master have a training schedule? How long and how deep can this master teach me? Will this master teach me everything he knows or will he keep secrets when I approach a certain level? After I have studied for many years, will I be able to find an advanced master to continue my study? In order to answer these questions, you have to survey and investigate. You have to know the historical background of the style and the master's experience. Once you have answered the above questions, then you can begin your taijiquan study without any doubt or confusion.

The first step in learning taijiquan is to understand the fundamental theory and principles through discussion with your master, reading the available books, studying with classmates, and then pondering on your own. You should ask yourself: How does taijiquan benefit the body and improve health? How can taijiquan be used for martial purposes? What are the differences between taijiquan and other martial styles? Once you have answers to these questions, you should have a picture of the art and an idea of where you are going. The next question to arise should be: How do I train the relaxation, calmness, and concentration which are the most basic and important aspects of taijiquan? This leads you to the second step of the training.

Usually, if you have the right methods and concepts, you can train your mind to be calm and concentrated and can relax physically in a short time. Keeping this meditative attitude is very important for beginning training. The next step is to train your breathing. The breathing must be deep, natural, and long. If you are interested in health only, you can use Buddhist or normal abdominal breathing. However, if you want to advance to martial applications, you should train and master Daoist, or reverse abdominal breathing (read Chapter 2). You should be able to expand and withdraw the muscles of the abdomen area easily. After you have trained your breath correctly, you should then begin to sense the qi in your abdomen and dan tian. This will lead to the fourth step—generating and experiencing qi. If you are interested in knowing more about taijiquan and breathing, please refer to the book, *The Essence of Taiji Qigong*, published by YMAA.

Usually, qi can be generated in two ways: externally and internally. To generate qi externally is called wai dan (外丹), and when it is generated internally it is called nei dan (內丹). Through training qi generation you will gradually realize what qi is and why smooth qi circulation benefits the body. You will also build up your sensitivity to the movement of qi. The more you train, the more sensitive you will become. After a time, you should then go to the next step—circulating qi. This is best practiced through still meditation, which will enhance your qi generation and circulation. Qi circulation is guided by the calm mind and made possible by a relaxed body. You must train your mind to guide the qi wherever you wish in coordination with correct breathing. First you should develop small circulation, which moves the qi up the spine and down the center of the front of the body (i.e., governing and conception vessels, 任脈，督脈). Eventually you should develop grand circulation whereby qi is circulated to every part of your body. When you have completed the above six steps, you should have built a firm foundation for taijiquan practice. With correct instruction, it should take less than six months to complete the above training (except for grand circulation).

The above six steps are purely mental training. When you practice these, you can simultaneously practice the fundamental stances that build the root for the taijiquan forms. You should be familiar with all the stances and should practice them statically to strengthen your legs. Also, at this stage you can begin fundamental breath coordination drills. These drills are designed for the beginning student to train: 1. coordination of breathing and movement; 2. coordination of qi circulation and the forms; 3. smoothness and continuity; 4. relaxation; and 5. calmness and concentration of the mind. These drills will help you experience qi circulation and the mood or atmosphere of taijiquan practice. After you have mastered the fundamental stances and fundamental drills, you should then go on to the fundamental moving drills.

The taijiquan solo sequence is constructed with about thirty-seven apparent techniques and more than two hundred hidden techniques. It is practiced to enhance qi circulation and improve health, and it is the foundation of all taijiquan martial techniques. It usually takes from six months to three years to learn this sequence, depending on the instructor, the length of the sequence, the student's talent, and most importantly, his or her commitment to practice. After a student has learned this sequence, it will usually take another three years to attain a degree of calmness and relaxation and to internalize the proper coordination of the breathing. When practicing, not only the whole of your attention, but also your feelings, emotions, and mood should be on the sequence. It is just like when musicians or dancers perform their art—their emotions and total being must be melded into the art. If they hold anything back, then even if their skill is very great, their art will be dead.

When you finish learning the solo sequence, you should then start discussing and investigating the martial applications of the postures. This is a necessary part of the training of a martial arts practitioner, but it will also help the non-martial artist to better understand the sequence and circulate qi. With the instruction of a qualified master, it will take at least two or three years to understand and master the techniques. While this stage of analysis is going on, you should begin to pick up fundamental (fixed step) pushing hands.

Pushing hands trains you to listen to and to feel the opponent's jin, understand it, neutralize it, and then counterattack. There are two aspects of pushing hands training. The first emphasizes feeling the opponent's jin and then neutralizing it, and the second emphasizes understanding the emitting of jin and its applications. Therefore, when you start the fundamental pushing hands, you should also start fundamental jin training that is usually difficult to practice and understand. For this, a qualified master is extremely important. While training jin, the coordination of the sounds "hen" and "ha" become very important. Uttering "hen" and "ha" can enable you to emit or withdraw your jin to the maximum and coordinate the qi with it, and can also help to raise your spirit of vitality.

When you finish your analysis of the sequence, you have established the martial foundation of taijiquan. You should then start to train speeding up the solo sequence, training jin in every movement. In fast taiji training, practice emitting jin in pulses with a firm root, proper waist control, and qi support. In addition, develop the feeling of having an enemy in front of you while you are doing the form. This will help you learn to apply the techniques naturally and to react automatically. After practicing this for a few years, you should have grasped the basics of jin and should start advanced pushing hands and jin training.

Advanced (moving step) pushing hands will train you to step smoothly and correctly in coordination with your techniques and fighting strategy. This training builds the foundation of free-pushing hands and free fighting. Advanced jin training enables you to understand the higher level of jin application and covers the entire range of jin. During these two steps of training, you should continue your qi enhancement, expansion, and transportation training to strengthen the qi support of your jin. The martial applications of pushing hands should be analyzed and discussed. This is the bridge that connects the techniques learned in the sequence to the real applications. When you understand all the techniques thoroughly, you should then get involved in free-pushing hands and learn the two-person fighting set.

The Taiji Fighting Set was designed to train the use of techniques in a way that resembles real fighting. Proper footwork is very important. Once you are moving and interacting fluidly, you can begin to use jin. The final step in training is free fighting with different partners. The more partners you practice with, the more experience you will gain. The more time and energy you spend, the more skillful you will become.

The most important thing in all this training is your attitude. Remember to study widely, question humbly, investigate, discriminate, and work perseveringly. This is the way to success.

1-9. Becoming a Proficient Taijiquan Artist

Once you have mastered the basic theory and fundamental techniques, you have reached a level where you are qualified to share and discuss your knowledge with others. You should be capable of teaching someone else without too much deviation from the right path. The best way to start your teaching career is to be an assistant instructor for an experienced master for several years. Under his supervision you will learn how to teach, but most importantly, you can access his experience and pick up the many small points that do so much to fill out your knowledge. After a few years you should start teaching on your own. Teaching is the best way to learn and become a proficient taijiquan artist. Through teaching, you learn how to analyze, how to explain, and how to set up a training schedule. After a few years of doing this, you can create something of value and add to the store of taijiquan knowledge.

LECTURE
TAIJIQUAN
LECTURE

It is the urge to teach that has been responsible for taijiquan's art being passed down from generation to generation. A master earns respect from sharing his knowledge with his students. Through his teaching and research he also gains the friendship of those who share his interest and enthusiasm.

If you are hoping and planning to become a taijiquan master, there are several points you should always remember:

Know the History. History is experience. If you do not know the past, you will be lost in the future. The past gives spiritual stimulation. From the past, you know your source and root. Knowing the history of Taijiquan is the obligation of every practitioner who is willing to carry the responsibility of continuing the long tradition of the art.

A desire to know the history of the art indicates enthusiasm and a depth of interest in the art, which will lead to a deep and profound knowledge. Remember, history is like a mirror that helps you to see through yourself. It shows you the right way to the future.

Know the Theory and Principles. Every martial style is based on its own theory and principles. Taijiquan has its own unique principles, and if you disobey them you are no longer doing taijiquan. Fortunately, these theories and principles have been passed down for generations through oral instruction or written documents. In order to be qualified as a taijiquan instructor, you must study all these documents and understand them. They, along with commentary, are presented in the book *Tai Chi Theory and Martial Power*, published by YMAA.

Know What You are Doing. Once you know the history and principles, you should ask yourself a few questions: Have I practiced these martial applications long enough so that I can use them naturally whenever necessary? Do I have a good training schedule for myself and my students? How well do I know what I am doing? All in all, am I qualified to be a taijiquan instructor?

If your answers to these questions are negative, your teaching may earn you more shame than honor. When your qualifications are limited, you must work to improve yourself and your teaching. Be humble and keep researching and pondering. Practice and discuss with your taijiquan friends, participate in seminars and workshops, and most important of all, make friends with all taijiquan stylists. Never be afraid to be humble and ask for other people's ideas and experiences. When you practice, keep digging and plowing, and never be satisfied with what you have already done. Look forward and not behind, and one day you will harvest more than others. Then you will become a master.

Know What Other Instructors are Doing. In order to become a real master, you need to know not only yourself, but also others. When you understand others' styles you can understand your own style better and evaluate it more objectively. You can evaluate how good it is and where its limitations are. Every style has its own specialties, so if you think some style is not as good as yours, it might just be that your knowledge of that style is still shallow. Also, when you see a style that seems better than yours, don't give up your style for it. That would be throwing away all the time and effort you have spent on it. After all, once you have invested a lot of time in this new style, you may find that there is nothing beneath the surface glitter that initially attracted you. If you believe that your style and your personal level of ability are superior to others, you must beware of losing your humility, for this may cause you to lose your enthusiasm for learning.

Sometimes you may hear of a martial artist who has studied only ten years, but claims to have mastered five or even ten styles. Since it usually takes at least ten years of daily practice to master one style, such a person has probably only studied each style very superficially. Consider carefully whether you want to master one or two styles, or whether you prefer learning a limited portion of ten or more styles. It is best to pick a style you believe is best for you and to dig in and really learn it. If you learn one style to its fullest, you can understand other styles more deeply and can add substantial elements from other styles.

Know Your Students. Knowing your students is almost as important as knowing yourself. These are the questions you must ask about each student: What is his motivation in learning taijiquan? Can I trust this student? Is this student patient and persevering enough to fulfill his goals? If I teach him will I be wasting my time? When this student has finished learning from me, will he continue his study from other sources? Will he become a good master in the future? Does he have good morality?

You must ask yourself these questions before you invest time and energy in any student. A student must first show interest, enthusiasm, respect, and loyalty. Then he must demonstrate strong will, patience, and perseverance to carry on the training. In other words, a student must show that he is worthy of your trust and teaching. And once he does this, you must respect the difficult sacrifices that he has made and teach him from your heart.

Notes

1. *The Complete Arts of Shaolin Wushu,* 少林武術大全, 德虔編著。北京体育出版社, 1991.

2. 中國武術大辭典, *(Chinese Wushu Great Dictionary),* 人民体育出版社 (People's Athletic Publications), Beijing, 1990.

3. 一膽，二力，三功夫。

4. "太極拳，刀、劍、杆、散手合編" (*Tai Chi Chuan: Saber, Sword, Staff, and Sparring*), Chen, Yan-lin (陳炎林). Reprinted in Taipei, Taiwan, 1943.

5. 外練筋骨皮，內練一口氣。

6. 外家由硬而軟，內家由軟而硬，其法雖異，其的則同。

7. 外家由外而內，內家由內而外，其途雖異，其終的則一致。

8. 外家先力爾氣，內家先氣后力。

9. 練拳不練功，到老一場空。

10. 師父領進門，修行在自身。

11. 大道不過三兩句，說破不值三文錢。

12. 南雷集王征南墓志銘:"宋之張三豐為武當丹士。徽宗召之,路梗不得進。夜夢元帝授之拳法,厥明以單丁殺賊百余。"

13. 明史方妓傳:"張三豐遼東懿州人,名全一。一名君寶。三豐其號也。 以不修邊幅,又號張邋遢。頎而偉,龜形鶴背。大耳圓目,鬚髯如戟。 寒暑惟一衲簑,所啖升斗輒盡。或數日不食,或數月不食,一日千里。 善嬉戲,旁若無人。嘗与其徒游武當。筑草盧而居之,洪武二十四年, 太祖聞其名,遣使覓之不得。"

14. 明郎瑛七修類稿: " 張仙名君寶,字全一。別號玄玄, 時人又稱張邋遢 。天順三年,曾來謁帝。予見其像,鬚鬢豎立,一髻背垂,紫面大腹, 而攜笠者。上為錫誥之文,封為通微顯化真人。"

15. 解剖生理學 (*A Study of Anatomic Physiology*), 李文森編著。 華杏出版股份有限公司。Taipei, 1986.

16. *Tai Chi Theory and Martial Power*, Dr. Yang Jwing-Ming. YMAA, Boston, 1987.

17. 太極生兩儀，兩儀生四象，四象生八卦，八卦生六十四卦。

18. 徒訪師三年，師考徒三年。

19. 入門引路須口授，功夫無息法自然。

20. 名師出高徒。

21. 要喉頭永不拋，問盡天下眾英豪。如訊大功因何得，表里精粗無不到。

CHAPTER 2

Qi, Qigong, and Taijiquan
氣、氣功、太極拳之關係

2-1. Introduction

Qigong has always been an important part of Chinese martial arts training. Without qigong training, a martial artist will have lost the origin of martial power, and what he or she uses will be only muscular power. This will make Chinese martial arts no different from the Western fighting arts. The most unique elements of Chinese martial arts are in the qigong training and the buildup of internal energy (i.e., qi). Moreover, through mental concentration, qi can be led throughout the physical body to boost its functioning to a higher level. However, the most important aspect of qigong training is to learn to feel yourself, to understand yourself, and to deal with your own mind. This is the path of self-discipline and spiritual cultivation. From this training, you will begin to understand the way of your life more deeply. From this, you can see that the way of Chinese martial arts is a way of life, and your life can be built upon an understanding of Chinese martial arts. This bridge between these two mountains is the practice of qigong.

Qigong has been studied and developed in China for more than four thousand years. It is not easy for any person to achieve a deep, profound understanding and feeling for such arts in a short time. To help you grasp the concepts of martial qigong training, you must first build the foundation of knowledge and understanding. This will provide you with a baseline reference for all your further study and evaluation.

This chapter will provide you with a simple qigong practice "road map" that can guide you to the garden of qigong practice. You should study it carefully. If you can understand this chapter, you will soon grasp the rationale of every training method in this book. In the next section, first I will define the terminology of qi, qigong, and their relationship to humanity. Having this definition, we will not treat qi as mysterious. Then, in order to help you understand the historical background of qigong, different categories of qigong will be briefly summarized in section 2-3. Next, in section 2-4, the theoretical foundations of qigong training will be discussed. From comprehension of this section, you will have less doubt in your qigong practice. Finally, we will discuss and summarize the relationship between qigong and taijiquan. If you wish to learn more about qigong, please refer to these books: *The Root of Chinese Qigong* and *Qigong the Secret of Youth, Da Mo's Muscle/Tendon Changing and Marrow/Brain Washing Classic*, published by YMAA.

2-2. Qi, Qigong, and Man

Before we discuss the relationship of qi with the human body, we should first define qi and qigong. We will first discuss the general concept of qi, including both the traditional understanding and the possible modern scientific paradigms, which allow us to use modern concepts to explain qigong.

A General Definition of Qi. Qi is the energy or natural force that fills the universe. The Chinese have traditionally believed that there are three major powers in the universe. These three powers (*san cai*, 三才) are heaven (*tian*, 天), earth (*di*, 地), and man (*ren*, 人). Heaven (the sky or universe) has heaven qi (*tian qi*, 天氣), the most important of the three, which is made up of the forces which the heavenly bodies exert on the earth, such as sunshine, moonlight, the moon's gravity, and the energy from the stars. In ancient times, the Chinese believed that weather, climate, and natural disasters were governed by heaven qi. Chinese people still refer to the weather as heaven qi (*tian qi*, 天氣). Every energy field strives to stay in balance, so whenever the heaven qi loses its balance, it tries to rebalance itself. The wind must blow, rain must fall, even tornadoes or hurricanes must happen in order for the heaven qi to reach a new energy balance.

Under heaven qi is earth qi. It is influenced and controlled by heaven qi. For example, too much rain will force a river to flood or change its path. Without rain, the plants will die. The Chinese believe that earth qi is made up of lines and patterns of energy, as well as the earth's magnetic field and the heat concealed underground. These energies must also balance; otherwise disasters such as earthquakes will occur. When the qi of the earth is balanced, plants will grow and animals thrive.

Finally, within the earth qi, each individual person, animal, and plant has its own qi field, which always seeks to be balanced. When any individual thing loses its qi balance, it will sicken, die, and decompose. All natural things, including mankind and our human qi, grow within and are influenced by the natural cycles of heaven qi and earth qi. Throughout the history of qigong, people have been most interested in human qi and its relationship with heaven qi and earth qi.

In China, qi is defined as any type of energy that is able to demonstrate power and strength. This energy can be electricity, magnetism, heat, or light. For example, electric power is called electric qi (*dian qi*, 電氣), and heat is called heat qi (*re qi*, 熱氣). When a person is alive, his body's energy is called human qi (*ren qi*, 人氣).

Qi is also commonly used to express the energy state of something, especially living things. As mentioned before, the weather is called heaven qi (*tian qi*, 天氣) because it indicates the energy state of the heavens. When something is alive it has vital qi (*huo qi*, 活氣), and when it is dead it has dead qi (*si qi*, 死氣) or ghost qi (*gui qi*, 鬼氣). When a person is righteous and has the spiritual strength to do good, he is said to have normal qi or righteous qi (*zheng qi*, 正氣). The spiritual state or morale of an army is called energy state (*qi shi*, 氣勢).

You can see that the word "qi" has a wider and more general definition than most people think. It does not refer only to the energy circulating in the human body, but instead can refer to a form of universal energy and can even be used to express the manifestation or state of this energy. It is important to understand this when you practice qigong, so that your mind is not channeled into a narrow understanding of qi, which would limit your future understanding and development.

A Narrow Definition of Qi. Now that you understand the general definition of qi, let us look at how qi is defined in qigong society today. As mentioned before, among the three powers, the Chinese have been most concerned with the qi that is related to our health and longevity. After four thousand years of emphasizing human qi, when people mention qi they usually mean the qi circulating in our bodies.

If we look at the Chinese medical and qigong documents that were written about two thousand years ago, the word "qi" was written (炁). This character is constructed of two words, (无) on the top, which means "nothing," and (灬) on the bottom, which means "fire." This means that the word qi was actually written as "no fire" in ancient times. If we go back through Chinese medical and qigong history, it is not hard to understand this expression.

In ancient times, the Chinese physicians or qigong practitioners were actually looking for the yin-yang balance of the qi, which was circulating in the body. When this goal was reached, there was "no fire" in the internal organs. This concept is very simple. According to Chinese medicine, each of our internal organs needs to receive a specific amount of qi to function properly. If an organ receives an improper amount of qi (usually too much, i.e., too yang), it will start to malfunction, and, in time, physical damage will occur. Therefore, the goal of the medical or qigong practitioner was to attain a state of "no fire," which eventually became the word qi.

However, in more recent publications, the qi of "no fire" has been replaced by the word 氣 which is again constructed of two words, 气 meaning "air," and 米 meaning "rice." This shows that later practitioners realized that the qi circulating in our bodies is produced mainly by the inhalation of air and the consumption of food (rice). Air is called kong qi (空氣), which means literally "space energy."

For a long time, people were confused about just what type of energy was circulating in our bodies. Many people believed that it was heat, others considered it to be electricity, and many others assumed that it was a mixture of heat, electricity, and light.

This confusion lasted until the early 1980s when the concept of qi gradually became clear. If we think carefully about what we know from science, we can see that (except possibly for gravity) there is actually only one type of energy in this universe, and that is electromagnetic energy. This means that light (electromagnetic waves) and heat (infrared waves) are also part of electromagnetic energy. This makes it very clear that the qi circulating in our bodies is actually "bioelectricity," and that our body is a "living electromagnetic field."[1] This field is affected by our thoughts, feelings, activities, the food we eat, the quality of the air we breathe, our lifestyle, the natural energy that surrounds us, and also the unnatural energy that modern science inflicts upon us.

Next, let us define qigong. Once you understand what qigong is, you can better understand the role that Chinese martial qigong plays in Chinese martial arts and qigong societies.

A General Definition of Qigong. We have explained that qi is energy and that it is found in the heavens, in the earth, and in every living thing. As mentioned in the first chapter, in China, the word "gong" (功) is often used instead of "gongfu" (or *kung fu*, 功夫), which means energy and time. Any study or training that requires a lot of energy and time to learn or to accomplish is called gongfu. The term can be applied to any special skill or study as long as it requires time, energy, and patience. Therefore, the correct definition of qigong is any training or study dealing with qi that takes a long time and a lot of effort. You can see from this definition that qigong is a science that studies the energy in nature. The main difference between this energy science and Western energy science is that qigong focuses on the inner energy of human beings while Western energy science pays more attention to the energy outside of the human body. When you study qigong, it is worthwhile to also consider the modern, scientific point of view and not restrict yourself to only the traditional beliefs.

The Chinese have studied qi for thousands of years. Some of the information on the patterns and cycles of nature has been recorded in books, one of which is the *Book of Changes (Yi Jing,* 易經*)*, 1122 B.C. When the *Yi Jing* was written, the Chinese people, as mentioned earlier, believed that natural power included heaven (*tian*, 天), earth (*di*, 地), and man (*ren*, 人). These are called the three powers (*san cai*, 三才) and are manifested by the three qi's: heaven qi, earth qi, and human qi. These three facets of nature have their definite rules and cycles. The rules never change, and the cycles repeat regularly. The Chinese people used an understanding of these natural principles and the *Yi Jing* to calculate the changes of natural qi. This calculation is called the eight trigrams (*bagua*, 八卦). From the eight trigrams are derived the 64 hexagrams. Therefore, the *Yi Jing* was probably the first book that taught the Chinese people about qi and its variations in nature and man. The relationship of the three natural powers and their qi variations were later discussed extensively in the book *Theory of Qi's Variation (Qi Hua Lun*, 氣化論*)*.

Understanding heaven qi is very difficult, and it was especially so in ancient times when the science was just developing. But since nature is always repeating itself, the experiences accumulated over the years have made it possible to trace the natural patterns. Understanding the rules and cycles of heavenly timing (*tian shi*, 天時) will help you to understand natural changes of the seasons, climate, weather, rain, snow, drought, and all other natural occurrences. If you observe carefully, you can see many of these routine patterns and cycles caused by the rebalancing of the qi fields. Among the natural cycles are those which repeat every day, month, or year, as well as cycles of twelve years and sixty years.

Earth qi is a part of heaven qi. If you can understand the rules and the structure of the earth, you can understand how mountains and rivers are formed, how plants grow, how rivers move, what part of the country is best for someone to live, where to build a house and which direction it should face so that it is a healthy place to live, and many other things related to the earth. In China today there are people called geomancy teachers (*di li shi*, 地理師) or wind water teachers (*feng shui shi*, 風水師), who make their living this way. The term "wind water" (*feng shui*) is commonly used because the location and character of the wind and water in a landscape are the most important factors in evaluating a location. These experts use the accumulated body of geomantic knowledge and the *Yi Jing* to help people make important decisions, such as where and how to build a house, where to bury their dead, and how to rearrange or redecorate homes and offices so they are better places to live and work in. Many people even believe that setting up a store or business according to the guidance of feng shui can make them more prosperous.

Among the three qi's, human qi is probably the one studied most thoroughly. The study of human qi covers a large number of different subjects. The Chinese people believe that human qi is affected and controlled by heaven qi and earth qi, and that they in fact determine your destiny. Therefore, if you understand the relationship between nature and people, in addition to understanding human relations (*ren shi*, 人事), you can predict wars, the destiny of a country, a person's desires and temperament, and even his or her future. The people who practice this profession are called "calculate life teachers" (*suan ming shi*, 算命師).

However, the greatest achievement in the study of human qi is in regard to health and longevity. Since qi is the source of life, if you understand how qi functions and know how to regulate it correctly, you should be able to live a long and healthy life. Remember that you are part of nature and you are channeled into the cycles of nature. If you go against this natural cycle, you may become sick, so it is in your best interest to follow the way of nature. This is the meaning of "Dao," which can be translated as "the natural way."

Many different aspects of human qi have been researched, including acupuncture, acupressure, massage, herbal treatment, meditation, and qigong exercises. The use of acupuncture, acupressure, and herbal treatment to adjust human qi flow has become the root of Chinese medical science. Meditation and moving qigong exercises are used widely by the Chinese people to improve their health or even to cure certain illnesses. In addition, Daoists and Buddhists use meditation and qigong exercises in their pursuit of enlightenment.

In conclusion, the study of any of the aspects of qi including heaven qi, earth qi, and human qi should be called qigong. However, since the term is usually used today only in reference to the cultivation of human qi through meditation and exercises, we will only use it in this narrower sense to avoid confusion.

A Narrow Definition of Qigong. As mentioned earlier, the narrow definition of qi is "the energy circulating in the human body." Therefore, the narrow definition of qigong is "the study of the qi circulating in the human body." Because our bodies are part of nature, the narrow definition of qigong should also include the study of how our bodies relate to heaven qi and earth qi. Chinese qigong consists today of several different fields: acupuncture, herbs for regulating human qi, martial arts qigong, qigong massage, qigong exercises, qigong healing, and religious enlightenment qigong. Naturally, these fields are mutually related and in many cases cannot be separated.

The Chinese have discovered that the human body has twelve major channels (*shi er jing*, 十二經) and eight vessels (*ba mai*, 八脈) through which the qi circulates. The twelve channels are like rivers that distribute qi throughout the body and also connect the extremities (fingers and toes) to the internal organs. Here you should understand that the internal organs of Chinese medicine do not necessarily correspond to the physical organs as understood in the West, but rather to a set of clinical functions similar to each other and related to the organ system. The eight vessels, which are often referred to as the extraordinary vessels, function like reservoirs and regulate the distribution and circulation of qi in your body.

When the qi in the eight reservoirs is full and strong, the qi in the rivers is strong and will be regulated efficiently. When there is stagnation in any of these twelve channels or rivers, the qi that flows to the body's extremities and to the internal organs will be abnormal, and illness may develop. You should understand that every channel has its particular qi flow strength, and every channel is different. All of these different levels of qi strength are affected by your mind, the weather, the time of day, the food you have eaten, and even your mood. For example, when the weather is dry, the qi in the lungs will tend to be more positive than when it is moist. When you are angry, the qi flow in your liver channel will be abnormal. The qi strength in the different channels varies throughout the day in a regular cycle, and at any particular time one channel is strongest. For example, between 11 A.M. and 1 P.M. the qi flow in the heart channel is the strongest. Furthermore, the qi level of the same organ can be different from one person to another.

Whenever the qi flow in the twelve rivers or channels is not normal, the eight reservoirs will regulate the qi flow and bring it back to normal. For example, when you experience a sudden shock, the qi flow in the bladder immediately becomes deficient. Normally, the reservoir will immediately regulate the qi in this channel so that you recover from the shock. However, if the reservoir qi is also deficient or if the effect of the shock is too great and there is not enough time to regulate the qi, the bladder will suddenly contract, causing unavoidable urination.

When a person is sick, his qi level tends to be either too positive (excessive yang) or too negative (deficient yin). A Chinese physician would use either a prescription of herbs to adjust the qi, or else he would insert acupuncture needles at various spots on the channels to inhibit the flow in some channels and stimulate the flow in others so that balance could be restored. However, there is another alternative and that is to use certain physical and mental exercises to adjust the qi: in other words, to use qigong.

The above discussion is only to offer an idea of the narrow definition of qigong. In fact, when people talk about qigong today, most of the time they are referring to the mental and physical exercises that work with the qi.

A Modern Definition of Qi. It is important that you know about the progress that has been made by modern science in the study of qi. This will keep you from getting stuck in the ancient concepts and the level of understanding.

In ancient China, people had very little knowledge of electricity. They only knew from acupuncture that when a needle was inserted into the acupuncture cavities, some kind of energy other than heat was produced, which often caused a shock or a tickling sensation. It was not until the last few decades, when the Chinese people were more acquainted with electromagnetic science that they began to recognize that this energy circulating in the body, which they called qi, might be the same thing as what today's science calls "bioelectricity."

It is understood now that the human body is constructed of many different electrically conductive materials and that it forms a living electromagnetic field and circuit. Electromagnetic energy is continuously being generated in the human body through the biochemical reaction in food and air assimilation and circulated by the electromotive forces (EMF) generated within the body.

In addition, you are constantly being affected by external electromagnetic fields such as that of the earth, or the electrical fields generated by clouds. When you practice Chinese medicine or qigong, you need to be aware of these outside factors and take them into account.

Countless experiments have been conducted in China, Japan, and other countries to study how external magnetic or electrical fields can affect and adjust the body's qi field. Many acupuncturists use magnets and electricity in their treatments. They attach a magnet to the skin over a cavity and leave it there for a period of time. The magnetic field gradually affects the qi circulation in that channel. Alternatively, they insert needles into cavities and then run an electric current through the needle to reach the qi channels directly. Although many researchers have claimed a degree of success in their experiments, none have been able to publish any detailed and convincing proof of the results or give a good explanation of the theory behind the experiment. As with many other attempts to explain the *how* and *why* of acupuncture, conclusive proof is elusive and many unanswered questions remain. Of course, this theory is quite new, and it will probably take a great deal more study and research before it is verified and completely understood. At present, there are many conservative acupuncturists who are skeptical.

To untie this knot, we must look at what modern Western science has discovered about bioelectromagnetic energy. Many bioelectricity-related reports have been published, and frequently the results are closely related to what is experienced in Chinese qigong training and medical science. For example, during the electrophysiological research of the 1960s, several investigators discovered that bones are piezoelectric; that is, when they are stressed, mechanical energy is converted to electrical energy in the form of electric current.[1] This might explain one of the practices of Marrow Washing Qigong in which the stress on the bones and muscles is increased in certain ways to increase the qi circulation.

Dr. Robert O. Becker has done important work in this field. His book, *The Body Electric*,[2] reports on much of the research concerning the body's electric fields. It is presently believed that food and air are the fuels that generate the electricity in the body through biochemical reaction. This electricity, which is circulated throughout the entire body by means of electrically conductive tissue, is one of the main energy sources that keep the cells of the physical body alive.

Whenever you have an injury or are sick, your body's electrical circulation is affected. If this circulation of electricity stops, you die. But bioelectric energy not only maintains life; it is also responsible for repairing physical damage. Many researchers have sought ways of using external electrical or magnetic fields to speed up the body's recovery from physical injury. Richard Leviton reports: "Researchers at Loma Linda University's School of Medicine in California have found, following studies in sixteen countries with over 1,000 patients, that low-frequency, low-intensity magnetic energy has been successful in treating chronic pain related to tissue ischemia and has also worked in clearing up slow-healing ulcers, and in 90 percent of patients tested, raised blood flow significantly."[3]

Mr. Leviton also reports that every cell of the body functions like an electric battery and is able to store electric charges. He reports that "Other biomagnetic investigators take an even closer look to find out what is happening, right down to the level of the blood, the organs, and the individual cell, which they regard as 'a small electric battery.'"[3] This has convinced me that our entire body is essentially a big battery that is assembled from millions of small batteries. All of these batteries together form the human electromagnetic field.

Furthermore, much of the research on the body's electrical field relates to acupuncture. For example, Dr. Becker reports that the conductivity of the skin is much higher at acupuncture cavities, and it is now possible to locate them precisely by measuring the skin's conductivity (Figure 2-1).[2] Many of these reports prove that the acupuncture that has been done in China for thousands of years is reasonable and scientific.

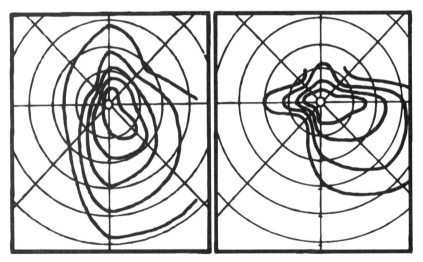

Figure 2–1. Electrical Conductivity Maps of the Skin Surface over Acupuncture Points

Some researchers use the theory of the body's electricity to explain many of the ancient miracles that have been attributed to the practice of qigong. A report by Albert L. Huebner states: "These demonstrations of body electricity in human beings may also offer a new explanation of an ancient healing practice. If weak external fields can produce powerful physiological effects, it may be that fields from human tissues in one person are capable of producing clinical improvements in another. In short, the method of healing known as the laying on of hands could be an especially subtle form of electrical stimulation."[1]

Another frequently reported phenomenon is that when a qigong practitioner has reached a high level of development, a halo would appear behind and/or around his head during meditation. This is commonly seen in paintings of Jesus Christ, the Buddha, and various Oriental immortals. Frequently the light is pictured as surrounding the whole body. This phenomenon may again be explained by the "body electric theory." When a person has cultivated his qi (electricity) to a high level, the qi may be led to accumulate in the head. This qi may then interact with the oxygen molecules in the air and ionize them, causing them to glow.

Although the link between the theory of the "body electric" and the Chinese theory of qi is becoming more accepted and better proven, there are still many questions to be answered. For example, how does the mind actually generate an EMF (electromotive force) to circulate the electricity in the body? How is the human electromagnetic field affected by the multitude of other electric fields that surround us, such as radio wiring or electrical appliances? How can we readjust our electromagnetic fields and survive in outer space or on other planets where the magnetic field is completely different from the earth's? You can see that the future of qigong and bioelectric science is a challenging and exciting one. It is my hope that we begin to use modern technology to understand the inner energy world.

A Modern Definition of Qigong. If you now accept that the inner energy (qi) circulating in our bodies is bioelectricity, then we can now formulate a definition of qigong based on electrical principles.

Let us assume that the circuit shown in Figure 2-2 is similar to the circuit in our bodies. Unfortunately, although we now have a certain degree of understanding of this circuit from acupuncture, we still do not know in detail exactly what the body's circuit looks like. We know that there are twelve primary qi channels (*qi* rivers, 經) and eight vessels (*qi* reservoirs, 脈) in our body. There are also thousands of small qi channels (*luo*, 絡) which allow the qi to reach the skin and the bone marrow. In this circuit, the twelve internal organs are connected and mutually related through these channels.

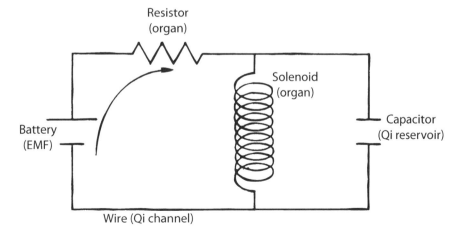

Figure 2–2. The Human Bioelectric Circuit is Similar to an Electric Circuit

If you look at the electrical circuit in the illustration, you will see:
  1. The qi channels are like the wires that carry electric current.
  2. The internal organs are like electrical components, such as resistors and solenoids.
  3. The qi vessels are like capacitors, which regulate the current in the circuit.

How do you keep this electrical circuit functioning most efficiently? Your first concern is the resistance of the wire that carries the current. In a machine, you want to use a wire that has a high level of conductivity and low resistance; otherwise the current may melt the wire. Therefore, the wire should be of a material like copper or perhaps even gold. In your body, you want to keep the current flowing smoothly. This means that your first task is to remove anything that interferes with the flow and causes stagnation. Fat has low conductivity, so you should use diet and exercise to remove excess fat from your body. You should also learn how to relax your physical body because this opens all of the qi channels. This is why relaxation is the first goal in taijiquan and many qigong exercises.

Your next concern in maintaining a healthy electrical circuit is the components—your internal organs. If you do not have the correct level of current in your organs, they will either burn out from too much current (yang) or malfunction because of a deficient level of current (yin). In order to avoid these problems in a machine, you use a capacitor to regulate the current. Whenever there is too much current, the capacitor absorbs and stores the excess, and whenever the current is weak, the capacitor supplies current to raise the level. The eight qi vessels are your body's capacitors. Qigong is concerned with learning how to increase the level of qi in these vessels so they can supply current when needed and keep the internal organs functioning smoothly. This is especially important as you get older and your qi level is generally lower.

In addition, in order to have a healthy circuit, you have to be concerned with the components themselves. If any of them are not strong and of good quality, the entire circuit will have problems. This means that the final concern in qigong practice is how to maintain or even rebuild the health of your internal organs. Before we go any further, we should point out that there is an important difference between the circuit shown in the diagram and the qi circuit in our bodies. This difference is that the human body is alive, and with the proper qi nourishment, all of the cells can be regrown and the state of health improved. For example, if you can jog about three miles today and if you keep jogging regularly and gradually increase the distance, eventually you can easily jog five miles. This is because your body rebuilds and readjusts itself to fit the circumstances.

This means that if we can increase the qi flow through our internal organs, they can become stronger and healthier. Naturally, the increase in qi must be slow and gradual so that the organs can adjust to it. In order to increase the qi flow in your body, you need to work with the EMF (electromotive force) in your body. If you do not know what EMF is, imagine two containers filled with water and connected by a tube. If both containers have the same water level, then the water will not flow. However, if one side is higher than the other, the water will flow from that container to the other. In electricity, this potential difference is called electromotive force. Naturally, the higher the EMF, the stronger the current will flow.

You can see from this discussion that the key to effective qigong practice is, in addition to removing resistance from the qi channels, learning how to increase the EMF in your body. Now let us see what the sources of EMF in the body are so that we may use them to increase the flow of bioelectricity. Generally speaking, there are five major sources:

1. **Natural Energy.** Since your body is constructed of electrically conductive material, its electromagnetic field is always affected by the sun, the moon, clouds, the earth's magnetic field, and by the other energies around you. The major influences are the sun's radiation, the moon's gravity, and the earth's magnetic field. These affect your qi circulation significantly and are responsible for the pattern of your qi circulation since you were formed. We are now also being greatly affected by the energy generated by modern technology, such as the electromagnetic waves generated by radio, TV, microwave ovens, computers, and many other things.

2. **Food and Air.** In order to maintain life, we take in food and air essence through our mouth and nose. These essences are then converted into qi through a biochemical reaction in the chest and digestive system (called the triple burner in Chinese medicine). When qi is converted from the essence, an EMF is generated that circulates the qi throughout the body. Consequently, a major part of qigong is devoted to getting the proper kinds of food and fresh air.

3. **Thinking**. The human mind is the most important and efficient source of bioelectric EMF. Any time you move to do something, you must first generate an idea (*yi*). This idea generates the EMF and leads the qi to energize the appropriate muscles to carry out the desired motion. The more you can concentrate, the stronger the EMF you can generate and the stronger the flow of qi you can lead. Naturally, the stronger the flow of qi you lead to the muscles, the more they will be energized. Because of this, the mind is considered the most important factor in qigong training.

4. **Exercise**. Exercise converts the food essence (fat) stored in your body into qi and therefore builds up the EMF. Many qigong styles have been created that utilize movement for this purpose.

5. **Converting Pre-Birth Essence into Qi.** The hormones produced by our endocrine glands are referred to as "pre-birth essence" in Chinese medicine. They can be converted into qi to stimulate the functioning of our physical body, thereby increasing our vitality. Balancing hormone production when you are young and increasing its production when you are old are important subjects in Chinese qigong.

From the foregoing, you can see that within the human body there is a network of electrical circuitry. In order to maintain the circulation of bioelectricity, there must be a battery wherein to store a charge. Where then, is the battery in our body?

Chinese qigong practitioners believe that there is a place which is able to store qi (bioelectricity). This place is called the elixir field (*dan tian*, 丹田). According to such practitioners, there are three dan tians in the human body. One is located at the abdominal area, one or two inches below the navel and called the lower dan tian (*xia dan tian*, 下丹田). The second is in the area of the lower sternum and is called the middle dan tian (*zhong dan tian*, 中丹田). The third is the lower center of forehead (or the third eye) connected to the brain and is called the upper dan tian (*shang dan tian*, 上丹田).

The lower dan tian is considered to be the residence of the water qi, or the qi that is generated from the original essence (*yuan jing*, 元精). Therefore, qi stored here is called original qi (*yuan qi*, 元氣). According to Chinese medicine, in this same area there is a cavity called "qihai" (Co-6, 氣海) that means "qi ocean." This is consistent with the conclusions drawn by qigong practitioners, who also call this area the lower dan tian (lower elixir field). Both groups agree that this area is able to produce qi or elixir like a field and that here the qi is abundant like an ocean.

In qigong practice, it is commonly known that in order to build up the qi to a higher level in the lower dan tian, you must move your abdominal area (i.e., the lower *dan tian*) up and down through abdominal breathing. This kind of up and down abdominal breathing exercise is called "qi huo" (起火) and means "start the fire." It is also called "back to childhood breathing" (*fan tong hu xi*, 返童呼吸). Normally, after you have exercised the lower dan tian for about ten minutes, you will have a feeling of warmth in the lower abdomen, which implies the accumulation of qi or energy.

Theoretically and scientifically, what is happening when the abdominal area is moved up and down? If you look at the structure of the abdominal area, you will see that there are about six layers of muscle and fasciae sandwiching each other in this area (Figure 2-3). In fact, what you actually see is the sandwich of muscles and fat accumulated in the fasciae layers. When you move your abdomen up and down, you are actually using your mind to move the muscles, not the fat. Whenever there is a muscular contraction and relaxation, the fat slowly turns into bioelectricity. When this bioelectricity encounters resistance from the fasciae layers, it turns into heat. From this, you can see how simple the theory might be for the generation of qi. Another thing you should know is that according to our understanding today, fat and fasciae are poor electrical

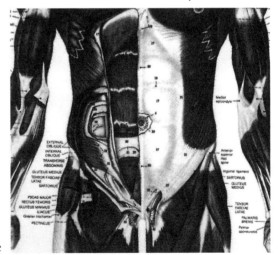

Figure 2–3. Anatomic Structure of the Abdominal Area

conductors, while the muscles are relatively good electrical conductors.[1,2,3] When these good and poor electrical materials are sandwiched together, they act like a battery. This is why, through up and down abdominal movements, the energy can be stored temporarily and generate warmth.

However, through nearly two thousand years of experience, Daoists have said that the front abdominal area is not the real dan tian, but is in fact a "false dan tian" (*jia dan tian*, 假丹田). Their argument is that although this lower dan tian is able to generate qi and build it up to a higher level, it does not store it for a long time. This is because the lower dan tian is located on the path of the conception vessel, so whenever qi is built up to a higher energy state, it will circulate in the conception and governing vessels. This lower dan tian therefore cannot be a battery as we understand the term. A real battery should be able to store the qi. Where then, is the "real dan tian" (*zhen dan tian*, 真丹田)?

Daoists teach that the real dan tian is at the center of the abdominal area, at the physical center of the gravity located in the large and small intestines (Figure 2-4). Now, let us analyze this from two different points of view.

First, let us take a look at how a life is started. It begins with a sperm from the father entering an egg from the mother, thus forming the original human cell (Figure 2-5).[4] This cell next divides into two cells, then four cells, etc. When this group of cells adheres to the internal wall of the uterus, the umbilical cord starts to develop. Nutrition and energy for further cell multiplication is absorbed through the umbilical cord from the mother's body. The baby keeps growing until maturation. During this nourishing and growing process, the baby's abdomen is moving up and down, acting like a pump drawing in nutrition and energy into his or her body. Later, immediately after the birth, air and nutrition are taken in

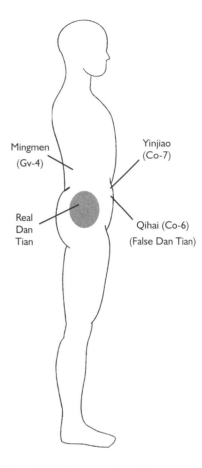

Figure 2–4. The Real Dan Tian and the False Dan Tian

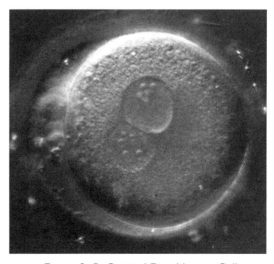

Figure 2–5. Original First Human Cell

from the nose and mouth through the mouth's sucking action and the lungs' breathing. As the child grows, it slowly forgets the natural movements of the abdomen. This is why the abdomen's up and down movement is called "back to the childhood breathing."

Think carefully: if your first human cell is still alive, where is this cell? Most likely, this cell has already died a long time ago. It is understood that approximately one trillion (10^{12}) cells die in a human body each day.[5] However, if we assume that this first cell is still alive, then it should be located at our physical center, that is, our center of gravity. If we think carefully, we can see that it is from this center that the cells could multiply evenly outward until the body is completely constructed. In order to maintain this even multiplication physically, the energy or qi must be centered at this point and radiate outward. When we are in an embryonic state, this is the gravity center and also the qi center. As we grow after birth, this center remains.

The above argument adheres solely

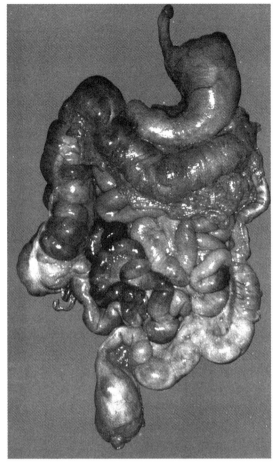

Figure 2–6. Anatomic Structure of the Real Dan Tian—Large and Small Intestines

to the traditional point of view of the physical development of our body. Next, let us analyze this center from another point of view.

If we look at the physical center of gravity, we can see that the entire area is occupied by the large and the small intestines (Figure 2-6). We know that there are three kinds of muscles existing in our body and we can examine them in ascending order of our ability to control them. The first kind is the heart muscle, in which the electrical conductivity among muscular groups is the highest. The heart beats all the time, regardless of our attention, and through practice and discipline, we are able to regulate only its beating, not start and stop it. If we supply electricity to even a small piece of this muscle, it will pump like the heart. The second category is those muscles that contract automatically but over which we can exert significant control if we make the effort. The diaphragm that controls breathing, our eyelids, our stomach (and large and small intestines) and reproductive organs are examples of this muscle type, and their electrical conductivity is lower than the first type. The third kind is those muscles that are directly controlled by our conscious mind. The electric conductivity of these muscles is the lowest of the three groups.

If you look at the structure of the large and small intestines, the first thing you notice is that the total length of your large and small intestines is approximately six times your body's height (Figure 2-7). With such long electrically conductive tissues sandwiched between all the mesentery, water, and outer casings (which it is reasonable to believe are poor electrical conductive tissues), the intestines act like a huge battery in our body (Figure 2-8).[6] From this, you can see that it makes sense both logically and scientifically that the center of gravity, rather than the false dan tian, is the real battery in our body.

Furthermore, the discovery by scientists in early 1996 that humans actually have two "brains" is of special interest.[7] According to their finding, we each have one brain in our head, exactly in accordance with classical anatomy. The second "brain," however, is located in the lower torso (i.e., the digestive system). Although these two brains are physically separate, they are connected by the spinal cord, the highly electrically conductive tissue, i.e., the Chinese thrusting vessel, (衝脈). This connection allows them to function as a single organ for the purpose of cognitive functions and memory.

The discoverers of this phenomenon explain that the upper brain (in the head) has both the powers of thought and memory, while the lower brain (in the torso) has only the power of memory. As a matter of fact, it really has only the ability to store and retrieve information. The upper brain still must process this information into what we think of as memory. Needless to say, the lower brain does not have the ability to think. The most amazing aspect of this discovery is that it confirms the Chinese belief that the real dan tian (i.e., large and small intestines) is able to store qi, while the upper dan

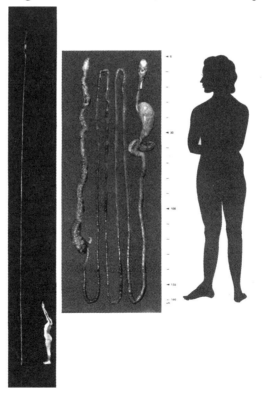

Figure 2–7. The large and small intestines are about six times your height.

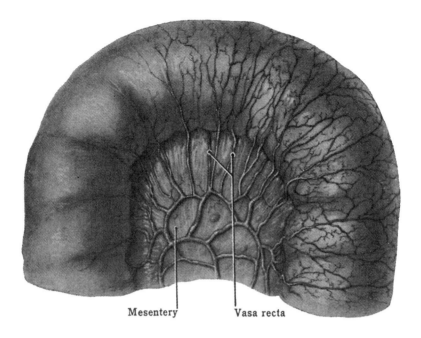

Mesentery   Vasa recta

Figure 2–8. Low Electrically Conductive Materials Such as Mesentery, Outer Casing, and Water in and Around the Intestines Make the Entire Area Act Like a Battery.

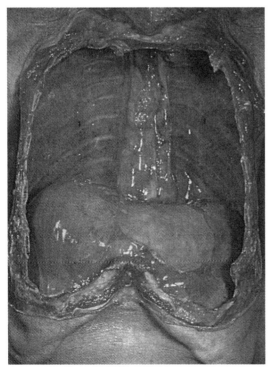

Figure 2–9. The Middle Dan Tian is Connected to the Diaphragm

tian governs thought and directs the qi. Expanding on our theory of qi's bioelectric component, when the upper brain thinks and forms intentions, this generates an electromotive force (EMF). The lower brain has the capability of storing information in the form of electrical charges. In other words, the lower brain might be the human battery wherein the life force resides. Once the upper brain generates an intention (i.e., an EMF), the change in state will immediately be directed from the lower brain through the spinal cord and nervous system to the desired area to activate the physical body for function. It is indeed even possible that what the Chinese called the lower dan tian is actually a "biobattery," which stores charges in our body. Electrical circulation in the body would require both an EMF and an energy source, or battery.

Next, let us examine the structure of the middle dan tian area. The middle dan tian is located next to the diaphragm (Figure 2-9). We know that the diaphragm is a membranous muscular partition separating the abdominal and the thoracic cavities. It functions in respiration and is a good electrically conductive material. On the top and the bottom of the diaphragm there are the fasciae, which isolate the internal organs from the diaphragm. We see again a good electrical conductor isolated by a poor one. That means it is capable of storing electricity or qi. Since this place is between the lungs and the stomach, which absorbs the post-birth essence (air and food) and converts it into energy, the qi accumulated in the middle dan tian is classified as fire qi. The reason for this name is that the qi converted from the contaminated air and the food can affect qi status and make it yang. Naturally, this fire qi can also agitate your emotional mind.

Finally, let us analyze the brain, which is considered the upper dan tian. We already know that the brain and the spinal cord are considered to be the central nervous system, in which the electrical conductivity is highest in our body. If we examine the brain's structure, we can see that it is segregated by the *arachnoid mater* (i.e., a delicate membrane of the spinal cord and brain, lying between the *pia mater* and *dura mater*) (Figure 2-10). It is reasonable to assume that these materials are low electrically conductive tissues. Again, it is another giant battery that consumes qi in great amounts. However, since the brain does not produce qi or bioelectricity, its function as a dan tian cannot be considered to be the same as the lower dan tian.

From the above discussion, you may have gained a better idea of how we can link ancient experience with modern scientific understanding. In order to make the scientific concept of qigong even clearer, let us look at qigong from another scientific point of view, this time chemical.

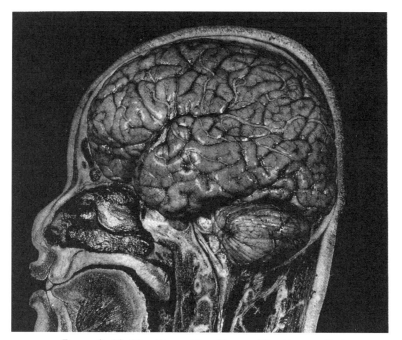

Figure 2–10. The Upper Dan Tian — The Human Brain

If we examine how we breathe, we can see that we inhale to take in oxygen, and we exhale to expel carbon dioxide (Figure 2-11). Thus, every minute we expel a great deal of carbon from our body through exhalation. Carbon is a material in a physical form that can be seen. The questions are where is the carbon in our body coming from? And through breathing, how much carbon is actually expelled?

The first source of carbon is from the food (glucose) we eat. When this food is converted into energy through chemical reaction during our daily activities, carbon dioxide is produced.[8]

$$\text{glucose} + 6O_2 \longrightarrow 6CO_2 + 6H_2O$$
$$\Delta G^{\circ\prime} = -686 \text{ kcal}$$

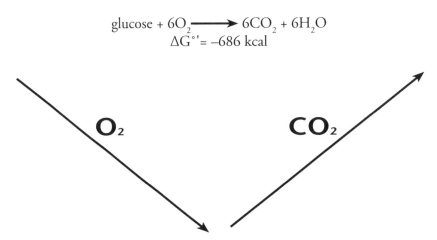

Figure 2–11. We Inhale to Absorb Oxygen and Exhale to Expel Carbon Dioxide.

The second source of this carbon is from the dead cells in our body. We already know that 96 percent of our body is constructed from the elements carbon, hydrogen, oxygen, and nitrogen, while other elements such as calcium (Ca), phosphorous (P), and potassium (K) that contribute 3 percent, and chloride (Cl), sulfur (S), sodium (Na), magnesium (Mg), iodine (I), and iron (Fe) that total 1 percent, comprise much less of our body weight. This means that the cells in our body contain a great amount of carbon.

In addition, consider that every cell in our body has a lifetime. As many as a trillion (10^{12}) cells die in our body every 24 hours.[5] For example, we know that the life span of a skin cell is 28 days. Naturally, every living cell, such as those of the bone, marrow, liver, has its own individual lifetime. We rely on our respiration to bring the carbon (i.e., dead cells) out and to supply living cells with new oxygen through inhalation and new carbon sources, water, and other minerals from eating. All this aids in the formation of new cells and the continuation of life.

From the foregoing, we can conclude that the cell replacement process is ongoing at all times in our life. Health during our lifetime depends on how smoothly and how quickly this replacement process is carried out. If there are new healthy cells to replace the old cells, you live and grow. If the cells replaced are as healthy as the original cells, you remain young. However, if there are fewer cells produced or if the new cells are not as healthy as the original cells, then you age. Now, let us analyze qigong from the point of view of cell replacement.

In order to produce a healthy cell, first you must consider the materials that are needed. From the structure of a cell, we know that we will need hydrogen, oxygen, carbon, and other minerals that we can absorb either from air or food. Therefore, air quality, water purity, and the choice of foods become critical factors for your health and longevity. Naturally, this has also been a big component of qigong study.

However, we know that air and water quality today has been contaminated by pollution. This is especially bad in urban and industrial areas. The quality of the food we eat depends on its source and processing methods. Naturally, it is not easy to find the same pristine environments as in ancient times. So we must learn how to fit into our new environment and choose the way of our life wisely.

Since carbon comprises such a major part of our body, how to absorb good quality carbon is an important issue in modern health. You may obtain carbon from animal products or from plants. Generally speaking, the carbon taken from plants is more pure and clean than that taken from animals.

According to past experience and analysis, red meat is generally more contaminated than white meat and is able to disturb and stimulate your emotional mind and confuse your thinking. Another source from which animal products can be obtained is fish. Again, some fish are good and others may be bad. For example, shrimp is high in cholesterol, which may increase the risk of high blood pressure.

Due to the impurities contained in most animal products, ancient qigong practitioners learned how to absorb protein from plants, especially from peas or beans. Soybean is one of the best of these sources; it is both inexpensive and easy to grow. However, if you are not a vegetarian originally, then it can be difficult for your body to produce the enzymes to digest an all-vegetable diet immediately. Humans evolved as omnivores, and the craving for meat can be strong. Even today, we all still have canine teeth, which were used to tear off raw meat in ancient times. Therefore, the natural enzymes existing in our body are more tailored to digesting meat. As an experiment, if we place a piece of meat and some corn in human digestive enzymes, we will see that the meat will be dissolved in a matter of minutes, while the corn will take many hours. This means it is generally easier for a human to absorb meat rather than plants as a protein source.

However, the above discussion does not mean you cannot absolutely absorb plant protein efficiently. The key is that if it is present to begin with, the enzyme production can be increased within your body, but it will take time. For example, if you cannot drink milk due to insufficient lactate in your stomach, you may start by drinking a little bit of milk every day and slowly increase it as days pass by. Six months later, you will realize that you can absorb milk. This means that if you wish to become a vegetarian, you must reduce the intake of meat products slowly and allow your body to adjust to it; otherwise you may experience protein deficiency.

In addition to a protein source, you must also consider minerals. Although they do not comprise a large proportion of our body, their importance in some ways is more significant than carbon. We know that calcium is an important element for bones, and iron is crucial for blood cells. Therefore, when we eat we must consume a variety of foods instead of just a few. How to absorb nutrition from food has always been an important part of Chinese qigong study.

In order to produce healthy cells, other than the concerns of the material side, you must also consider energy. You should understand that when a person ages quickly, often it is not because he or she is malnourished, but instead is due to the weakening of qi storage and circulation. Without an abundant supply of qi (bioelectricity), qi circulation will not be regulated efficiently, and therefore your life force will weaken and the physical body will degenerate. In order to have abundant qi storage, you must learn qigong in order to build up the qi in your eight vessels and also to help you understand how to lead the qi circulating in your body. This kind of qigong training includes wai dan (external elixir) and nei dan (internal elixir) practice, which we will discuss in the next section.

Other than the concern for materials needed and the qi required for cell production and replacement, the next thing you should ask yourself is how this replacement process is carried out. Then you will see that the entire replacement process depends on the blood cells. From Western medicine, we know that a blood cell is the carrier of water, oxygen, and nutrients to everywhere in the body through the blood circulatory network. From arteries and capillaries, the components for new cells are brought to every tiny place in the body. The old cells then absorb everything required from the blood stream and divide to produce new cells. The dead cells are brought back through veins to the lungs. Through respiration, the dead cell materials are expelled as carbon dioxide.

However, there is one thing missing from the last process. This is the qi or bioelectricity that is required for the biochemical process of cell division. It has been proven that every blood cell is actually like a dipole or a small battery, which is able to store bioelectricity and also to release it.[1] This means that each blood cell is actually a carrier of qi. In Chinese medicine, the blood and the qi are always together. Where there is blood, there is qi, and where there is qi, the blood will also be there. Therefore, the term "qi-xue" (i.e., *qi* blood, 氣血) is often used in Chinese medicine.

If you understand the above discussion and if we take a look at our blood circulatory system, then we can see that the arteries are located deeply underneath the muscles, while the veins are situated near the skin's surface. The color of the blood is red in the arteries because of the presence of oxygen, and its color is blue in the veins because of the absence of this oxygen and the presence of carbon. This implies that cell replacement actually happens from inside the body, moving outward. This can also offer us a hint that if we tense more, the blood circulation will be more stagnant and cell replacement will be slower. We can also conclude that most cell replacement occurs at night when we are at our most relaxed state during sleep. This can further lead us to conclude the importance of sleeping. We will discuss later how cell replacement is further related to our breathing.

If we already know that blood cells are the carriers of everything that is required for cell replacement, then we must also consider the healthy condition of our blood cells. If you have good health and a sufficient quantity of blood cells, then nutrition and qi can be carried to every part of the body efficiently. You will be healthy. However, if you do not have sufficient blood cells or the quality of the cells is poor, then the entire cell replacement process will be stagnant. Naturally, you will degenerate swiftly.

According to modern medical science, blood cells also have a life span. When the old ones die, new ones must be produced from the bone marrow. Bone marrow is the major blood factory. From medical reports, we know that normally, after a person reaches thirty, the marrow near the end side of the bone cavity turns yellow. This indicates that fat has accumulated there. It also means that red blood cells are no longer being produced in the yellowed area (Figure 2-12).[9] Chinese qigong practitioners believe that the degeneration of the bone marrow is due to insufficient qi supply. Therefore, Bone Marrow Washing Qigong was developed. From experience, through Marrow Washing Qigong practice, health can be improved and life can be extended significantly. If you are interested in this subject, please read *Qigong the Secret of Youth, Da Mo's Muscle/Tendon Changing and Marrow/Brain Washing Classic*, published by YMAA.

In addition to the above, the next thing that is highly important in human life is hormone production within your body. We already know from today's medical science that hormones act as a catalyst in the body. When the hormone levels are high, we are more energized and cell replacement can happen faster and more smoothly. When hormone production is slow and its level is low, then the cell replacement will be slow and we will age quickly. It was only in the last few years that scientists have discovered that by increasing the hormone levels in the body, we may be able to extend our life significantly.[10]

Maintenance of hormone production in a healthy manner has also been a major concern in Chinese qigong practice. According to Chinese medicine, glands that produce hormones were recognized since ancient times, but hormones were not understood. However, throughout a thousand years of practice and experience, the Chinese understood that the essence of life is stored in the kidneys. Today, we know that this essence is actually the hormones produced from the adrenal glands on the top of the kidneys. The Chinese also believed that through stimulation of the testicles and

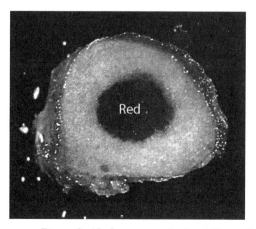 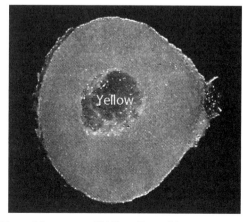

Figure 2–12. Structure of a Long Bone. Red Bone Marrow and Yellow Bone Marrow

ovaries, the life force could be increased. In addition, from still meditation practice, they learned how to lead the qi to the brain and raise the "spirit of vitality." It has also been found that through practice, bioelectricity can be led to the pituitary gland to stimulate growth hormone production. All of these practices are believed to be effective paths to longevity.

From medical science, we know that our hormone levels are significantly reduced when the last pieces of our bones are completed, between ages 29 and 30. Theoretically, when our body has completed constructing itself, it somehow triggers the reduction of our hormone levels. From this, you can see that maintaining the hormone levels in our body may be a key to longevity.

Finally, in order to prevent ourselves from getting sick, we must also consider our immune system. According to Chinese medicine and qigong, when qi storage is abundant, you get sick less. If we take a careful look, we can realize that every white blood cell is just like a fighting soldier. If we do not have enough qi to supply it, its fighting capability will be low. It is just like a soldier who needs food to maintain his strength. When the qi is strong, the immune system is strong. Therefore, the skin breathing technique has been developed, which teaches a practitioner to lead the qi to the surface of the skin to strengthen the "guardian qi" (*wei qi*, 衛氣) the energetic component of the immune system near the skin surface.

From the foregoing, hopefully I have offered you a challenge for profound thought and understanding. Although most of these conclusions are drawn from my personal research, further study and verification is still needed. I deeply believe that if we can all open our minds and share our opinions together, we can make our lives more healthy and meaningful.

2-3. Categories of Qigong

Often, people ask me the same question: Is jogging, weight lifting, or dancing a kind of qigong practice? To answer this question, let us trace back qigong history to before the Chinese Qin and Han dynastic periods (秦漢) (A.D. 255–223 B.C.). We can see that the origins of many qigong practices were actually in dancing. Through dancing, the physical body was exercised and the healthy condition of the physical body was maintained. Also, through dancing and matching movements with music, the mind was regulated into a harmonious state. From this harmonious mind, the spirit can be raised to a more energized state or can be calmed down to a peaceful level. This qigong dancing later passed to Japan during the Chinese Han dynasty and became a very elegant, slow, and high style of dancing in the Japanese royal court. This taijiquan-like dancing is still practiced in Japan today.

The ways of African or Native American dancing in which the body is bounced up and down is also known as a means of loosening up the joints and improving qi circulation. Naturally, jogging, weight lifting, or even walking is a kind of qigong practice. Therefore, we can say that any activity that is able to regulate the qi circulation in the body is a qigong practice.

Let us define it more clearly. In Figure 2-13, if the left vertical line represents the amount of usage of the physical body (yang), and the right vertical line is the usage of the mind (yin), then we can see that the more you practice toward the left, the more physical effort and the less mind is needed. This can be aerobic dancing, walking, or jogging in which the mind usage is relatively little compared to physical action. In this kind of qigong practice, normally you do not need special training, and it is classified as layman qigong. In the middle point, the mind and the physical activity are almost equally important. This kind of qigong will be the slow-moving qigong commonly practiced, in which the mind is used to lead the qi in coordination with the movements. For example, in taiji qigong, the Eight Pieces of Brocade, the Five Animal Sports, and many others are very typical qigong exercises, especially in Chinese medical and martial arts societies.

However, when you reach a profound level of qigong practice, the mind becomes more critical and important. When you reach this high level, you are dealing with your mind while you are sitting still. Most mental qigong training was practiced by the scholar and religious qigong practitioners. In this practice, you may have a little physical movement in the lower abdomen. However, the main focus of this qigong practice is in the peaceful mind or spiritual enlightenment that originates from the cultivation of your mind. This kind of qigong practice includes sitting chan (*ren*) (坐禪，忍), Small Circulation meditation (*Xiao Zhou Tian*, 小周天), Grand Circulation meditation (*Da Zhou Tian*, 大周天), or Brain Washing Enlightenment Meditation (*Xi Sui Gong*, 洗髓功).

Theoretically speaking, in order to have good health, you will need to maintain your physical condition and also build up abundant qi in your body. The best qigong for health is actually located in the middle of our model, where you learn how to regulate

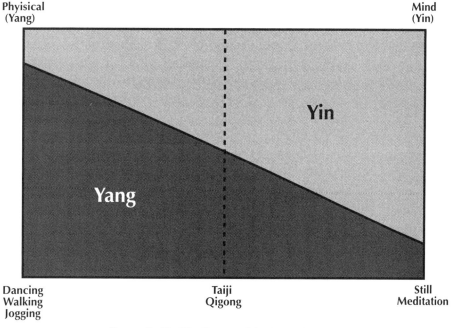

Figure 2–13. The Range of Defined Qigong

your physical body and also your mind. From this yin and yang practice, your qi can be circulated smoothly in the body.

Let us now review the traditional concepts of how qigong was categorized. Generally speaking, all qigong practices can be divided, according to their training theory and methods, into two general categories: external elixir (*wai dan*, 外丹) and internal elixir (*nei dan*, 內丹). Understanding the differences between them will give you an overview of most Chinese qigong practice.

External and Internal Elixirs

External Elixir (Wai Dan, 外丹). Wai means external or outside, and dan means elixir. External here means the skin surface of the body or the limbs, as opposed to the torso or the center of the body, which includes all of the vital organs. Elixir is a hypothetical, life-prolonging substance for which Chinese Daoists have been searching for several millennia. They originally thought that the elixir was something physical that could be prepared from herbs or chemicals purified in a furnace. After thousands of years of study and experimentation, they found that the elixir is in the body. In other words, if you want to prolong your life, you must find the elixir in your body and then learn to cultivate, protect, and nourish it. Actually, the elixir is what we have understood the inner energy or qi circulating in the body to be.

There are many ways of producing elixir or qi in the body. For example, in wai dan qigong practice, you may exercise your limbs such as dancing or even walking. As you exercise, the qi builds up in your arms and legs. When the qi potential in your limbs builds to a high enough level, the qi will flow through the channels, clearing any obstructions and flowing into the center of the body to nourish the organs. This is the main reason that a person who works out or has a physical job is generally healthier than someone who sits around all day.

Naturally, you may simply massage your body to produce the qi. Through massage, you may stimulate the cells of your body to a higher energized state and therefore the qi concentration will be raised and the circulation enhanced. Then, after the massage you relax and the higher levels of qi on the skin surface and muscles will flow into the center of the body and thereby improve the qi circulatory conditions in your internal organs. This is the theoretical foundation of the tui na qigong massage (pushing and grabbing massage, 推拿).

Through acupuncture, you may also bring the qi level near the skin surface to a higher level and from this stimulation, the qi condition of the internal organs can be regulated through qi channels. Therefore, acupuncture can also be classified as wai dan qigong practice. Naturally, the herbal treatments are a way of wai dan practice as well.

From this, we can briefly conclude that any possible stimulation or exercises that accumulate a high level of qi on the surface of the body and then flow inward toward the center of the body can be classified as wai dan (external elixir) (Figure 2-14).

Internal Elixir (Nei Dan, 內丹). Nei means internal and dan again means elixir. Thus, nei dan means to build the elixir internally. Here, internally means in the body instead of in the limbs. Normally, the qi is built in the qi vessels instead of the primary qi channels. Whereas in wai dan, the qi is built up in the limbs or skin surface and then moved into the body through primary qi channels, nei dan exercises build up qi in the body and lead it out to the limbs (Figure 2-15).

Generally, speaking, nei dan theory is deeper than wai dan theory, and it is more difficult to understand and practice. Traditionally, most of the nei dan qigong practices have been passed down more secretly than those of the wai dan. This is especially true of the highest levels of nei dan, such as marrow/brain washing, that were passed down to only a few trusted disciples.

Schools of Qigong Practice

We can also classify qigong into four major categories according to the purpose or final goal of the training: A. maintaining health; B. curing sickness; C. martial arts; D. enlightenment or Buddhahood. This is only a rough breakdown, however, since almost every style of qigong serves more than one of the above purposes. For example, although martial qigong focuses on increasing fighting effectiveness, it can also improve your health. Daoist qigong aims for longevity and enlightenment, but to reach this goal you need to be in good health and know how to cure sickness. Because of this multi-purpose aspect of the categories, it will be simpler to discuss their backgrounds rather than the goals of their training. Knowing the history and basic principles of each category will help you to understand their qigong more clearly.

Scholar Qigong—for Maintaining Health. In China before the Han dynasty, there were two major schools of scholarship. One of them was created by Confucius (孔子) (551-479 B.C.) during the Spring and Autumn period. Later, his philosophy was popularized and enlarged by Mencius (孟子) (372-289 B.C.) in the Warring States

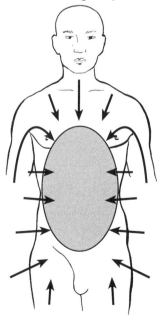

Figure 2–14. External Elixir (Wai Dan)

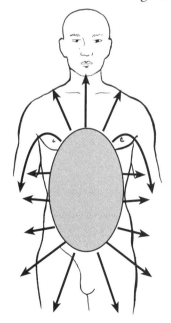

Figure 2–15 Internal Elixir (Nei Dan)

Period. The scholars who practice his philosophy are commonly called Confucians or Confucianists (*Ru Jia*, 儒家). The key words to their basic philosophy are loyalty (zhong, 忠), filial piety (*xiao*, 孝), humanity (*ren*, 仁), kindness (*ai*, 愛), trust (*xin*, 信), justice (*yi*, 義), harmony (*he*, 和), and peace (*ping*, 平). Humanity and human feelings are the main subjects of study. Ru Jia philosophy has become the center of much of Chinese culture.

The second major school of scholarship was called Dao Jia (*Daoism*, 道家) and was created by Lao Zi (老子) in the 6th century B.C. Lao Zi is considered to be the author of a book called the *Classic on the Virtue of the Dao* (*Dao De Jing*, 道德經), which describes human morality. Later, in the Warring States Period, his follower, Zhuang Zhou (莊周), wrote a book called *Zhuang Zi* (莊子) which led to the forming of another strong branch of Daoism. Before the Han dynasty, Daoism was considered a branch of scholarship. However, in the East Han dynasty (東漢) (A.D. 25-221), traditional Daoism was combined with the Buddhism imported from India by Zhang, Dao-ling (張道陵), and it began gradually to be treated as a religion. Therefore, the Daoism before the Han dynasty should be considered scholarly Daoism rather than religious.

With regard to their contribution to qigong, both schools emphasized maintaining health and preventing disease. They believed that mental and emotional excesses cause many illnesses. When a person's mind is not calm, balanced, and peaceful, the organs will not function normally. For example, depression can cause stomach ulcers and indigestion. Anger will cause the liver to malfunction. Sadness will cause stagnation and tightness in the lungs, and fear can disturb the normal functioning of the kidneys and bladder. They realized that if you want to avoid illness, you must learn to balance and relax your thoughts and emotions. This is called "regulating the mind" (*tiao xin*, 調心).

Therefore, the scholars emphasize gaining a peaceful mind through meditation. In their still meditation, the main part of the training is getting rid of thoughts so that the mind is clear and calm. When you become calm, the flow of thoughts and emotions slows down, and you feel mentally and emotionally neutral. This kind of meditation can be thought of as practicing emotional self-control. When you are in this "no thought" state, you become very relaxed, and can even relax deep down into your internal organs. When your body is this relaxed, your qi will naturally flow smoothly and strongly. This kind of still meditation was very common in ancient Chinese scholar society.

In order to reach the goal of a calm and peaceful mind, their training focused on regulating the mind, body, and breath. They believed that as long as these three things were regulated, the qi flow would be smooth and sickness would not occur. This is why the qi training of the scholars is called "xiu qi" (修氣), which means, "cultivating qi." "Xiu" in Chinese means to regulate, to cultivate, or to repair. It means to maintain in good condition. This is very different from the religious Daoist qi training after the East Han dynasty, which was called "lian qi" (練氣), and is translated as "train qi." "Lian" means to drill or to practice to make stronger.

Many of the qigong documents written by the Confucians and Daoists were limited to the maintenance of health. The scholar's attitude in qigong was to follow his natural destiny and maintain his health. This philosophy is quite different from that of the religious Daoist after the East Han dynasty who believed that one's destiny could be changed. They believed that it is possible to train your qi to make it stronger and to extend your life. It is said in scholarly society: "in human life, seventy is rare."[11] You should understand that few of the common people in ancient times lived past seventy because of the lack of good food and modern medical technology. It is also said: "peace with heaven and delight in your destiny" (安天樂命); and "cultivate the body and await destiny" (修身俟命). Compare this with the philosophy of the later Daoists who said: "one hundred and twenty means dying young."[12] They believed and have proven that human life can be lengthened and destiny can be resisted and overcome.

Confucianism and Daoism were the two major scholarly schools in China, but there were many other schools which were also more or less involved in qigong practices. We will not discuss them here because there are only a very limited number of qigong documents from these schools.

Medical Qigong—for Healing. In ancient Chinese society, most emperors respected the scholars and were affected by their philosophy. Doctors were not regarded highly because they made their diagnosis by touching the patient's body, which was considered characteristic of the lower classes in society. Although the doctors developed a profound and successful medical science, they were commonly looked down on. However, they continued to work hard and study, and quietly passed down the results of their research to following generations.

Of all the groups studying qigong in China, the doctors have been at it the longest. Since the discovery of qi circulation in the human body about four thousand years ago, the Chinese doctors have devoted a major portion of their efforts to studying the behavior of qi. Their efforts resulted in acupuncture, acupressure or cavity press massage, and herbal treatment.

In addition, many Chinese doctors used their medical knowledge to create different sets of qigong exercises either for maintaining health or for curing specific illnesses. Chinese medical doctors believed that doing only sitting or still meditation to regulate the body, mind, and breathing as the scholars did was not enough to cure sickness. They believed that in order to increase the qi circulation, you must move. Although a calm and peaceful mind was important for health, exercising the body was more important. They learned through their medical practice that people who exercised properly got sick less often, and their bodies degenerated less quickly than was the case with people who just sat around. They also realized that specific body movements could increase the qi circulation in specific organs. They reasoned from this that these exercises could also be used to treat specific illnesses and to restore the normal functioning of these organs.

Some of these movements are similar to the way in which certain animals move. It is clear that in order for an animal to survive in the wild, it must have an instinct for how to protect its body. Part of this instinct is concerned with how to build up its qi, and how to keep its qi from being lost. We humans have lost many of these instincts over the years that we have been separating ourselves from nature.

Many doctors developed qigong exercises which were modeled after animal movements to maintain health and cure sickness. A typical, well-known set of such exercises is Five Animal Sports (*Wu Qin Xi*, 五禽戲), created by Dr. Jun Qing (君倩) and later modified and publicized by the well-known medical qigong doctor, Hua Tuo (華佗) during the Chinese Three Kingdoms Period (三國) (A.D. 221-265). Another famous set, based on similar principles, is called the Eight Pieces of Brocade (*Ba Duan Jin,* 八段錦), and was created by Marshal Yue Fei (岳飛) during the Chinese Southern Song dynasty (南宋) (A.D. 1127-1280). Interestingly enough, Yue Fei was a soldier rather than a doctor.

In addition, using their medical knowledge of qi circulation, Chinese doctors researched until they found which movements could help cure particular illnesses and health problems. Not surprisingly, many of these movements were not unlike the ones used to maintain health, since many illnesses are caused by unbalanced qi. When an imbalance continues for a long period of time, the organs will be affected and may be physically damaged. This is like running a machine without supplying the proper electrical current, over time the machine will be damaged. Chinese doctors believe that before physical damage to an organ shows up in a patient's body, there is first an abnormality in the qi balance and circulation. Abnormal qi circulation is the very beginning of illness and organ damage. When qi is too positive (yang) or too negative (yin) in a specific organ's qi channel, your physical organ is beginning to suffer damage. If you do not correct the qi circulation, that organ will malfunction or degenerate. The best way to heal someone is to adjust and balance the qi even before there is any physical problem. Therefore, correcting or improving the normal qi circulation is the major goal of acupuncture or acupressure treatments. Herbs and special diets are also considered important treatments in regulating the qi in the body.

As long as the illness is limited to the level of qi stagnation and there is no physical organ damage, the qigong exercises used for maintaining health can be used to readjust the qi circulation and treat the problem. However, if the sickness is already so serious that the physical organs have started to fail, then the situation has become critical and a specific treatment is necessary. The treatment can be acupuncture, herbs, or even an operation, as well as specific qigong exercises designed to speed up the healing or even to cure the sickness. For example, ulcers and asthma can often be cured or helped by some simple exercises. Recently in both mainland China and Taiwan, certain qigong exercises have been shown to be effective in treating certain kinds of cancer.

Over the thousands of years of observing nature and themselves, some qigong practitioners went even deeper. They realized that the body's qi circulation changes with the seasons and that it is a good idea to help the body out during these periodic adjustments. They noticed also that in each season different organs have characteristic problems. For example, at the beginning of fall, your lungs have to adapt to the colder air you are breathing. While this adjustment is going on, the lungs are susceptible to disturbance, so your lungs may feel uncomfortable and you may catch colds easily. Your digestive system is also affected during seasonal changes. Your appetite may increase, or you may have diarrhea. When the temperature goes down, your kidneys and bladder will start to give you trouble. For example, because the kidneys are stressed, you may feel pain in your back. Focusing on these seasonal qi disorders, the meditators created a set of movements that can be used to speed up the body's adjustment. These qigong exercises are commonly called "four seasons gong" (*si ji gong*, 四季功).

In addition to Marshal Yue Fei, many people who were not doctors also created sets of medical qigong. These sets were probably created originally to maintain health and later were also used for curing sickness.

Martial Qigong—for Fighting. Chinese martial qigong was probably not developed until Da Mo (達磨) wrote the *Muscle/Tendon Changing Classic* in the Shaolin Temple during the Liang dynasty (梁) (A.D. 502-557). When Shaolin monks trained Da Mo's Muscle/Tendon Changing Qigong, they found that they could not only improve their health but also greatly increase the power of their martial techniques. Since then, by following Da Mo's qigong theories and concepts, many martial styles have developed qigong sets to increase their effectiveness. In addition, many martial styles have been created based on qigong theory. Martial artists have played a major role in Chinese qigong society.

When qigong theory was first applied to the martial arts, it was used to increase the power and efficiency of the muscles. The theory is very simple—the mind (*yi*) is used to lead qi to the muscles to energize them so that they function more efficiently. The average person generally uses his muscles at about 40 percent maximum efficiency. But if he can train his concentration and use his strong yi (the mind generated from clear thinking) to lead qi to the muscles effectively, then he can energize the muscles to a higher level and therefore, increase his fighting effectiveness.

As acupuncture theory became better understood, fighting techniques were able to reach even more advanced levels. Martial artists learned to attack specific areas, such as vital acupuncture cavities, to disturb the enemy's qi flow and create imbalances that cause injury or even death. In order to do this, the practitioner must understand the route and timing of the qi circulation in the human body. He also has to train so that he can strike the cavities accurately and to the correct depth. These cavity strike techniques are called pointing cavities (*dian xue,* 點穴) or pointing vessels (*dian mai,* 點脈).

Most of the martial qigong practices help to improve the practitioner's health. However, there are other martial qigong practices which, although they build up some special skill that is useful for fighting, also damage the practitioner's health. An example of this is iron sand palm (*tie sha zhang,* 鐵砂掌). Although this training can build up amazing destructive power, it can also harm your hands and affect the qi circulation in the hands and internal organs.

As mentioned in Chapter 1, since the 6th century, many martial styles have been created that were based on qigong theory. They can be roughly divided into external and internal styles.

The external styles emphasize building qi in the limbs to coordinate with the physical martial techniques. They follow the theory of wai dan (external elixir) qigong, which usually generates qi in the limbs through special exercises. The concentrated mind is used during the exercises to energize the qi. This increases muscular strength significantly and therefore increases the effectiveness of the martial techniques. Qigong can also be used to train the body to resist punches and kicks. In this training, qi is led to energize the skin and the muscles, enabling them to resist a blow without injury. This training is commonly called iron shirt (*tie bu shan*, 鐵布衫) or golden bell cover (*jin zhong zhao*, 金鐘罩). The martial styles that use wai dan qigong training are normally called external styles (*wai jia*, 外家) or hard qigong training that is called hard gong (*ying gong*, 硬功). Shaolin Gongfu is a typical example of a style that uses wai dan martial qigong.

Although wai dan qigong can help the martial artist increase his power, there is a disadvantage. Because wai dan qigong emphasizes training the external muscles, it can cause over-development. This can cause a problem called "energy dispersion" (*san gong*, 散功) when the practitioner gets older. In order to remedy this, when an external martial artist reaches a high level of external qigong training he will start training internal qigong, which specializes in curing the energy dispersion problem. That is why it is said: "Shaolin Gongfu from external to internal."

Internal martial qigong is based on the theory of nei dan (internal elixir). In this method, qi is generated in the body instead of the limbs, and this qi is then led to the limbs to increase power. In order to lead qi to the limbs, the techniques must be soft and muscle usage must be kept to a minimum. The training and theory of nei dan martial qigong is much more difficult than those of wai dan martial qigong. Interested readers should refer to the book: *Tai Chi Theory and Martial Power* published by YMAA

Several internal martial styles were created in the Wudang (武當山) and Emei (峨嵋山) mountains. Popular styles are Taijiquan, Baguazhang, Liu He Ba Fa, and Xingyiquan. However, you should understand that even the internal martial styles, which are commonly called soft styles, must on some occasions use muscular strength while fighting. That means in order to have strong power in the fight, the qi must be led to the muscular body and manifested externally. Therefore, once an internal martial artist has achieved a degree of competence in internal qigong, he or she should also learn how to use harder, more external techniques. That is why it is said: "The internal styles are from soft to hard."

In the last fifty years, some of the taiji qigong or taijiquan practitioners have developed training that is mainly for health, and is called "wuji qigong" (無極氣功) which means "no extremities qigong." Wuji is the state of neutrality—it precedes taiji, which is the state of complementary opposites. When there are thoughts and feelings in your mind, there is yin and yang, but if you can still your mind you can return to the emptiness of wuji. When you achieve this state, your mind is centered and clear, your body relaxed, and your qi is able to flow naturally and smoothly to reach the proper balance by itself. Wuji qigong has become very popular in many parts of China, especially Shanghai and Canton.

You can see that, although qigong is widely studied in Chinese martial society, the main focus of training was originally on increasing fighting ability rather than health. Good health was considered a by-product of training. It was not until the twentieth century that the health aspect of martial qigong started receiving greater attention. This is especially true in the internal martial arts.

Religious Qigong—for Enlightenment or Buddhahood. Religious qigong, though not as popular as other categories in China, is recognized as having achieved the highest accomplishments of all the qigong categories. It used to be kept secret in the monastic society, and it is only in the twentieth century that it has been revealed to laymen.

In China, religious qigong includes mainly Daoist and Buddhist qigong. The main purpose of their training is striving for enlightenment, or what the Buddhists refer to as Buddhahood. They are looking for a way to lift themselves above normal human suffering and to escape from the cycle of continual reincarnation. They believe that all human suffering is caused by the seven emotions and six desires (*qi qing liu yu*, 七情六欲). The seven emotions are happiness (*xi*, 喜), anger (*nu*, 怒), sorrow (*ai*, 哀), joy (*le*, 樂), love (*ai*, 愛), hate (*hen*, 恨), and desire (*yu*, 欲). The six desires are the six sensory pleasures derived from the eyes, ears, nose, tongue, body, and mind. If you are still bound to these emotions and desires, you will reincarnate after your death. To avoid reincarnation, you must train your spirit to reach a very high stage where it is strong enough to be independent after your death. This spirit will enter the heavenly kingdom and gain eternal peace. This training is hard to do in the everyday world, so practitioners frequently flee society and move into the solitude of the mountains where they can concentrate all of their energies on self-cultivation.

Religious qigong practitioners train to strengthen their internal qi to nourish their spirit (*shen*, 神) until the spirit is able to survive the death of the physical body. Marrow/Brain Washing Qigong training is necessary to reach this stage. It enables them to lead qi to the forehead, where the spirit resides, and raise the brain to a higher energy state. This training used to be restricted to only a few priests who had reached an advanced level. Tibetan Buddhists were also involved heavily in this training. Over the last two thousand years the Tibetan Buddhists, the Chinese Buddhists, and the Daoists have followed the same principles to become the three major religious schools of qigong training.

This religious striving toward enlightenment or Buddhahood is recognized as the highest and most difficult level of qigong. Many qigong practitioners reject the rigors of this religious striving and practice marrow/brain washing qigong solely for the purpose of longevity. It was these people who eventually revealed the secrets of marrow/brain washing to the outside world. If you are interested in knowing more about this training, you may refer to *Qigong, The Secret of Youth*, published by YMAA.

From the above brief summary, you may obtain a general concept of how Chinese qigong can be categorized. From the understanding of this general concept, you should not have further doubt about any qigong you are training.

In the next section, we will discuss general qigong training theory. This theoretical discussion of qigong practice will offer you a foundation upon which to build your training. Without this scientific theoretical support, your mind will continue wondering and wandering. Understanding the theory is like learning how to read a map. It can direct you to the final goal of practice without confusion.

2-4. Qigong Training Theory

Many people think that qigong is a difficult subject to comprehend. In some ways, this is true. However, you must understand one thing: regardless of how difficult the qigong theory and practice of a particular style is, the basic theory and principles are very simple and remain the same for all qigong styles. They are the root of the entire qigong practice. If you understand these roots, you can grasp the key to the practice and grow. All of the qigong styles originated from these roots, but each one has blossomed differently.

In this section we will discuss these basic qigong training theories and principles. With this knowledge as a foundation, you can understand not only what you should be doing, but also why you are doing it. Naturally, it is impossible to discuss all of the basic qigong ideas in such a short section. However, it will offer you the key to open the gate into the spacious, four thousand years old garden of Chinese qigong. If you wish to know more about the theory of qigong, please refer to *The Root of Chinese Qigong*, published by YMAA.

The Concept of Yin and Yang, Kan and Li. The concept of yin (陰) and yang (陽) is the foundation of Chinese philosophy. From this philosophy, Chinese culture was developed. Naturally, this includes Chinese medicine and qigong practice. Therefore, in order to understand qigong, first you should study the concept of yin and yang. In addition, you should also understand the concept of kan (坎) and li (離) that, unfortunately, has been commonly confused with the concept of yin and yang even in China.

The Chinese have long believed that the universe is made up of two opposite forces—yin and yang—that must balance each other. When these two forces begin to lose their balance, nature finds a way to re-balance them. If the imbalance is significant, disaster will occur. However, when these two forces interact with each other smoothly and harmoniously, they manifest power and generate millions of living things.

As mentioned earlier, yin and yang theory is also applied to the three great natural powers: heaven, earth, and man. For example, if the yin and yang forces of heaven (i.e., energy which comes to us from the sky) are losing balance, there can be tornadoes, hurricanes, or other natural disasters. When the yin and yang forces lose their balance on earth, rivers can change their paths and earthquakes can occur. When the yin and yang forces in the human body lose their balance, sickness and even death can occur. Experience has shown that the yin and yang balance of the earth and heaven affects the yin and yang balance in man. Similarly, the yin and yang balance of the earth is influenced by the heaven's yin and yang. Therefore, if you wish to have a healthy body and live a long life, you need to know how to adjust your body's yin and yang and how to coordinate your qi with the yin and yang energy of heaven and earth. The study of yin and yang in the human body is the root of Chinese medicine and qigong.

Furthermore, the Chinese have also classified everything in the universe according to yin and yang. Even feelings, thoughts, strategy, and the spirit are covered. For example, female is yin and male is yang, night is yin and day is yang, weak is yin and strong is yang, backward is yin and forward is yang, sad is yin and happy is yang, defense is yin and offense is yang, and so on.

Practitioners of Chinese medicine and qigong believe that they must seek to understand the yin and yang of nature and the human body before they can adjust and regulate the body's energy balance into a more harmonious state. Only then can health be maintained and the causes of sicknesses be corrected.

Another thing that you should understand is that the concept of yin and yang is relative instead of absolute. For example, the number seven is yang compared with three. However, if seven is compared with ten, then it is yin. That means in order to decide yin or yang, a reference point must first be chosen. Therefore, if five is the yin and yang balance number, then seven is yang and three is yin. If we choose zero as the yin and yang balance number, then any positive number is yang and any negative number is yin.

However, if what we are interested in is the most negative number, then we may choose the negative number as yang and positive number as yin with zero as the central number. For example, generally speaking, in qigong, techniques that can be seen physically and are the manifestation of qi are considered yang, and the techniques that cannot be seen but are felt are treated as yin. When the yin and yang concept is applied in Chinese medicine, qi is considered yang, since it plays such a major role in diagnosis and treatment, while the blood (physical) is considered yin.

Now let us discuss how the concept of yin and yang is applied to the qi circulating in the human body. Many people, even some qigong practitioners, are still confused by this. When it is said that qi can be either yin or yang, it does not mean that there are two different kinds of qi like male and female, fire and water, or positive and negative charges. Qi is energy, and energy itself does not have yin and yang. It is like the energy that is generated from the sparking of negative and positive charges. Charges have the potential for generating energy, but are not the energy itself.

When it is said that qi is yin or yang, it means that the qi is too strong or too weak for a particular circumstance. Again, it is relative and not absolute. Naturally, this implies that the potential that generates the qi is strong or weak. For example, the qi from the sun is yang qi, and qi from the moon is yin qi. This is because the sun's energy is yang in comparison to human qi, while the moon's is yin. In any discussion of energy where people are involved, human qi is used as the standard. People are always especially interested in what concerns them directly, so it is natural that we are interested primarily in human qi and tend to view all qi from the perspective of human qi. This is not unlike looking at the universe from the physical perspective of the earth.

When we look at the yin and yang of qi within the human body, however, we must redefine our point of reference. For example, when a person is dead, his residual human qi or ghost qi, (gui qi, 鬼氣) is weak compared to a living person's. Therefore, the ghost qi is yin as it dissipates, while the living person's qi is yang. When discussing qi within the body, in the lung channel for example, the reference point is the normal, healthy status of the qi there. If the qi is stronger than it is in the normal state, it is yang, and, naturally, if it is weaker than this, it is yin. There are twelve parts of the human body that are considered organs in Chinese medicine, and six of them are yin and six are yang. The yin organs are the heart, lungs, kidneys, liver, spleen, and pericardium, and the yang organs are the large intestine, small intestine, stomach, gall bladder, urinary bladder, and triple burner. Generally speaking, the qi level of the yin organs is lower than that of the yang organs. The yin organs store original essence and process the essence obtained from food and air, while the yang organs handle digestion and excretion.

When the qi in any of your organs is not in its normal state, you feel uncomfortable. If it is very much off from the normal state, the organ will start to malfunction and you may become sick. The qi in your entire body will also be affected and you will feel too yang, perhaps feverish, or too yin, such as the weakness after diarrhea.

The natural environment, such as weather, climate, and seasonal changes, also affects your body's qi level. Therefore, when the body's qi level is classified, the reference point is the level that feels most comfortable for those particular circumstances. Naturally, each of us is a little bit different, and what feels best and most natural for one person may be a bit different from what is right for another. That is why the doctor will usually ask "How do you feel?" It is according to your own standard that you are judged.

Breathing is closely related to the state of your qi, and is therefore also considered yin or yang. When you exhale you expel air from your lungs, your mind moves outward, and the qi around the body expands. In the Chinese martial arts, the exhale is generally used to expand the qi to energize the muscles during an attack. Therefore, the exhale is yang—it is expanding, offensive, and strong. Naturally, based on the same theory, the inhale is considered yin.

Your breathing is closely related to your emotions. When you lose your temper, your breathing is short and fast, i.e., yang. When you are sad, your body is more yin, and you inhale more than you exhale in order to absorb qi from the air to balance the body's yin and bring the body back into balance. When you are excited and happy your body is yang, and your exhale is longer than your inhale to get rid of the excess yang that is caused by the excitement.

As mentioned before, your mind is also closely related to your qi. Therefore, when your qi is yang, your mind is usually also yang (excited) and vice versa. The mind can also be classified according to the qi that generated it. The mind (yi, 意) that is generated from the calm and peaceful qi obtained from the original essence is considered yin. The mind (xin, 心) that originates with the food and air essence is emotional, scattered, and excited, and it is considered yang. The spirit, that is related to the qi, can also be classified as yang or yin based on its origin.

Do not confuse yin qi and yang qi with fire qi and water qi. When the yin and yang of qi are mentioned, it refers to the level of qi according to some reference point. However, when water and fire qi are mentioned, it refers to the quality of the qi. If you are interested in reading more about the yin and yang of qi, please refer to these books: *The Root of Chinese Qigong* and *Qigong, The Secret of Youth—Da Mo's Muscle/Tendon Changing and Marrow/Brain Washing Classic*, published by YMAA.

The terms kan and li occur frequently in qigong documents. In the eight trigrams, kan represents "water" while li represents "fire." However, the everyday terms for water and fire are also often used. Kan and li training has long been of major importance to qigong practitioners. In order to understand why, you must understand these two words, and the theory behind them.

First, you should understand that though kan-li and yin-yang are related, kan and li are not yin and yang. Kan is water, which is able to cool your body down and make it more yin, while li is fire, which warms your body and makes it more yang. Kan and li are the methods or causes, while yin and yang are the results. When kan and li are adjusted and regulated correctly, yin and yang will be balanced and interact harmoniously.

Qigong practitioners believe that your body is always too yang, unless you are sick or have not eaten for a long time, in which case your body may be more yin. Since your body is always yang, it is degenerating and burning out. It is believed that this is the cause of aging. If you can use water to cool down your body, you can slow down the degeneration process and thereby lengthen your life. This is the main reason why Chinese qigong practitioners have been studying ways of improving the quality of the water in their bodies, and of reducing the quantity of the fire. I believe that as a taijiquan and qigong practitioner you should always keep this subject at the top of your list for study and research. If you earnestly ponder and experiment, you can grasp the trick of adjusting them.

If you want to learn how to adjust them, you must understand that water and fire mean many things in your body. The first concerns your qi. As mentioned earlier, qi is classified as fire and water. When your qi is not pure and causes your physical body to heat up and your mental/spiritual body to become unstable (yang), it is classified as fire qi. The qi that is pure and is able to cool both your physical and spiritual bodies (make them more yin) is considered water qi. However, your body can never be purely water. Water can cool down the fire, but it must never totally quench it, because then you would be dead. It is also said that fire qi is able to agitate and stimulate the emotions, and from these emotions generate a "mind." This mind is called xin (心) and is considered the fire mind, yang mind, or emotional mind. On the other hand, the mind that water qi generates is calm, steady, and wise. This mind is called yi (意) and is considered to be the water mind or wisdom mind. If your spirit is nourished by the fire qi, although your spirit may be high, it will be scattered and confused (a yang spirit). Naturally, if the spirit is nourished and raised up by water qi, it will be firm and steady (a yin mind). When your yi is able to govern your emotional xin effectively, your will (strong emotional intention) can be firm.

You can see from this discussion that your qi is the main cause of the yin and yang of your physical body, your mind, and your spirit. To regulate your body's yin and yang, you must learn how to regulate your body's water and fire qi, but in order to do this efficiently you must know their sources.

Once you have grasped the concepts of yin-yang and kan-li, then you have to think about how to adjust kan and li so that you can balance the yin and yang in your body.

Theoretically, a qigong practitioner would like to keep his body in a state of yin-yang balance, which means the center point of the yin and yang forces. This center point is commonly called wuji (無極) (no extremities). It is believed that wuji is the original, natural state where yin and yang are not distinguished. In the wuji state, nature is peaceful and calm. In the wuji state, all of the yin and yang forces have gradually combined harmoniously and disappeared. When this wuji theory is applied to human beings, it is the final goal of qigong practice where your mind is neutral and absolutely calm. The wuji state makes it possible for you to find the origin of your life and to combine your qi with the qi of nature.

The ultimate goal and purpose of qigong practice is to find this peaceful and natural state. In order to reach this goal, you must first understand your body's yin and yang so that you can balance them by adjusting your kan and li. Only when your yin and yang are balanced will you be able to find the center balance point, the wuji state.

Theoretically, between the two extremes of yin and yang are millions of paths (i.e., different kan and li methods) that can lead you to the neutral center. This accounts for the hundreds of different styles of qigong that have been created over the years. You can see that the theory of yin and yang and the methods of kan and li are the root of training all Chinese qigong styles. Without this root, the essence of qigong practice would be lost.

Qigong Training Theory. Every qigong form or practice has its special training purpose and theory. If you do not know the purpose and theory, you have lost the root (meaning) of the practice. Therefore, as a qigong practitioner, you must continue to ponder and practice until you understand the root of every set or form.

Remember that getting the gold is not enough. Like the boy in the old Chinese story, you should concern yourself with learning the trick of turning the rock into gold. You can see that getting the gold is simply gaining the flowers and branches, and there can be no growth. However, if you have the trick, which is the theory, then you will have the root and you may continue to grow by yourself.

Now that you have learned the basic theory of the qigong practice, let us discuss the general training principles. In Chinese qigong society, it is commonly known that in order to reach the goal of qigong practice, you must learn how to regulate the body (*tiao shen,* 調身), regulate the breathing (*tiao xi,* 調息), regulate the emotional mind (*tiao xin,* 調心), regulate the qi (*tiao qi,* 調氣), and regulate the spirit (*tiao shen,* 調神). Tiao in Chinese is constructed from two words, 言 (*yan,* means speaking or talking) and 周 (*zhou,* means round or complete). That means the roundness (i.e., harmony) or the completeness is accomplished by negotiation. Like an out-of-tune in piano, you must adjust it and make it harmonize with others. This implies that when you are regulating one of the above five processes, you must also coordinate and harmonize the other four regulating elements.

Regulating the body includes understanding how to find and build the root of the body, as well as the root of the individual forms you are practicing. To build a firm root, you must know how to keep your center, how to balance your body, and most important of all, how to relax so that the qi can flow.

To regulate your breathing, you must learn how to breathe so that your respiration and your mind mutually correspond and cooperate. When you breathe this way, your mind can attain peace more quickly and, therefore, concentrate more easily on leading the qi.

Regulating the mind involves learning how to keep your mind calm, peaceful, and centered so that you can judge situations objectively and lead qi to the desired places.

The mind is the main key to success in qigong practice.

Regulating the qi is one of the ultimate goals of qigong practice. In order to regulate your qi effectively you must first have regulated your body, breathing, and mind. Only then will your mind be clear enough to sense how the qi is distributed in your body and understand how to adjust it.

For Buddhist and Daoist priests who seek enlightenment or Buddhahood, regulating the spirit (*shen*) is the final goal of qigong. This enables them to maintain a neutral, objective perspective of life, and this perspective is the eternal life of the Buddha. The average qigong practitioner has lower goals. He raises his spirit in order to increase his concentration and enhance his vitality. This makes it possible for him to lead qi effectively throughout his entire body so that it carries out the managing and guarding duties. This maintains health and slows the aging process.

If you understand these few things you can quickly enter into the field of qigong. Without all of these important elements, your training will be ineffective and your time will be wasted.

Before you start training, you must first understand that all of the training originates in your mind. You must have a clear idea of what you are doing, and your mind must be calm, centered, and balanced. This also implies that your feeling, sensing, and judgment must be objective and accurate. This requires emotional balance and a clear mind. This takes a lot of hard work, but once you have reached this level you will have built the root of your physical training, and your yi (mind) can lead your qi throughout your physical body.

Regulating the Body (Tiao Shen, 調身)

When you learn any qigong, either moving or still, the first step is to learn the correct postures or movements. After you have learned the postures and movements, learn how to improve them until you can perform the forms accurately. Then you start to regulate your body until it has reached the stage that could provide the best condition for the qi to build up or to circulate.

In still qigong practice or soft qigong movement, this means to adjust your body until it is in the most comfortable and relaxed state. This implies that your body must be centered and balanced. If it is not, you will be tense and uneasy, and this will affect the judgment of your yi and the circulation of your qi. In Chinese medical society it is said: "[When] shape [body's posture] is not correct, then the qi will not be smooth. [When] the qi is not smooth, the yi [wisdom mind] will not be peaceful. [When] the yi is not peaceful, then the qi is disordered."[13] You should understand that the relaxation of your body originates with your yi. Therefore, before you can relax your body, you must first relax or regulate your mind (*yi*). This is called "*shen xin ping heng*," (身心平衡) which means "body and heart [i.e., mind] balanced." The body and the mind are mutually related. A relaxed and balanced body helps your yi to relax and concentrate. When your yi is at peace and can judge things accurately, your body will be relaxed, balanced, centered, and rooted. Only when you are rooted can you raise up your spirit of vitality.

Relaxation. Relaxation is one of the major keys to success in qigong. You should re-member that only when you are relaxed will all your qi channels be open. In order to be relaxed, your yi must first be relaxed and calm. When the yi coordinates with your breathing, your body can relax.

In qigong practice there are three levels of relaxation. The first level is the external physical relaxation, or postural relaxation. This is a very superficial level, and almost anyone can reach it. It consists of adopting a comfortable stance and avoiding un-necessary strain in how you stand and move. The second level is the relaxation of the muscles and tendons. To do this your yi must be directed deep into the muscles and tendons. This relaxation will help open your qi channels, and will allow the qi to sink and accumulate in the dan tian.

The final stage is the relaxation that reaches the internal organs and the bone mar-row. Remember, only if you can relax deep into your body will your mind be able to lead the qi there. Only at this stage will the qi be able to reach everywhere. Then you will feel transparent—as if your whole body had disappeared. If you can reach this level of relaxation, you can communicate with your organs and use qigong to adjust or regu-late the qi disorders that are giving you problems. You will also be able to protect your organs more effectively, and therefore slow down their degeneration.

Rooting. In all qigong practice it is very important to be rooted. Being rooted means to be stable and in firm contact with the ground. If you want to push a car you have to be rooted; the force you exert into the car needs to be balanced by the force into the ground. If you are not rooted, when you push the car you will only push yourself away and not move the car. Your root is made up of your body's sinking, centering, and balance.

Before you can develop your root, you must first relax and let your body "settle." As you relax, the tension in the various parts of your body will dissolve, and you will find a comfortable way to stand. You will stop fighting the ground to keep your body up and will learn to rely on your body's structure to support itself. This lets the muscles relax even more. Since your body isn't struggling to stand up, your yi won't be push-ing upward, and your body, mind, and qi will all be able to sink. If you let dirty water sit quietly, the impurities will gradually settle to the bottom, leaving the water above it clear. In the same way, if you relax your body enough to let it settle, your qi will sink to your dan tian and the bubbling wells (*yongquan*, K-1, 湧泉) in your feet, and your mind will become clear. Then you can begin to develop your root.

To root your body you must imitate a tree and grow an invisible root under your feet. This will give you a firm root to keep you stable in your training. Your root must be wide as well as deep. Naturally, your yi must grow first because it is the yi that leads the qi. Your yi must be able to lead the qi to your feet and be able to communicate with the ground. Only when your yi can communicate with the ground will your qi be able to grow beyond your feet and enter the ground to build the root. The bubbling well cavity is the gate that enables your qi to communicate with the ground.

After you have gained your root, you must learn how to keep your center. A stable center will make your qi develop evenly and uniformly. If you lose this center, your qi will not be led evenly. In order to keep your body centered, you must first center your yi and then match your body to it. Only under these conditions will the qigong forms you practice have their root. Your mental and physical centers are the keys that enable you to lead your qi beyond your body.

Balance is the product of rooting and centering. Balance includes balancing the qi and the physical body. It does not matter which aspect of balance you are dealing with; first, you must balance your yi, and only then can you balance your qi and your physical body. If your yi is balanced, it can help you to make accurate judgments and therefore to correct the path of the qi flow.

Rooting includes not just rooting the body, but also the form or movement. The root of any form or movement is found in its purpose or principle. For example, in certain qigong exercises you want to lead the qi to your palms. In order to do this you may imagine that you are pushing an object forward while keeping your muscles relaxed. In this exercise, your elbows must be down to build the sense of root for the push. If you raise the elbows, you lose the sense of "intention" of the movement because the push would be ineffective if you were really pushing something. Since the intention or purpose of the movement is its reason for being, you now have a purposeless movement, and you have no reason to lead qi in any particular way. Therefore, in this case, the elbow is the root of the movement.

Regulating the Breath (Tiao Xi, 調息)

Regulating the breath means to regulate your breathing until it is calm, smooth, and peaceful. Only when you have reached this point will you be able to make the breathing deep, slender, long, and soft, which is required for successful qigong practice.

Breathing is affected by your emotions. For example, when you are angry or excited you exhale more strongly than you inhale. When you are sad, you inhale more strongly than you exhale. When your mind is peaceful and calm, your inhalation and exhalation are relatively equal. In order to keep your breathing calm, peaceful, and steady, your mind and emotions must first be calm and neutral. Therefore, in order to regulate your breathing, you must first regulate your mind.

The other side of the coin is that you can use your breathing to control your yi. When your breathing is uniform, it is as if you were hypnotizing your yi, which helps to calm it. You can see that yi and breathing are interdependent and that they cooperate with each other. Deep and calm breathing relaxes you and keeps your mind clear. It fills your lungs with plenty of air so that your brain and entire body have an adequate supply of oxygen. In addition, deep and complete breathing enables the diaphragm to move up and down, which massages and stimulates the internal organs. For this reason, deep breathing exercises are also called "internal organ exercises."

Deep and complete breathing does not mean that you inhale and exhale to the maximum. This would cause the lungs and the surrounding muscles to tense up, which in turn would keep the air from circulating freely and hinder the absorption of oxygen. Without enough oxygen, your mind becomes scattered, and the rest of your body tenses up. In correct breathing, you inhale and exhale to about 70 or 80 percent of capacity so that your lungs stay relaxed.

You can conduct an easy experiment. Inhale deeply so that your lungs are completely full, and time how long you can hold your breath. Then try inhaling to only about 70 percent of your capacity, and see how long you can hold your breath. You will find that with the latter method you can last much longer than the first one. This is simply because the lungs and the surrounding muscles are relaxed. When they are relaxed, the rest of your body and your mind can also relax, which significantly decreases your need for oxygen. Therefore, when you regulate your breathing, the first priority is to keep your lungs relaxed and calm.

When training, your mind must first be calm so that your breathing can be regulated. When the breathing is regulated, your mind is able to reach a higher level of calmness. This calmness can again help you to regulate the breathing, until your mind is deep. After you have trained for a long time, your breathing will be full and slender, and your mind will be very clear. It is said: "xin xi xiang yi," (心息相依) which means "heart [mind] and breathing [are] mutually dependent." When you reach this meditative state, your heartbeat slows down, and your mind is very clear: you have entered the sphere of real meditation.

An Ancient Daoist named Li, Qing-an (李清庵) said: "Regulating breathing means to regulate the real breathing until [you] stop."[14] This means that correct regulating means regulating is no longer necessary. Real regulating is no longer a conscious process but has become so natural that it can be accomplished without conscious effort. In other words, although you start by consciously regulating your breath, you must get to the point where the regulating happens naturally, and you no longer have to think about it. When you breathe, if you concentrate your mind on your breathing, then it is not true regulating because the qi in your lungs will become stagnant. When you reach the level of true regulating, you don't have to pay attention to it, and you can use your mind efficiently to lead the qi. Remember, wherever the yi is, there is the qi. If the yi stops in one spot, the qi will be stagnant. It is the yi that leads the qi and makes it move. Therefore, when you are in a state of correct breath regulation, your mind is free. There is no sound, stagnation, urgency, or hesitation, and you can finally be calm and peaceful.

You can see that when the breath is regulated correctly, the qi will also be regulated. They are mutually related and cannot be separated. This idea is explained frequently in the Daoist literature. The Daoist Guang Cheng Zi (廣成子) said: "One exhale, the earth qi rises; one inhale, the heaven qi descends; real man's [meaning one who has attained the real Dao] repeated breathing at the navel, then my real qi is naturally connected."[15] This says that when you breathe you should move your abdomen as if you were breathing from your navel. The earth qi is the negative (yin) energy from your kidneys, and the sky qi is the positive (yang) energy that comes from the food you eat and the air you breathe. When you breathe from the navel, these two qi's will connect and combine. Some people think that they know what qi is, but they really don't. Once you connect the two qi's, you will know what the "real" qi is, and you may become a "real" man, which means to attain the Dao.

The Daoist book *Sing [of the] Dao [with] Real Words (Chang Dao Zhen Yan, 唱道真言)* says: "One exhale one inhale to communicate qi's function, one movement one calmness is the same as [i.e., is the source of] creation and variation."[16] The first part of this statement again implies that the functioning of qi is connected with the breathing. The second part of this sentence means that all creation and variation comes from the interaction of movement (yang) and calmness (yin). The *Yellow Yard Classic (Huang Ting Ching,* 黃庭經) says: "Breathe original qi to seek immortality."[17] In China, the traditional Daoists wore yellow robes, and they meditated in a yard or hall. This sentence means that in order to reach the goal of immortality, you must seek to find and understand the original qi that comes from the dan tian through correct breathing.

Moreover, the Daoist Wu Zhen Ren (伍真人) said: "Use the post-birth breathing to look for the real person's [i.e. the immortal's] breathing place."[18] In this sentence it is clear that in order to locate the immortal breathing place, the dan tian, you must rely on and know how to regulate your post-birth, or natural, breathing. Through regulating your post-birth breathing you will gradually be able to locate the residence of the qi, the dan tian, and eventually you can use your dan tian to breathe like the immortal Daoists. Finally, in the Daoist song, *The Great Daoist Song of the Spirit's Origin (Ling Yuan Da Dao Ge,* 靈源大道歌) it is said: "The originals [original *jing, qi,* and *shen*] are internally transported peacefully, so that you can become real [immortal]; [if you] depend on [only] external breathing [you] will not reach the end [goal]."[19] From this song, you can see the internal breathing (breathing at the dan tian) is the key to training your three treasures and finally reaching immortality. However, you must first know how to regulate your external breathing correctly.

All of these emphasize the importance of breathing. There are eight key words for air breathing that a qigong practitioner should follow during his practice. Once you understand them you can substantially shorten the time needed to reach your qigong goals. These eight key words are 1. calm (*jing,* 靜); 2. slender (*xi,* 細); 3. deep (*shen,* 深); 4. long (*chang,* 長); 5. continuous (*you,* 悠); 6. uniform (*yun,* 勻); 7. slow (*huan,* 緩), and 8. soft (*mian,* 綿). These key words are self-explanatory, and with a little thought you should be able to understand them.

Regulating the Mind (Tiao Xin, 調心)

It is said in Daoist society that "[When] large Dao is taught, first stop thought; when thought is not stopped, [the lessons are] in vain."[20] This means that when you first practice qigong, the most difficult training is to stop your thinking. The final goal for your mind is "the thought of no thought" (無念之念). Your mind does not think of the past, the present, or the future. Your mind is completely separated from influences of the present such as worry, happiness, and sadness. Then your mind can be calm and steady and can finally gain peace. Only when you are in the state of "the thought of no thought" will you be relaxed and able to sense calmly and accurately.

Regulating your mind means using your consciousness to stop the activity in your mind in order to set it free from the bondage of ideas, emotion, and conscious thought. When you reach this level, your mind will be calm, peaceful, empty, and light. Then your mind has truly reached the goal of relaxation. Only when you reach this stage will you be able to relax deep into your marrow and internal organs. Only then will your mind be clear enough to see (feel) the internal qi circulation and to communicate with your qi and organs. In Daoist society it is called, "nei shi gongfu" (內視功夫), which means the gongfu of internal vision.

When you reach this real relaxation, you may be able to sense the different elements that make up your body: solid matter, liquids, gases, energy, and spirit. You may even be able to see or feel the different colors that are associated with your five organs: green (liver), white (lungs), black (kidneys), yellow (spleen), and red (heart).

Once your mind is relaxed and regulated and you can sense your internal organs, you may decide to study the five-element theory. This is a very profound subject, and sometimes interpreted differently by Oriental physicians and qigong practitioners. But when understood properly, it can give you a method of analyzing the interrelationships between your organs and help you devise ways to correct imbalances.

For example, the lungs correspond to the element *metal*, and the heart to the element *fire*. *Metal* (the lungs) can be used to adjust the heat of the *fire* (the heart) because metal can take a large quantity of heat away from fire, (and thus cool down the heart). When you feel uneasy or have heartburn (excess fire in the heart), you may use deep breathing to calm down the uneasy emotions or cool off the heartburn.

Naturally, it will take a lot of practice to reach this level. In the beginning, you should not have any ideas or intentions because they will make it harder for your mind to relax and empty itself of thoughts. Once you are in a state of "no thought," place your attention on your dan tian. It is said: "Yi shou dan tian" (意守丹田), which means "The mind is kept on the dan tian." The dan tian is the origin and residence of your qi. Your mind can build up the qi here, i.e., start the fire, (*qi huo*, 起火), then lead the qi anywhere you wish, and finally lead the qi back to its residence. When your mind is on the dan tian, your qi will always have a root. When you keep this root, your qi will be strong and full, and it will go where you want it to. You can see that when you practice qigong, your mind cannot be completely empty and relaxed. You must find the firmness within the relaxation, and then you can reach your goal.

In qigong training, it is said: "Use your yi [mind] to lead your qi" (*yi yi yin qi*)(以意引氣). Notice the word 'lead.' Qi behaves like water—it cannot be pushed, but it can be led. When qi is led, it will flow smoothly and without stagnation. When it is pushed, it will flood and enter the wrong paths. Remember, wherever your yi goes first, the qi will naturally follow. For example, if you intend to lift an object, this intention is your yi. This yi will lead the qi to the arms to energize the physical muscles, and then the object can be lifted.

It is said: "Your yi cannot be on your qi. Once your yi is on your qi, the qi is stagnant."[21] When you want to walk from one spot to another, you must first mobilize your intention and direct it to the goal, and then your body will follow. The mind must always be ahead of the body. If your mind stays on your body, you will not be able to move.

In qigong training, the first thing is to know what qi is. If you do not know what qi is, how will you be able to lead it? Once you know what qi is and experience it, then your yi will have something to lead. The next thing in qigong training is to know how your yi communicates with your qi. That means that your yi should be able to sense and feel the qi flow and understand how strong and smooth it is. In taiji qigong society, it is commonly said that your yi must "listen" to your qi and "understand" it. Listen means to pay careful attention to what you sense and feel. The more you pay attention, the better you can understand. Only after you understand the qi situation will your yi be able to set up the strategy. In qigong your mind or yi must generate the idea (visualize your intention), which is like an order to your qi to complete a certain mission.

The more your yi communicates with your qi, the more efficiently the qi can be led. For this reason, as a qigong beginner you must first learn about yi and qi, and also learn how to help them communicate efficiently. Yi is the key in qigong practice. Without this yi you would not be able to lead your qi, let alone build up the strength of the qi or circulate it throughout your entire body.

Remember when the yi is strong, the qi is strong, and when the yi is weak, the qi is weak. Therefore, the first step of qigong training is to develop your yi. The first secret of a strong yi is calmness. When you are calm, you can see things clearly and not be disturbed by surrounding distractions. With your mind calm, you can concentrate.

Confucius said: "First you must be calm, then your mind can be steady. Once your mind is steady, then you are at peace. Only when you are at peace, are you able to think and finally gain."[22] This procedure is also applied in meditation or qigong exercise: First calm, then steady, peace, think, and finally gain. When you practice qigong, first you must learn to be emotionally calm. Once calm, you can see what you want and firm your mind (steady). This firm and steady mind is your intention or yi (it is how your yi is generated). Only after you know what you really want will your mind gain peace and be able to relax emotionally and physically. Once you have reached this step, you must then concentrate or think in order to execute your intention. Under this thoughtful and concentrated mind, your qi will follow and you can gain what you wish.

However, the most difficult part of regulating the mind is learning how to neutralize the thoughts that keep coming back to bother you. This is especially true in still meditation practice. In still meditation, once you have entered a deep, profound meditative state, new thoughts, fantasies, your imagination, or any guilt from what you have done in the past that is hidden behind your mask will emerge and bother you. Normally, the first step of the regulating process is to stop new fantasies and images. To do this, you must come to an understanding of both the concious and subconcious aspects of your mind. That means you must learn how to remove the mask from your face. Only then will you see yourself clearly. Therefore, the first step is to know yourself. Then, you must learn how to handle the problem instead of continuing to avoid it.

There are many ways of regulating your mind. However, the most important key to success is to use your wisdom mind to analyze the situation and find the solution. Do not let your emotional mind govern your thinking. Here, I would like to share with you a few stories about regulating the mind. Hopefully these stories can provide you with a guideline for your own regulation.

In China many centuries ago, two monks were walking side by side down a muddy road when they came upon a large puddle that completely blocked the road. A very beautiful lady in a lovely gown stood at the edge of the puddle, unable to go farther without spoiling her clothes.

Without hesitation, one of the monks picked her up and carried her across the puddle, set her down on the other side, and continued on his way. Many hours later when the two monks were preparing to camp for the night, the second monk turned to the first and said, "I can no longer hold this back. I'm quite angry at you! We are not supposed to look at women, particularly pretty ones, never mind touch them. Why did you do that?" The first monk replied, "Brother, I left the woman at the mud puddle; why are you still carrying her?"

From this story, you can see that often, the thoughts that bother you are created by none other than yourself. If you can use your wisdom mind to govern yourself, many times you can set your mind free from emotional bondage regardless of the situation.

It is true that frequently the mind bothers or enslaves you to the desire for material enjoyment or money. From this desire, you misunderstand the meaning of life. A really happy life comes from satisfaction of both material and spiritual needs.

Have you ever thought about what the real meaning of your life is? What is the real goal for your life? Are you enslaved by money, power, or love? What will make you truly happy?

I remember a story one of my professors at Taiwan University told me: "There was a jail with a prisoner in it," he said, "who was surrounded by mountains of money. He kept counting the money and feeling so happy about his life, thinking that he was the richest man in the whole world. A man passing by saw him and said through the tiny window: "Why are you so happy? You are in prison? Do you know that?" The prisoner laughed: "No! No! It is not that I am inside the jail. It is that you are outside of the jail!"

How do you feel about this story? Do you want to be a prisoner and a slave to money, or do you want to be the real you and feel free internally? Think and be happy.

There is another story that was told to me by one of my students. Since I heard this story, it has always offered me a new guideline for my life. This new guideline is to appreciate what you have; only then will you have a peaceful mind. This does not mean you should not be aggressive in pursuing a better life. Keep pursuing by creating a new target and a new path for your life. It is yang. However, often you will be depressed and discouraged by the obstacles on this path. Therefore, you must also learn how to comfort yourself and appreciate what you already have. This is yin. Only if you have both yin and yang can your life be happy and meaningful.

Long ago, there was a servant who served a bad tempered and impatient master. It did not matter how he tried, he was always blamed and beaten by this master. However, it was the strange truth that the servant was always happy, and his master was always sad and depressed.

One day, there was a kind man who could not understand this phenomenon, and finally he decided to ask this servant why he was always happy even though he was treated so badly. The servant replied: "Everyone has one day of life each day; half of the day is spent awake and the other half is spent sleeping. Although in the daytime, I am a servant and my master treats me badly, in the nighttime, I always dream that I am a king and there are thousands of servants serving me luxuriously. Look at my master:

In the daytime, he is mad, depressed, greedy, and unhappy. In the nighttime, he has nightmares and cannot even have one night of nice rest. I really feel sorry for my master. Comparing me to him, I am surely happier than he is."

Friends, what do you think about this story? You are the only one responsible for your happiness. If you are not satisfied and always complain about what you have obtained, you will be on the course of forever-unhappiness. It is said in the West: "If you smile, the whole world smiles with you, but if you cry, you cry alone." What an accurate saying!

Regulating the Qi (Tiao Qi, 調氣)

Before you can regulate your qi you must first regulate your body, breath, and mind. If you compare your body to a battlefield, then your mind is like the general who generates ideas and controls the situation, and your breathing is the strategy. Your qi is like the soldiers who are led to the most advantageous places on the battlefield. All four elements are necessary and all four must be coordinated with each other if you are to win the war against sickness and aging.

If you want to arrange your soldiers most effectively for battle, you must know which area of the battlefield is most important, and where you are weakest (where your qi is deficient) and need to send reinforcements. If you have more soldiers than you need in one area (excessive qi), then you can send them somewhere else where the ranks are thin. As a general, you must also know how many soldiers are available for the battle, and how many you will need for protecting yourself and your headquarters. To be successful, not only do you need good strategy (breathing), but you also need to communicate and understand the situation with your troops effectively, or all of your strategy will be in vain. When your yi (the general) knows how to regulate the body (knows the battlefield), how to regulate breathing (set up the strategy), and how to effectively regulate qi (direct your soldiers), you can reach the final goal of qigong training.

In order to regulate your qi so that it moves smoothly in the correct paths, you need more than just efficient yi-qi communication. You also need to know how to generate qi. If you do not have enough qi in your body, how can you regulate it? In a battle, if you do not have enough soldiers to set up your strategy, you have already lost.

When you practice qigong, you must first train to make your qi flow naturally and smoothly. There are some qigong exercises in which you intentionally hold your yi, and thus hold your qi, in a specific area. As a beginner, however, you should first learn how to make the qi flow smoothly instead of building a qi dam, which is commonly done in external martial qigong training.

In order to make qi flow naturally and smoothly, your yi must first be relaxed. Only when your yi is relaxed will your body be relaxed and the qi channels open for the qi to circulate. Then you must coordinate your qi flow with your breathing. Breathing regularly and calmly will make your yi calm and allow your body to relax even more.

Regulating the Spirit (Tiao Shen, 調神)

There is one thing that is more important than anything else in a battle, and that is fighting spirit. You may have the best general who knows the battlefield well and is also an expert strategist, but if his soldiers do not have a high fighting spirit (morale), he might still lose. Remember, spirit is the center and root of a fight. When you keep this center, one soldier can be equal to ten soldiers. When his spirit is high, a soldier will obey his orders accurately and willingly, and his general can control the situation efficiently. In a battle, in order for a soldier to have this kind of morale, he must know why he is fighting, how to fight, and what he can expect after the fight. Under these conditions, he will know what he is doing and why, and this understanding will raise up his spirit, strengthen his will, and increase his patience and endurance.

Shen, which is the Chinese term for spirit, originates from the yi (the general). When the shen is strong, the yi is firm. When the yi is firm, the shen will be steady and calm. The shen is the mental part of a soldier. When the shen is high, the qi is strong and easily directed. When the qi is strong, the shen is also strong.

To the religious qigong practitioners, the goal of regulating the spirit is to set the spirit free from the bondage of the physical body, and thus reach the stage of Buddhahood or enlightenment. To the layman practitioners, the goal of regulating the spirit is to keep the spirit of living high to prevent the body from getting sick and degenerating. It is often seen that before a person retires, he has good health. However, once retired, he will get sick easily and his physical condition will deteriorate quickly. When you are working, your spirit remains high and alert. This keeps the qi circulating smoothly in the body.

All of these training concepts and procedures are common to all Chinese qigong. To reach a deep level of understanding and penetrate to the essence of any qigong practice, you should always keep these five training criteria in mind and examine them for deeper levels of meaning. This is the only way to gain the real mental and physical health benefits from your training. Always remember that qigong training is not just the forms. Your feelings and comprehension are the essential roots of the entire training. This yin side of the training has no limit, and the deeper you understand this, the better you will see how much more there is to know.

2-5. Qigong and Taijiquan

As previously explained, martial qigong is one of the four major qigong categories in Chinese qigong. Taijiquan is only one school of martial qigong. It was developed in Daoist monasteries and because of this, its ultimate goal is enlightenment. In order to reach this goal, a taijiquan practitioner must regularly follow the fundamental principles of qigong practice, which include regulating the body, the breathing, the mind, the qi, and finally the spirit. Taiji qigong is based on these training principles, and it was created to lead the beginning practitioner to more fully contemplate what it means to study qigong. Section 4-4, will introduce many taiji qigong practices. If you are interested in knowing more of this training, both the theory and practice, please refer to the book *The Essence of Taiji Qigong*, published by YMAA.

In addition, if you wish to grasp the root and comprehend the essence of taijiquan, you should study hundreds of written documents that are passed down to us from ancient times. These documents distill the accumulated experience of many well-known masters. If you are interested in these documents please refer to the book *Tai Chi Theory and Martial Power*, published by YMAA.

Regulating the Body in Taijiquan. When you learn taijiquan or taiji qigong , the first thing you learn is the correct forms, or the postures created by experienced masters in the past. Every form or posture has its meaning and purpose. Each was created from a deeply profound understanding of the style. It takes an enourmous amount of experience before you can create forms that are valuable for practice, either for martial purpose or for your health.

Once you become familiar with these forms, then you can learn the methods of relaxation. In order to reach a deep level of relaxation, you must learn to regulate both your breathing and your mind. Your breathing will be easier to regulate at first. The peace and comfort that this brings will make it possible to regulate the mind. The regulated mind will in turn help to relax the body and the breathing, creating a beneficial cycle. From this deep relaxation, the qi circulation will be smooth and free. This allows you to have a balanced and full feeling internally. From this feeling, you can find your root, both physically and mentally. Once you have this firm root, your spirit can be raised to a high level.

Moreover, once you can relax to a deep level, you must be able to perform your movements smoothly and naturally, until your mind does not have to focus on them. It is said in the ancient poem, *Taiji Classic:* "Every form of every posture follows smoothly; no forcing, no opposition, the entire body is comfortable. Each form smooth."[23] When you reach this stage, you will be in the state of "regulating without regulating." In addition, from one movement to next, you should remain relaxed, and every part of your body coordinates with all other parts harmoniously. Therefore, it is said: "Once in motion, every part of the body is light and agile and must be threaded together."[24] It is also said: "Top and bottom follow each other; the entire body should be harmonious."[25]

When you reach this goal, your physical and mental centers can be stable, and torso will be relaxed and stay upright comfortably. When this happens, you can be balanced and move agilely. It is said: "An insubstantial energy leads the head [upward]," (虛領頂 勁); "Body central and upright,"(身體中正), and "Stand like a balanced scale, [move] lively like a cartwheel."[26]

From this, you can see that in taijiquan, relaxation, balance, centering, harmony, and natural ease are emphasized in regulating the body. If you practice with these goals in mind, you will master the most essential keys to taijiquan practice.

Regulating the Breathing in Taijiquan. Breathing plays a very important role in qigong and taiji practice. Breathing correctly calms the mind and relaxes the body. This makes it possible for the qi to circulate smoothly, and helps the yi to focus and lead qi wherever desired. Breathing should be deep, relaxed, and regular. In qigong, there are two common methods of breathing. The Buddhist method uses normal breathing, in which the abdomen expands as you inhale, whereas the Daoist method uses "reverse" breathing, in which the abdomen expands as you exhale.[27-30] Taijiquan was developed according to the Daoist method and therefore uses reverse breathing.

When you coordinate your breathing with the forms, the breathing should be smooth and natural. It should also coordinate with the external movements. It is said: "Internal and external are mutually coordinated. Breathe naturally."[31] In the sequence, breathing coordinates with the forms. Since some of the forms are long and some are short, you must vary the length of your breaths to keep the speed of the sequence uniform. If a form in the sequence is too long for one breath, add another. Your breathing should be relaxed—do not hold it; do not force it. Don't hold your breath because your lungs will tighten and your body will tense. This not only slows the qi circulation, but also damages lung cells.

Once your breathing naturally coordinates with the movements, you should no longer pay attention to it. The reason for this is that the mind must be ahead of the qi in order to lead it, and you cannot do this if your mind is on your breathing. If you develop a sense of having an enemy in front of you, the spirit of vitality is raised and the mind is kept ahead of the qi, leading it naturally in support of your movements.

Finally, like pushing a car, right before we push we inhale deeply (reversed breathing), and when we push, we exhale. This is the natural way of manifesting the internal power into the physical form. That is why it is said: "Inhalation is storage, and exhalation is emitting. That is because inhalation lifts up naturally [the spirit of vitality]. It can also lift [control] the opponent. [When you] exhale, then [your qi] can sink naturally. [You] can also release [jin] out to the opponent. That means use yi [your mind] to move your qi; don't use li [strength]."[32]

Regulating the Mind in Taijiquan. The mind, both yi (mind) and xin (heart), controls the actions of the qi, and it is the qi which controls the actions of the body. It is said: "Use the heart [mind] to transport the qi; [the mind] must be sunk [steady] and calm; then [the qi] can condense [deep] into the bones. Circulate the qi throughout the body; it [qi must be smooth and fluid]; then it can easily follow the mind … yi [mind] and qi must exchange skillfully; then you have gained the marvelous trick of roundness and aliveness … The xin [heart, mind] is the order; the qi is the message flag."[33] It is also said: "If asked, what is the standard [criteria] of its [thirteen postures] application, [the answer is] yi [mind] and qi are the master, and the bones and muscles are the chancellor."[34]

From the above sayings, it is clear that the ancient masters placed great emphasis on the mind and the qi. A qigong proverb says: "Use your mind to lead your qi" (*yi yi yin qi*, 以意引氣). This is the key to using qi, because it tells you that if you want to move your qi somewhere, your mind must go there first. Remember: first there is yi; then there is qi.

When there is an action, we generate yi (idea or mind) first, and from this, yi; the qi is led to the muscles and nerves to activate or energize the muscles for contraction and relaxation. From this, you can see that the origin of any action is the yi.

From this, you can also see that in order for your body to have a higher functioning capability, you must have a concentrated, meditative mind, abundant qi storage in the lower dan tian, and knowledge of how to lead the qi to the required body area to en-ergize the physical body to a higher working efficiency. That is why, since A.D. 550, all Chinese martial styles have practiced qigong.

Since it is the yi which leads the qi and makes all of the actions happen, it is im-portant that you should not just have a concentrated mind, but also know the keys to leading. The first key is the mind of balance for your entire body, both externally and internally. It is said: "Up and down, forward and backward, left and right, it's all the same. All of this is done with the yi (mind), not externally. If there is a top, there is a bottom; if there is a front, there is a back; if there is a left, there is a right. If yi [mind] wants to go upward, this implies considering downward. [This means] if [you] want to lift and defeat an opponent, you must first consider his root. When the opponent's root is broken, he will inevitably be defeated quickly and certainly. Substantial and in-substantial must be clearly distinguished. Every part [of the body] has a substantial and an insubstantial aspect. The entire body and all the joints should be threaded together without the slightest break."[35] The second key is to have a sense of enemy. This means that you must apply your yi to the purpose of each movement. Every taijiquan move-ment had a martial purpose when it was created. If you cannot manifest this purpose, from yi to external action, you have lost the essence of the movement.

Finally, the most important factor for regulating the mind in taijiquan is mental calmness. When the mind is excited, it will be scattered, not concentrated. When this happens, your mental and physical bodies will be tensed. You will also be uprooted and spiritualy confused. Therefore, it is said: "First Saying: The xin [heart, mind] is quiet [calm]. When the heart [mind] is not quiet [calm], then [I am] not concentrated on one [thing]. When I lift hands, forward and backward, left and right, [I am] totally without direction [purpose]. In the beginning the movements do not follow the mind. Put the heart on recognizing and experiencing. Follow the opponent's movements, follow the curve, and then expand. Don't lose [him], don't resist, don't extend or with-draw by yourself. [If the] opponent has li [power], I also have li, but my li is first. [If the] opponent is without power, I also am without power; however my yi [mind] is still first. One must be careful in every movement. Wherever I am in contact, there the heart [mind] must be. One must seek information from not losing and not resisting; if I do that from now on, in one year or in half a year, I will be able to apply this with my body. All of this is using yi [the mind], not using jin. If I practice longer and longer, then the opponent is controlled by me, and I am not controlled by the opponent."[36]

Regulating the Qi in Taijiquan. The first task of regulating the qi in taijiquan prac-tice is knowing the location of the dan tian (丹田). Knowledge of the dan tian is fun-damental to taijiquan practice. Therefore, it is said: "Grasp and hold the dan tian to train internal gongfu."[37] Once you have knowledge of the dan tian, you must learn the embryo breathing technique, which allows you to use your mind to lead the qi to the dan tian, to keep it full and strong. It is said: "Qi should be full and stimulated."(氣宜 鼓蕩) When you lead the qi downward to store it in the lower dan tian, you should, at the same time, raise up your spirit like there is an insubstantial energy leading your head upward. That is why it is said: "An insubstantial energy leads the head upward.

The qi is sunk to the dan tian."[38] This implies that when you have a highly raised spirit, you can store the qi in the lower dan tian more efficiently.

The second task of regulating the qi in taijiquan practice is learning how to use the mind to lead the qi smoothly, continuously, and naturally. In this case, there is no qi stagnation in the body, and consequently there is no tightness in the movements. That is why it is said: "Don't be broken and then continuous; refine your one qi."[39] It is also said: "[You] want the entire body's qi to circulate smoothly; [it] must be continuous and non-stop."[40] Again, another saying: "Qi [circulates] in the entire body without the slightest stagnation."[41] Once you reach this stage, you can lead the qi to any place in your body. It is said: "Transport qi as though through a pearl with a 'nine-curved hole'; not even the tiniest place won't be reached."[42]

However, the most important task of regulating the qi is to coordinate your mind and qi smoothly and harmoniously. When your mind is calm and steady, the status of your qi circulation will be strong, yet smooth and fluid. However, if your mind is excited, the qi will be floating. If this happens, you will be tense and have lost the most essential key to taijiquan practice. Therefore, it is said: "Use the xin [heart, mind] to transport the qi [the mind] must be sunk [steady] and calm; then [the qi] can condense [deep] into the bones. Circulate the qi throughout the body; it [the qi] must be smooth and fluid; then it can easily follow the mind.[43] It is also said: "Yi [mind] and qi must exchange skillfully; then you have gained the marvelous trick of roundness and aliveness. This means the substantial and insubstantial can vary and exchange.[44]

In order to regulate the qi to a smooth and natural state, not only must your mind be calm, but breathing must also be correct. Breathing is considered to be a strategy in qigong practice. With correct breathing, the qi can be led by the mind more efficiently and effectively. When your mind and breathing coordinate with each other, you can lead the qi to the skin surface to enhance your guardian qi (wei qi, 衛氣), and also to the bone marrow to nourish the marrow qi (sui qi, 髓氣). When you reach this stage, you will feel no stagation of the qi, and the entire body becomes transparent to the energy. It is said: "Third saying: qi condenses. When the appearance of qi is dispersed and diffused, then it is not conserved, and the body easily can be scattered and disordered. In order to make qi condense into the bones, your exhalation and inhalation must flow agilely (smoothly). The entire body is without gap."[45]

Once you have regulated your mind and breathing to the point of needing no concious effort, then your qi will circulate freely, smoothly, and naturally. When this happens, your mind should focus on the spirit of vitality. This means that your mind should be on your opponent (i.e., sense of enemy). When this happens, it allows you to lead the qi to the movements for physical manifestation. With this, you manifest the meaning or the essence of the taiji movement both internally and externally. It says in the classics: "[Throughout your] entire body, your mind is on the spirit of vitality (jing-shen, 精神), not on the qi. [If concentrated] on the qi, then stagnation. A person who concentrates on breath has no li [strength, 力]; a person who cultivates qi [develops] pure hardness [power]."[46]

All of the above quoted ancient sayings have been recorded, translated, and commented on in the book *Tai Chi Theory and Martial Power*, available from YMAA. If you are interested in knowing more about the essence of taiji, you should refer to this book. However, if you wish to know more about qigong theory and training in taijiquan, you should refer to these books: *The Essence of Taiji Qigong* and *The Essence of Shaolin White Crane*, published by YMAA.

Regulating the Spirit in Taijiquan. Once you have regulated your body, breathing, and mind, your qi should be circulating smoothly and naturally. When you have reached this stage, you are ready to regulate your spirit. The spirit is closely related to your mind. When your mind is calm and firm, the spirit can be retained internally. It is said: "Qi should be full and stimulated, shen (*spirit*) should be retained internally."[47] Retaining the spirit internally means to be centered and to avoid unnecessary actions of the body, mind, and eyes. Thus concentrated, you can use your mind to act quickly and efficiently, and you will avoid betraying your intentions to the opponent. When the spirit is raised to a high level, you will be so alert and agile that you can sense your opponent's slightest movement or intention. Your techinques will be skillful, smooth, and effective. Therefore it is said: "[If] the jing-shen (spirit of vitality) can be raised, then [there is] no delay or heaviness [clumsiness]. That means the head is suspended."[48]

As mentioned earlier, in order to raise your spirit of vitality, first your qi must be concentrated and sunk. Then it is possible for the spirit of vitality to rise to the top of your head. This clears the mind and allows the body to move lightly and without inhibition. The *Song of Five Key Words* talks of the importance of a calm heart (i.e., mind), an agile body, condensed qi, and integrated jin, and then goes on to say: "Fifth Saying: Spirit condenses. All in all, [if] the above four items [are] totally acquired, it comes down to condensing shen (spirit). When shen condenses, then one qi [can be] formed, like a drum. Training qi belongs to shen. Qi appears agitated [i.e., abundant] and smooth. The spirit of vitality is threaded and concentrated."[49]

The final goal of spiritual cultivation in taijiquan practice is reaching spiritual enlightenment. Through practicing taijiquan, you understand the meaning of life until you reach the stage of clarity about your life and the natural universe. When you have reached this stage, your actual taijiquan practice will no longer be important, since its essence will be infused into your very being.

Notes

1. "Life's Invisible Current," Albert L. Huebner. *East West Journal*, June, 1986.

2. *The Body Electric*, Robert O. Becker, M.D. and Gary Selden. Quill, William Morrow, New York, 1985.

3. "Healing with Nature's Energy," Richard Leviton. *East West Journal*, June, 1986.

4. *A Child is Born*, Lennart Nilsson. A DTP/Seymour Lawrence Book, 1990.

5. 解剖生理學 (*A Study of Anatomic Physiology*)，李文森編著。
   華杏出版股份有限公司。Taipei, 1986.

6. *Grant's Atlas of Anatomy 7th Edition*, James E. Anderson. Williams & Wilkins Co., 1978, pp. 9-92.

7. "Complex and Hidden Brain in the Gut Makes Cramps, Buttflies and Valium," Sandra Blakeslee. *The New York Times*, Science, January 23, 1996.

8. *Bioenergetics*, Albert L. Lehninger. W. A. Benjamin, Inc., Menlo Park, California, 1971, pp. 5-6.

9. *Photographic Anatomy of the Human Body*, J. W. Rohen. 邯鄲出版社， Taipei, Taiwan, 1984.

10. "Restoring Ebbing Hormones May Slow Aging," Jane E. Brody. *The New York Times*, July 18, 1995.

11. 人生七十古來稀。

12. 一百二十謂之夭。

13. 形不正，則氣不順。氣不順，則意不寧。意不寧，則氣散亂。

14. 調息要調無息息。

15. 廣成子曰：一呼則地氣上升，一吸則天氣下降，人之反覆呼吸于蒂，則
    我之真氣自然相接。

16. 唱道真言曰：一呼一吸通乎氣机，一動一靜同乎造化。

17. 黃庭經曰：呼吸元氣以求仙。

18. 伍真人曰：用后天之呼吸，尋真人呼吸處。

19. 靈源大道歌曰：元和內運即成真，呼吸外求終未了。

20. 大道教人先止念，念頭不住亦徒然。

21. 意不在氣，在氣則滯。

22. 孔子曰：先靜爾后有定，定爾后能安，安爾后能慮，慮爾后能得。

23. 式式勢順，不拗不背，周身舒适。

24. 一舉動，周身俱要輕靈，尤須貫穿。

25. 上下相隨，周身一致。

26. 立如平准，活似車輪。

27. *The Great Dictionary of Chinese Wushu*, 中國武術大辭典。人民体育出版社。Beijing, 1990. p. 354.

28. *Zhongguo Wushu*, 中國武術實用大全。康戈武。今日中國出版社。Beijing, 1990. p. 390 & p. 389.

29. *Practical Chinese Medical Qigong Study*, 實用中醫氣功學。馬濟 。人主編。上海科學技術出版社。1992. p. 192.

30. *Health Sitting Meditation Classic*, 健康靜坐經。唐經武編著。Taipei, Taiwan, 1986. pp. 52-54.

31. 內外相合，呼吸自然。

32. 吸為蓄，呼為發。蓋吸則自然提得起，亦拏得人起。呼則自然沉得下，
    亦放人得出，此是以意運氣，非以力運氣也。

33. 以心行氣，務令沈著，乃能收斂入骨。以氣運身，務令順遂，乃能便利
    從心。意氣須換得靈，乃有圓活之妙。所謂變轉虛實也。心為令，气為
    旗，腰為纛。

34. 若問体用何為准，意氣君來骨肉臣。

35. 上下前后左右皆然。凡此皆是意,不在外面。有上即有下,有前即有后,有左即有右。如意要向上,即寓下意。若將物掀起,而加以挫之之意。斯其根自斷,乃壞之速而無疑。虛實宜分清楚,一處有一處虛實,處處總此皆如是。周身節節貫串,無令絲毫間斷耳。

36. 一曰心靜。心不靜則不專一。一舉手,前后左右,全無定向。起初舉動,未能由己,要悉心体認,雖人所動,隨屈就伸,不丟不頂,勿自伸縮。彼有力,我亦有力,我力在先。彼無力,我亦無力,我意仍在先。要刻刻留心,挨何處,心須用在何處。須向不丟不頂中討消息;從此做去,一年半載,便能施于身,此全是用意,不是用勁,久之則人為我制,我不為人制矣。

37. 拿住丹田練內功。

38. 虛領頂勁,氣沈丹田。

39. 舉動輕靈神內斂,莫教斷續一氣研。

40. 要遍体氣流行,一定繼續不能停。

41. 氣遍身軀不少滯。

42. 行氣如九曲珠,無微不到。

43. 以心行氣,務令沈著,乃能收斂入骨。以氣運身,務令順遂,乃能便利從心。

44. 意氣須換得靈,乃有圓活之妙。所謂變轉虛實也。

45. 三曰氣斂。氣勢散漫,便無含蓄,身易散亂,務使氣斂入骨,呼吸通靈。周身罔間。

46. 全身意在精神,不在氣。在氣則滯,有氣者無力,養氣者純剛。

47. 氣宜鼓蕩,神宜內斂。

48. 精神能提得起,則無遲重之虞。所謂頂頭懸也。

49. 五曰神聚。上四者俱備,總歸神聚,神聚則一氣鼓鑄,練氣歸神,氣勢騰挪,精神貫注。

CHAPTER 3

Taijiquan Thirteen Postures (Eight Doors and Five Steppings)

太極拳十三勢 - 八門五步

3-1. Introduction

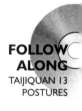

FOLLOW ALONG TAIJIQUAN 13 POSTURES

Philosophically, the major concepts of taijiquan are rooted in Daoism (道家). In particular, two major Daoist texts were, and are still today, important for the taijiquan practitioner: the *Dao De Jing* (道德經) and the *Yi Jing* (易經). While neither book is in any way a martial manual, both books firmly establish a way of thinking about the world that affected every aspect of taijiquan from breathing techniques to power development.

In the *Dao De Jing*, a book of poems reputedly written by Li Er (李耳) or Lao Zi (老子) around the fourth century B.C., one of its major themes that has come to dominate and influence taijiquan is the idea of Dao. As presented by Lao Zi, Dao is the ultimate reality from which all things evolved. Therefore, the goal of life is to follow, without contention, the natural order of the manifestations of Dao, and eventually Dao itself. The emphasis on doing the natural according to the laws of the universe, versus the forced or artificial, was very important to Lao Zi. The scholar Fung, Yu-lan has stated: "If one understands these laws and regulates one's actions in conformity with them, one can then turn everything to one's advantage."[1] It is out of this basic idea that taijiquan received its name, which means the Grand Ultimate Fist (i.e., fist means martial style) or the fist which manifests the Dao of taiji. The basic goal inherent in the idea of taiji, or the grand ultimate, is to return to the original source of the universe, the wuji state (無極). The closer you can get to the first principle or cause, the more you can complete yourself. Thus, taijiquan practitioners have taken this idea of the Grand Ultimate and have applied it to their martial system. For fighting or for health, the taijiquan artist will follow the natural inclination of things.

From the *Yi Jing*, a book over two thousand years older than Lao Zi's *Dao De Jing*, taijiquan martial artists took the concept of yin (陰) and yang (陽). In the natural flow of events, the operating principle that drives the universe is the interplay of two polar forces—yin and yang. The yin is considered the passive force while yang is considered the

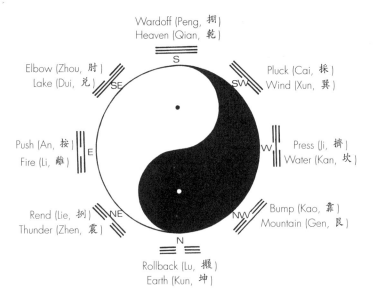

Figure 3-1. The directions of the eight basic techniques according to Chang, San-feng.

active one. Between the dynamic tension of yin and yang, all things find their nature.

In the *Yi Jing* the dynamic interplay of yin and yang is represented by a two dashed line (━ ━, *yin*) and a single solid line (━, *yang*). These lines are then arranged into groups of three (e.g., ☷) and six (e.g., ䷁). Traditionally, the discovery of the trigrams, of which there are eight, is attributed to Fu Xi (伏羲) around the period of 2852-2738 B.C. Later, King Wen of Zhou (周文王) combined the trigrams into hexagrams, of which there are sixty-four. Because yin and yang are fundamental principles, the eight trigrams and sixty-four hexagrams can be used to understand the mysteries of nature. These representations of yin and yang can then be used to predict everything from the birth of a child to the fate of a nation.

From the important and fundamental trigrams, taijiquan evolved its basic martial strategies. First, by looking at the arrangement of the bagua, the eight original trigrams that represent the eight fundamental directions of action, the trigrams correspond to the eight basic techniques of taijiquan. Each of the eight techniques was assigned a direction and a trigram to describe its fundamental nature, as shown in Figure 3-1. For example, the technique of "wardoff" (*peng*, 掤) is composed of three lines that are symbolic of the yang principle; therefore, this particular technique contains extreme energy and is used with a great explosion of power. The three yang lines indicate that its explosiveness requires exhalation to bring out the full power of the practitioner. On the other hand, the technique of "rollback" (*lu*, 攦) contains three yin lines; therefore, this technique is purely defensive and requires inhalation; it absorbs rather than attacks. A technique such as "push down" or "press down" (*an*, 按) is a mixture of offensive and defensive, although the offensive will dominate because there are two yang lines to the one yin line.

In addition to the various technical actions, the taiji theorists added five active

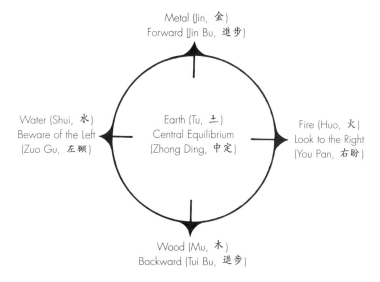

Figure 3-2. The directions of the Five Elements according to Chang, San-feng.

steppings or strategic movements that represented the five basic elements that compose the universe: metal (*jin*, 金), wood (*mu*, 木), water (*shui*, 水), fire (*huo*, 火), and earth (*tu*, 土). The five elements are called the *wuxing* (五行) and correspond to the movements of stepping forward (*jin*, 進步), stepping backward (*tui bu*, 退步), beware of the left (*zuo gu*, 左顧), look to the right (*you pan*, 右盼), and center equilibrium (*zhong ding*, 中定) (Figure 3-2). Taken together, as explained in Chapter 1, these thirteen elements are formally known as the thirteen postures (*shi san shi*, 十三勢). The thirteen postures are one of the foundation stones for taijiquan as a martial art. In fact, many people have called the art "shi san shi" in reference to its fundamental principles.

The *Yi Jing* also influenced taijiquan in other different and subtle ways. For example, as explained earlier, in terms of the overall style, taijiquan has two types of meditation that are considered yin and yang: conventional sitting meditation and the moving meditation of the taijiquan sequence. Taken together, both are needed to fully develop the yin and yang aspects of health and martial defense. On a smaller scale, the act of breathing has been broken down into a yin and yang relationship: inhaling is yin and exhaling is yang.

With this short introduction, you can hopefully have a general idea of the philosophical background of taijiquan. For a more complete discussion on the *Dao De Jing* and the *Yi Jing*, you can consult many good scholarly books on this subject. Once you have fully acquainted yourself with the principles of the two books, you can more clearly see the underlying general theory behind taijiquan.

In the next section, we will explore the concept of the eight trigrams, also known as the eight doors or the thirteen postures. From this, you will gain a clearer understanding of how taijiquan can be applied in personal combat. Then, in section 3-3, the five strategic movements, or five steppings, will be reviewed.

3-2. Eight Doors (八門)

In this section, we will define the eight basic taijiquan technical moving patterns: peng, lu, ji, an, cai, lie, zhou, and kao. These eight moving patterns are commonly called "eight trigrams" (*bagua*, 八卦) or "eight doors" (*ba men*, 八門). It is from these eight basic moving patterns and the five basic strategic steppings that the entire taijiquan was constructed. Therefore, these eight basic moving patterns are the foundation of the taijiquan. If you can comprehend the meaning of these eight movements and apply them into the practice, you will soon become a proficient taijiquan practitioner.

1. Peng (掤). Peng can be translated as "wardoff." Peng has the feeling of roundness and expansion. Generally, this round and expanding feeling is formed and generated from the chest and the arm(s). For example, when you use your arm to push people away with the support of the arcing chest (Figure 3-3), it is called "peng kai" (掤開) and means "open with wardoff." The expanding force can be upward, forward, or sideways (Figure 3-4). The force generated from peng is very offensive and forceful, just like a beach ball bouncing you away. Peng is often used to generate a round, circular defensive force by the chest and the arms. This allows you a chance to wardoff the opponent's power upward and thereby neutralize his attacking force (Figure 3-5).

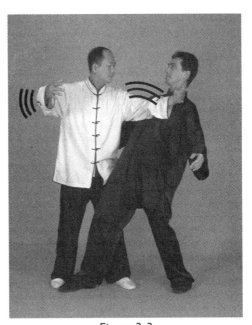

Figure 3-3

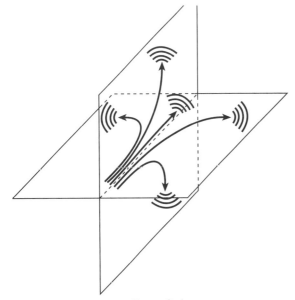

Figure 3-4

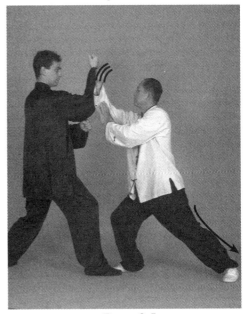

Figure 3-5

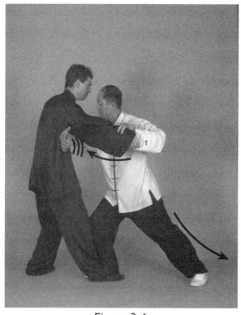

Figure 3-6

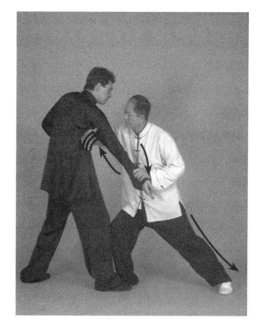

Figure 3-7

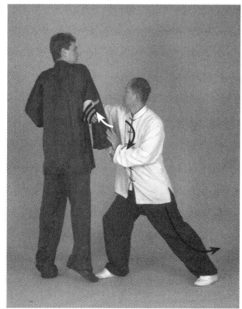

Figure 3-8

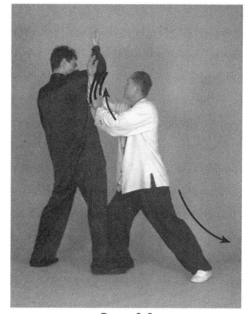

Figure 3-9

The typical examples in taijiquan postures are peng, (wardoff forward or slightly upward) (Figures 3-6, 3-7, and 3-8); grasp sparrow's tail (upward) (Figure 3-9); wave hands in the clouds

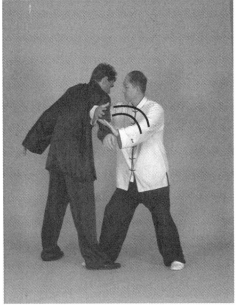

Figure 3-10

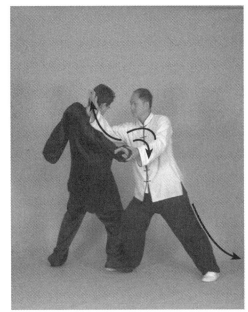

Figure 3-11

(sideways) (Figure 3-10); and crane spreads its wings (upward diagonally) (Figure 3-11).

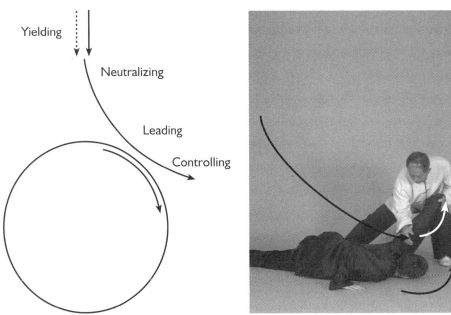

Figure 3-12

Figure 3-13

2. Lu (捋). Lu means to yield, lead and neutralize; it is commonly translated as "rollback." The main purpose of this movement is to yield to the force first, then to lead it backward and to the side for neutralizing (Figure 3-12). Theoretically, lu is a defensive strategic movement. However, occasionally lu can be aggressive when the timing and situation allows. For example, when you yield and lead, you may also lock or break the opponent's arm (Figure 3-13).

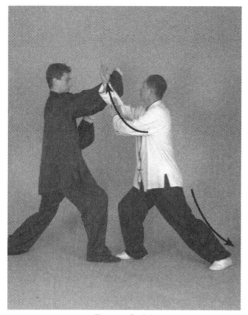

Figure 3-14

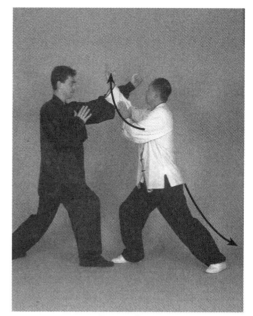

Figure 3-15

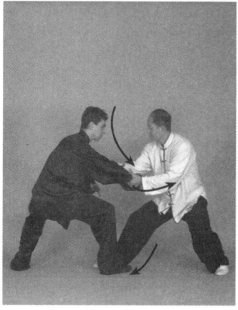

Figure 3-16

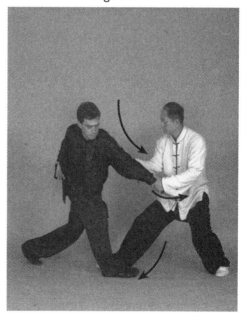

Figure 3-17

In Chinese martial arts, lu can be applied in two ways. One is to first wardoff the opponent's arm with your arm (Figures 3-14 and 3-15), and then to rollback his arm backward and to your side (Figures 3-16 and 3-17). This rollback action is also called "small rollback" (xiao lu, (小撠).

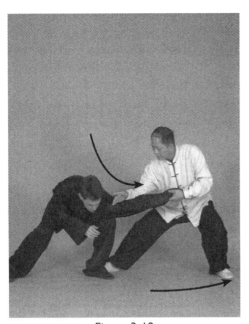

Figure 3-18

The other case is to use one of your hands to grab your opponent's wrist while using the forearm of the other arm to press and lock the rear side of his post-arm (upper-arm) (Figure 3-18). This kind of rollback is called "large rollback" (da lu, (大攦).

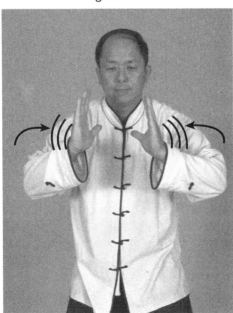

Figure 3-19

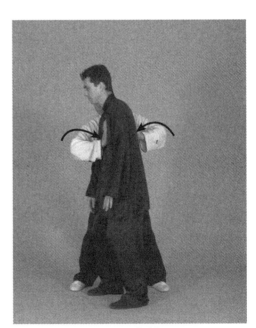

Figure 3-20

3. Ji (擠). Ji means to "squeeze" or to "press." This action can be performed with two hands, where the palms face and then press against each other (Figures 3-19 and 3-20).

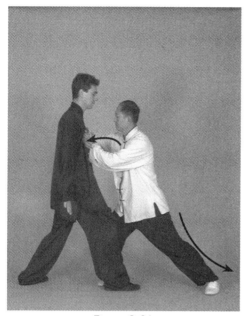

Figure 3-21

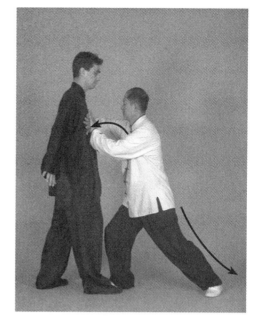

Figure 3-22

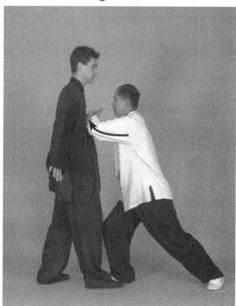

Figure 3-23

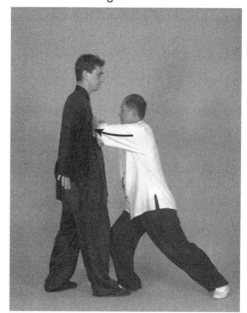

Figure 3-24

Alternatively, the ji action can also be done by "pressing forward" with both hands. For example, the rear hand presses the front wrist forward. This can be done with the front of the palm facing in (Figure 3-21) or facing out (Figure 3-22). The main pressing power is generated by pressing the rear palm into the front wrist, which is supported from the torso and legs. Alternatively, "press" can also be performed by pressing both forearms forward, again with the front palm either facing out (Figure 3-23) or facing in (Figure 3-24).

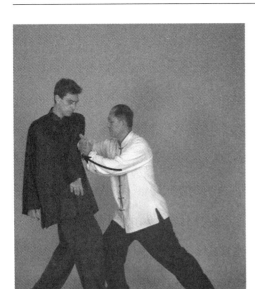

Figure 3-25

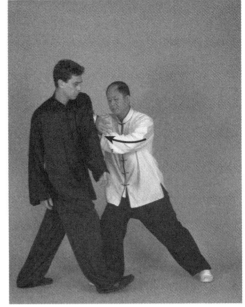

Figure 3-26

Press can also be done by pressing the forearm with the rear hand, with the front palm facing either out (Figure 3-25) or facing in (Figure 3-26).

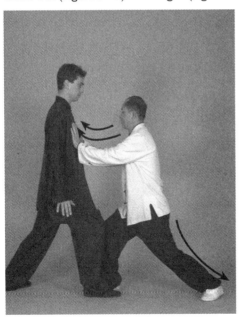

Figure 3-27

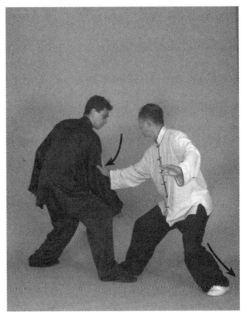

Figure 3-28

4. An (按). An means to "stamp," or to "press down, forward, or upward." An can be done with both hands (Figure 3-27) or with a single hand (Figure 3-28).

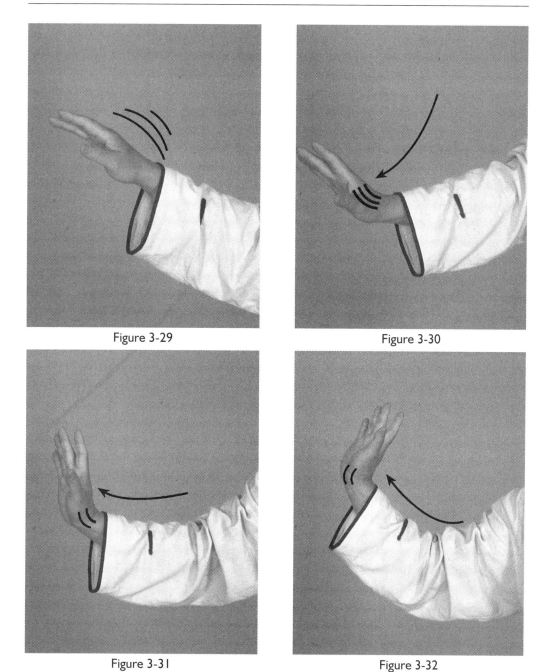

Figure 3-29

Figure 3-30

Figure 3-31

Figure 3-32

The An action is generally done with the fingers pointing forward first (Figure 3-29) and then, right before reaching the target, the wrist is angled downward (Figure 3-30), forward (Figure 3-31), or upward (Figure 3-32). This kind of action is called "settling the wrist" (zuowan, 坐腕), .

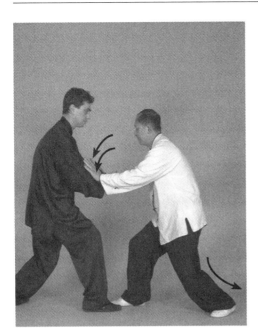

Figure 3-33

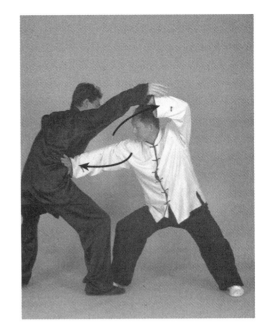

Figure 3-34

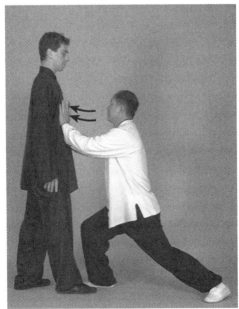

Figure 3-35

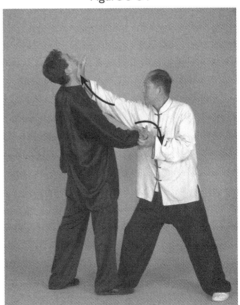

Figure 3-36

An is commonly used to seal the opponent's arm or joints (Figure 3-33), or for attacking his abdominal area (Figure 3-34) by "pressing downward." It is also often used to attack the opponent's chest by "pressing forward" (Figure 3-35) or "pressing upward" (Figure 3-36).

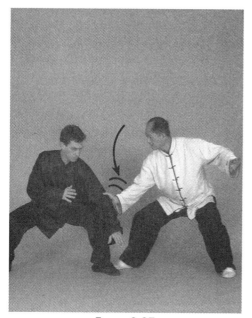

Figure 3-37

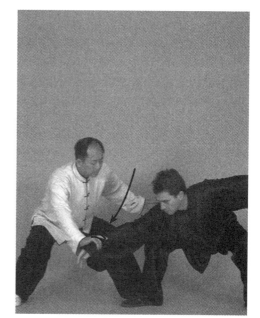

Figure 3-38

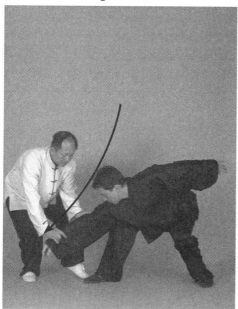

Figure 3-39

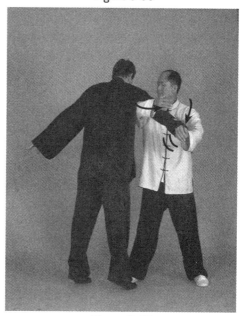

Figure 3-40

5. Cai (採). Cai means to "pluck" or to "grab." This is the action of locking the opponent's joints, such as the elbow (Figure 3-37) or wrist (Figure 3-38). Normally, after plucking or grabbing, the motion then leads either downward (e.g., pick up needle from sea bottom) (Figure 3-39), sideward (e.g., wave hands in clouds) (Figure 3-40), *(continued on next page)*

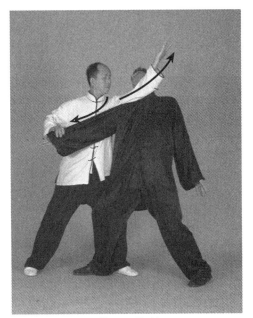

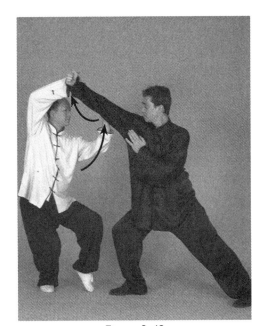

Figure 3-41   Figure 3-42

downward diagonally (e.g., diagonal flying) (Figure 3-41), or upward (e.g., stand high to search out the horse) (Figure 3-42). The main purpose of cai is to forcibly lead the opponent's arm in the desired direction. From this action, the opponent's balance can be destroyed, or the arm can be immobilized for further attack.

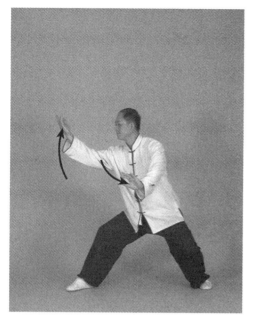

Figure 3-43

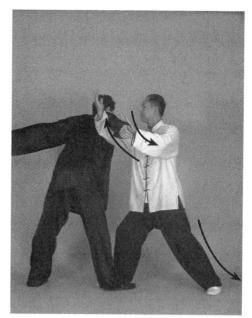

Figure 3-44

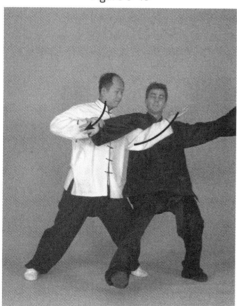

Figure 3-45

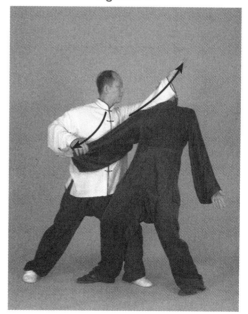

Figure 3-46

6. Lie (挒). Lie means to "rend" or to "split." This movement has the feeling of splitting a bamboo shaft or a piece of wood into two parts. Therefore, the action is forward and to the side (Figure 3-43). Lie is the action of using the arm to split or rend so as to put your opponent into a locked position or to make him fall. Very often it is considered a sideward peng. Lie can be used to lock the arm (e.g., wild horses share the mane) (Figure 3-44) or to bounce the opponent off balance (e.g., grasp the sparrow's tail or diagonal flying) (Figures 3-45 and 3-46).

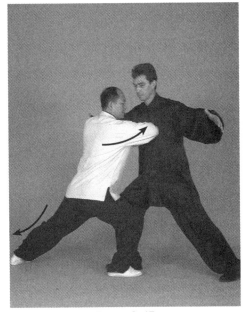

Figure 3-47

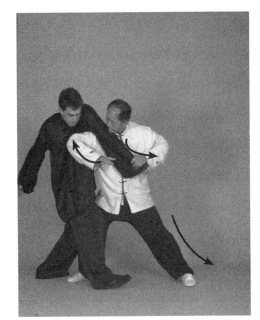

Figure 3-48

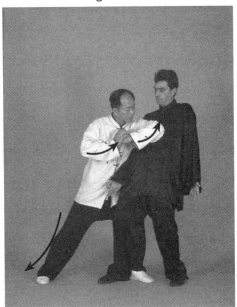

Figure 3-49

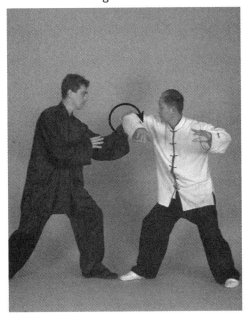

Figure 3-50

7. Zhou (肘). Zhou means to "elbow," and implies the use of the elbow to attack or to neutralize a lock of the elbow. It includes both offensive and defensive purposes. When the elbow is used to attack through striking (*da*, 打) or pressing (*ji*, 擠), the chest area is the main target (Figures 3-47 to 3-49). When the elbow is used to neutralize a lock, a circular yielding motion is generally applied. From the circular yielding motion, the elbow can neutralize the attack (*hua*, 化) (Figure 3-50) to wrap or coil your opponent's arm (*chan*, 纏) (Figure 3-51) or to seal the opponent's arm from further attack (*feng*, 封) (Figures 3-52 and 3-53).

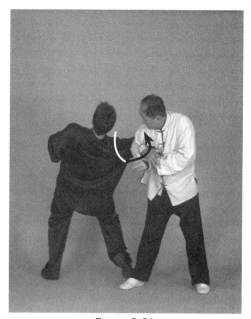

Figure 3-51

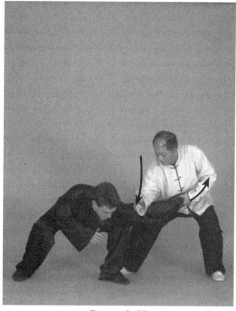

Figure 3-52

The elbow is like a steering wheel that directs its arm's movement. Therefore, it is very common that, in order to immobilize your arm movement, your opponent will lock or grab your elbow, and consequently your arm will be controlled. When this happens, you must know how to circle your elbow and how to coil your forearm to reverse the situation. From this, you can see that for defensive purposes, knowing how to maneuver your elbow is very important.

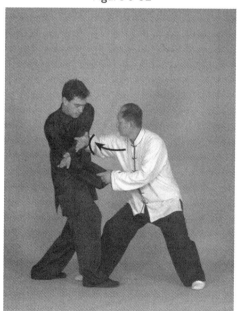

Figure 3-53

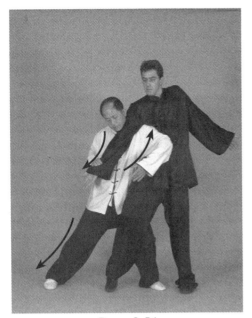

Figure 3-54

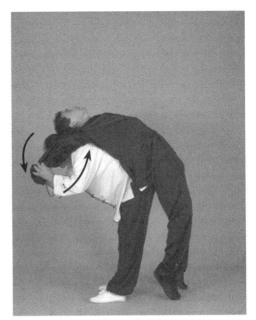

Figure 3-55

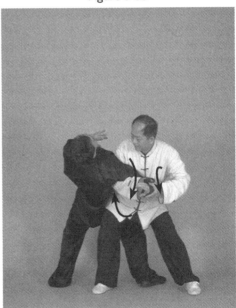

Figure 3-56

8. Kao (靠). Kao means to "bump," and implies using part of your body, such as your shoulder (*jian kao*, 肩靠) (Figure 3-54), back (*bei kao*, 背靠) (Figure 3-55), hip (*tun kao*, 臀靠) (Figure 3-56), thigh (*tui kao*, 腿靠) (Figures 3-57 and 3-58), knee (*xi kao*, 膝靠) (Figure 3-59), and chest (*xiong kao*, 胸靠) (Figure 3-60) to bump the opponent's body.

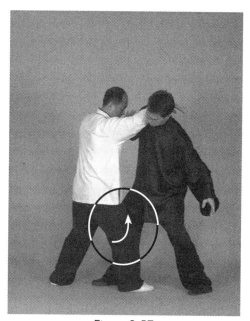

Figure 3-57

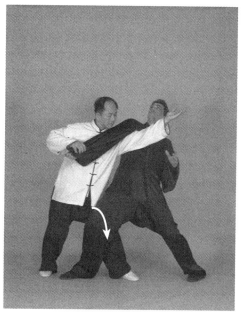

Figure 3-58

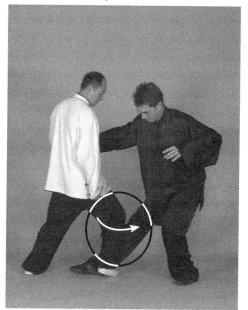

Figure 3-59

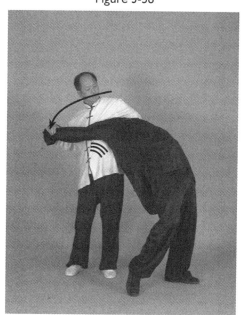

Figure 3-60

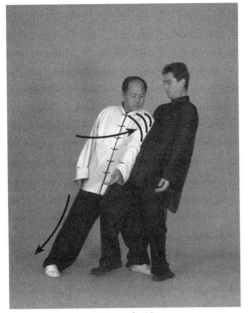

Figure 3-61

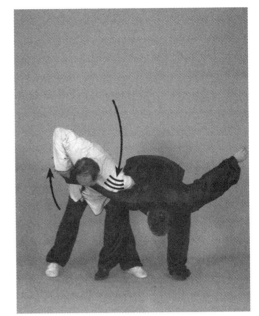

Figure 3-62

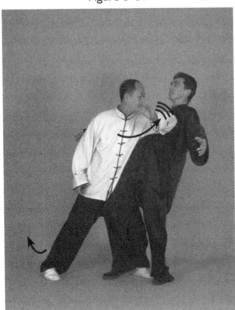

Figure 3-63

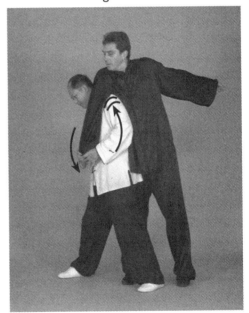

Figure 3-64

From the direction of kao, it can be classified as forward kao (*qian kao*, 前靠) (Figure 3-61), downward kao (*xia kao*, 下靠) (Figure 3-62), sideways kao (*ce kao*, 側靠) (Figure 3-63), and upward kao (*shang kao*, 上靠) (Figure 3-64). Kao is especially important in very close-range situations with your opponent. If you apply kao skillfully, you can destroy your opponent's rooting and balance and are therefore able to prevent him from further attack. Alternatively, whenever your opponent is attempting to regain his balance, you can take the opportunity to execute further action, such as kicking or striking. Naturally, you can also use kao to make your opponent fall when applied correctly. Kao is extremely powerful and destructive in some circumstances; you should be very careful in your training, and avoid using it on your opponent's vital areas, such as the solar plexus, unless you desire to cause serious injury.

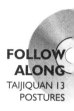

FOLLOW ALONG
TAIJIQUAN 13 POSTURES

3-3. Five Steppings (五步)

In this section, we will discuss the five important taijiquan strategic directional movements: forward, backward, left, right, and center. These five movements are commonly called "five elements" (*wuxing*, 五行) or "five steppings" (*wu bu*, 五步).

In a battle, it is very important to keep an advantageous distance between you and your opponent for your attack or defense. Because of this, all of the Chinese martial arts styles train students to move forward, backward, and sideways for advancing, retreating, and dodging. It is the same in taijiquan. In order to apply the techniques correctly, you must know how to set up a correct distance and angle that will allow you to have the most advantageous maneuvering. Therefore, how you step and direct your body naturally and automatically in a battle is an important factor in winning.

However, in taijiquan, due to the sticking and adhering strategy and techniques, you and your opponent are often in a stationary and urgent position. At that moment, you may not be able to step and move, since it could offer your opponent an opportunity to destroy your balance and rooting. Therefore, in taijiquan pushing hands training, stationary pushing hands has always been the first priority. In order to help you move beyond such limited training, here we will summarize the basic strategic movements in taijiquan.

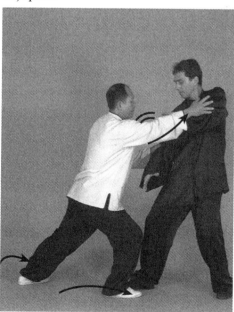
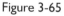

Figure 3-65

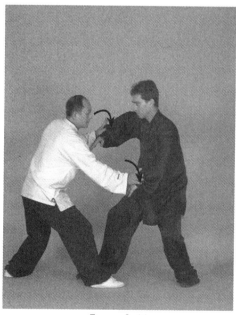

Figure 3-66

1. Jin Bu (Step Forward) (進步). Step forward (*jin bu*) is normally used to maintain distance when your opponent is retreating. In order to stick and adhere, you must keep a good distance. Often, when your opponent realizes that your techniques are better than his, he will try to retreat and free himself from your sticking and adhering. Therefore, in order to keep him in the same awkward situation, you must know how to step forward skillfully (Figure 3-65).
Step forward is also often used to close the distance between you and your opponent from the long range into the medium or short range, or from the medium range into the short range. For example, once your have neutralized your opponent's punch with sticking (Figure 3-66), in

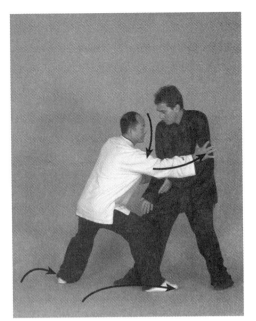

Figure 3-67

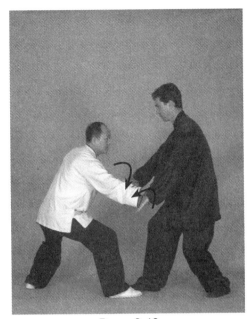

Figure 3-68

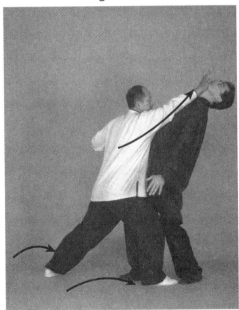

Figure 3-69

order to adhere to his arm, you must close from the medium range into the short range, which allows you to have better control for your taijiquan techniques (Figure 3-67). Naturally, when the opportunity allows, after you control your opponent's arms (Figure 3-68), you may step forward to gain advancing power for your striking (Figure 3-69).

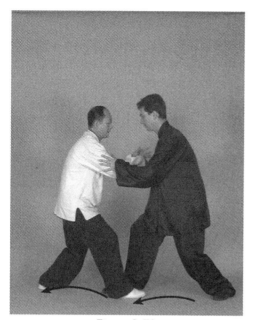

Figure 3-70

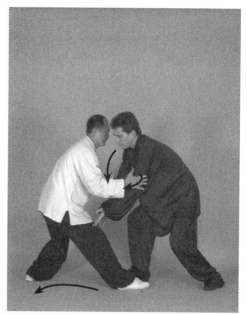

Figure 3-71

2. Tui Bu (Step Backward) (退步). The strategy of step backward is exactly opposite from that of step forward. With stepping backward, you can retreat from an urgent situation (Figure 3-70). Often, stepping backward is used to yield to oncoming power, providing you more time to lead and neutralize an attack. For example, when your opponent is pressing your chest with his palms, you may step backward to yield and at the same time squeeze both his arms inward (Figure 3-71). From this, you can see that generally speaking, step backward is a defensive maneuver.

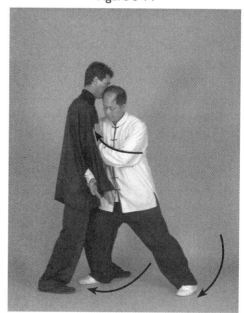

Figure 3-72

3. Zuo Gu (See the Left) (左顧). Zuo means "left" and gu means to "see" or to "look for." Therefore, zuo gu means "to see or to look for the opportunity on your left." While you are in a fighting situation, you should always be looking for an opportunity to step to your sides. Stepping to the side will offer you an advantageous opportunity to enter your opponent's empty door (Figure 3-72). Often, stepping to the left is part of a technique that could put your opponent into an awkward position.

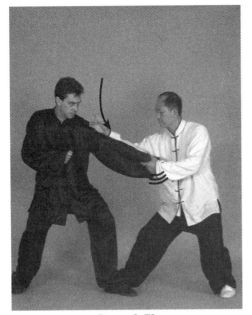

Figure 3-73

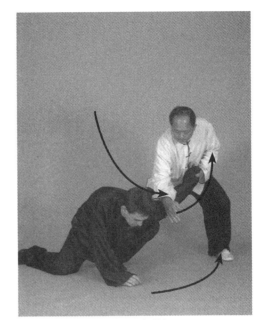

Figure 3-74

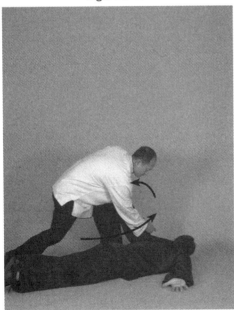

Figure 3-75

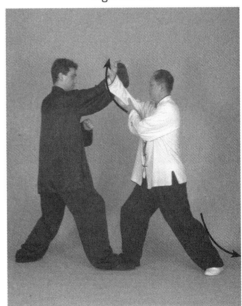

Figure 3-76

For example, when you apply the da lu "large rollback" technique, in order to make the technique effective, you must step your left leg to your left and put your opponent into a controlled position (Figures 3-73 to 3-75).

Naturally, stepping to the side is also commonly used to dodge or to avoid oncoming power. From sideways stepping, you may direct your opponent's power to the side and thereby stop him from further action. For example, in xiao lu "small rollback", once you have neutralized your opponent's power (Figure 3-76), you may step your right leg to his right (i.e., your left) and at the same time pull him off balance (Figure 3-77).

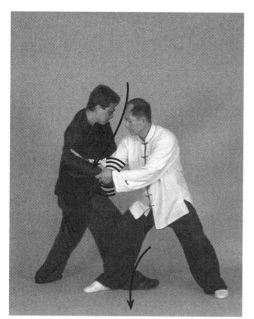

Figure 3-77

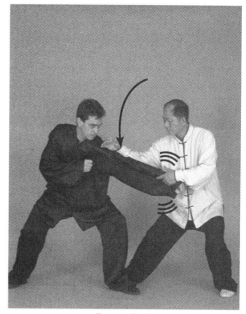

Figure 3-78

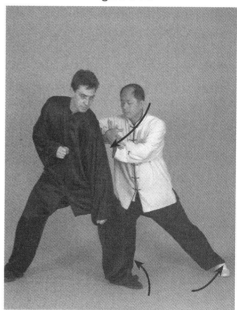

Figure 3-79

Often "zuo gu" is also translated as "beware of the left." This means to *beware* of the left-hand side attack from your opponent. This can also be interpreted as beware of an opportunity on your left.

4. You Pan (Look to the Right) (右盼). This is the same strategic movement as *see the left*. This time, you should keep looking for an opportunity for you to step to your right. The purposes are the same as those of see the left, and it serves for dodging and setting up advantageous angles for your attack. For example, in the da lu "large rollback" technique, once you have performed rollback on your opponent's arm (Figure 3-78), you may step both your legs to your right; this will offer you a good angle for your ji "pressing" (Figure 3-79).

5. Zhong Ding (Firm the Center) (中定).
Zhong means "center" and ding means to "stabilize" or to "firm." In taijiquan practice, zhong ding is probably one of the most important trainings on which a beginner should concentrate. In order to stabilize your center, you must first have firm root. In order to have a firm root, you must first have firmed your center. In order to firm your center, you must first have good balance. In order to balance yourself, you must first know how to relax yourself and to allow the qi to move smoothly and naturally in your body. This will offer you an accurate sensation of your balance. Only when you have a firm root can your spirit be raised (Figure 3-80).

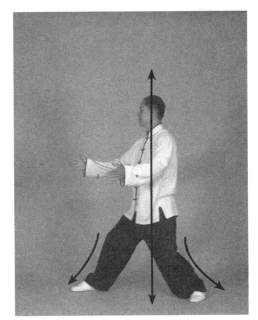

Figure 3-80

From this, you can see that to firm the center and root is not an easy task, especially for a beginner. Generally, zhong ding is learned from standing qigong and stationary pushing hands practice. In stationary pushing hands drills, you and your partner are looking for each other's center and root and are trying to destroy them. Naturally, you must also learn how to protect your center and root from being destroyed by your partner.

Notes

1. *A Short History of Chinese Philosophy*, Fung, Yu-lan. MacMillan, New York, 1961, p. 65.

CHAPTER 4

Traditional Yang Style Taijiquan
傳統楊氏太極拳套路

4-1. Introduction

Before we introduce and analyze the traditional Yang Style Taijiquan sequence, we would first like you to understand how martial sequences are created and what purposes they serve. Sometimes people who lack this understanding tend to view the taijiquan sequence as a dance or abstract movement. A proper understanding of the root of the art will help you practice in the most effective way.

A martial sequence, called *taolu* (套路) or *tan* (趟), is a combination of many techniques, constructed in the imagination of its creator to resemble a real fight. The creator of a sequence must be an expert in the style and experienced enough to see the advantages and disadvantages of a form, technique, or even just a step or stance. Within a martial sequence are hidden the secret techniques of a specific style. Chinese martial sequences commonly contain two or three levels of fighting techniques. The first level is the obvious applications of the movements and contains the fundamentals of the style.

The second level is deeper and is usually not obvious in the movements of a sequence. For example, a form might contain a false stance at a particular spot. This stance allows the practitioner to kick when necessary, but this kick may not actually be done in the sequence. Experienced martial artists can usually see through to this second level of applications.

The third level is the hardest to see, but it usually contains the most effective techniques of the style. These third-level techniques often require more movement or steps than are shown in the sequence and must be explained and analyzed by the master himself. In addition, when a proficient martial artist is able to understand to the depth of the third level, he or she can understand the secrets hidden "behind" the form of the four categories of fighting techniques. These categories were explained fully in the first chapter and include kicking, punching, wrestling, and qin na. Therefore, a Chinese martial sequence has several purposes:

1. A sequence is used to preserve the essence of a style and its techniques. It is just like a textbook that is the foundation of your knowledge of a style.

2. A sequence is used to train a practitioner in the particular techniques of a style. When a student practices a sequence regularly, he can master the techniques and build a good foundation in his style.

3. A sequence is used to train a student's patience, endurance, and strength, as well as stances, movements, and jin.

4. A sequence is also used to help the student build a sense of enemy. From routinely practicing with an imaginary opponent, he can make the techniques alive and effective in a real fight.

The taijiquan sequence was created for these same purposes. However, as an internal style it also trains the coordination of mind, breathing, qi, and the movements. Because of this, the yang aspect of taijiquan training comes slowly in the beginning and then gradually incorporates speed and an external manifestation of the inner essence. The yin side of the training is to practice taijiquan at a slower and slower speed, in order to cultivate a more deeply meditative mind that, in coordination with correct breathing, will develop stronger qi. This subject will be further explored in the next section.

Though Yang Style Taijiquan has many different versions that can have 24, 48, 81, 88, 105 or more postures depending, in part, upon the method of counting, it actually contains only 37 fundamental martial moving patterns, called the thirty-seven postures. These fundamental moving patterns form the basis of more than 250 martial applications or techniques. Within the sequence, many postures or fundamental techniques are repeated one or more times. There are two main reasons for this:

1. To increase the number of times you practice techniques that are considered more important and useful. This, naturally, will help you learn and master them more quickly. For example, wardoff, rollback, press (squeeze), and push (downward pressing), considered the most basic fighting forms, are repeated eight times in the long sequence.

2. To increase the duration of practice for each sequence. When early taijiquan practitioners found that the original short sequence was not long enough to satisfy their exercise and practice needs, they naturally increased the time of practice by repeating some of the forms. Doing this lengthened sequence once in the morning and/or evening is usually sufficient for health purposes. However, if you also intend to practice taijiquan for martial purposes, you should perform the sequence continuously three times, both morning and evening if possible. The first time is for warming up, the second is for qi transportation training, and the third time is for relaxed recovery.

In the next section, we will highlight methods of advancing your taijiquan practice from a shallow to a deep level, both in its martial arts yang aspect and its deeply meditative yin aspect. In section 4-3, the key points of taijiquan postures will be discussed. Then, fundamental taijiquan training practices will be summarized in section 4-4. Finally, traditional Yang Style Taijiquan will be introduced, along with the Yang Style Long Form, in section 4-5. If you have difficulty assimilating the movements of this sequence, you may refer to the video, *Tai Chi Chuan Classical Yang Style*, published by YMAA Publication Center. YMAA has also published several books that can add substantially to your understanding of the martial applications of this traditional sequence. These are *Tai Chi Theory and Martial Power*, *Tai Chi Chuan Martial Applications*, *The Essence of Taiji Qigong*, and *Taiji Chin Na*.

4-2. How to Practice the Taijiquan Sequence

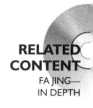

RELATED CONTENT
FA JING—
IN DEPTH

Normally, it takes at least three years to learn the taijiquan sequence and to circulate qi smoothly in coordination with the breathing and postures. You should then learn to transport qi and develop qi balance. Even after you have accomplished this, there is still more to learn before you can be considered a proficient taijiquan martial artist. You must learn how to strengthen your qi through practice, you must develop a sense of having an enemy in front of you during the sequence, and lastly, you must learn how to train jin during the sequence.

In taijiquan, qi plays a major role in jin. When qi is strong and full, then the jin will also be strong. An important way to strengthen and extend your qi is to practice the sequence slower and slower. This is the yin aspect of taijiquan practice, which helps you to build both a strong, concentrated mind and internal qi. If it usually takes 20 minutes to finish the entire sequence, increase the time to 25 minutes, then 30 minutes, and so on. Do not add any more breaths. Everything is the same except that every breath that is used to lead the qi gets longer and longer. In order to do this you must be very calm and relaxed, and your qi must be full like a drum or balloon, first in your abdomen and later in your whole body. If you can extend a sequence that normally takes 20 minutes to one hour, your qi will be very full and fluid, your mind calm, and the postures very relaxed. When you do the sequence at this speed, your pulse and heartbeat will slow down, and you will be in a deep self-hypnotic meditative state. You will hardly notice your physical body, but instead you will feel like a ball of energy. When this happens, you feel you are transparent.

Even when you can do the form very well, it may still be dead. To make it come alive you must develop a sense of enemy. When practicing the solo sequence, you must imagine there is an enemy in front of you, and you must clearly feel his movements and his interaction with you. Your ability to visualize realistically will be greatly aided if you practice the techniques with a partner. There are times when you will not use visualizations, but every time you do the sequence your movement must be flavored with this knowledge of how you interact with an opponent. The more you practice with this imaginary enemy before you, the more realistic and useful your practice will be. If you practice with a very vivid sense of enemy, you will learn to apply your qi and jin naturally, and your whole spirit will melt into the sequence. This is not unlike performing music. If one musician just plays the music and the other plays it with his whole heart and mind, the two performances are as different as night and day. In one case the music is dead, while in the other it is alive and touches us.

If you don't know how to incorporate jin into the forms, then even if you do the sequence for many years it will still be dead. In order for the sequence to be meaningful,

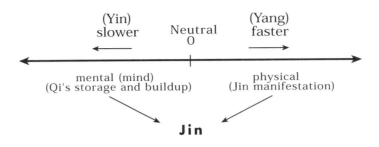

Figure 4–1

jin and technique must be combined. An important way to do this is to practice fast taijiquan. Practicing fast taijiquan is part of the Yang aspect of taijiquan, and it allows you to manifest your internal qi into external forms and power (Figure 4-1). Once you can do the sequence of movements automatically and can coordinate your breathing and qi circulation with the movements, you should practice doing the form faster and faster. Remember, if you ever get into a fight, things are likely to move pretty fast, so you have to be able to respond fast in order to defend yourself effectively. If you only practice slowly, then when you need to move fast your qi will be broken, your postures unstable, and your yi scattered. If any of this happens, you will not be able to use your jin to fight. Therefore, once you have developed your qi circulation you should practice the sequence faster until you can do it at fighting speed. Make sure you don't go too fast too soon, or you will sacrifice the essentials such as yi concentration, qi balance, breath coordination, and the storage of jin in the postures. When doing fast taiji, do not move at a uniform speed. Incorporate the pulsing movement of jin so that you are responding appropriately to the actions of your imaginary enemy. It is difficult to develop the pulsing movement of jin solely by doing the sequence, so you should also do jin training either before or concurrently with the fast taijiquan. If you are interested in knowing more about taijiquan jin development, you should refer to this book: *Tai Chi Theory and Martial Power*, published by YMAA.

4-3. Postures and Taijiquan

Since taijiquan is an internal qigong martial style, correct posture is essential. Incorrect postures can cause many problems: a tight posture can stagnate the internal qi circulation, wrong postures may expose your vital points to attack, floating shoulders and elbows will break the jin and reduce jin storage.

Taijiquan students are generally taught to make the postures large at first. This helps the beginner to relax, makes it easier to see and feel the movements, and also helps him or her to sense the qi flow. Furthermore, because large postures are more expanded and relaxed, the qi flow can be smoother. Large posture taijiquan was emphasized by Yang, Cheng-fu and has been popularly accepted as the best taijiquan practice for health since 1926.

Large postures also make it easier to train jin. It is more difficult to learn jin with small postures because the moves are smaller and quicker, and they require more subtle sensing jins. Large postures build the defensive circle larger and longer than small postures, which allows you more time to sense the enemy's jin and react. It is best to first master the large circles and only then to make the circles smaller and increase your speed. Thus, the poem of *Thirteen Postures: Comprehending External and Internal Training* states: "First look to expanding, then look to compacting, then you approach perfection."[1,2]

In addition, when you begin taijiquan, you should first train with low postures and then gradually get higher. When you first start training taijiquan, you will not understand how to build your root by leading your qi to the bubbling well cavity (*yongquan*, K-1, 湧泉) on the soles of your feet. Without this firm foundation you will tend to float and your jin will be weak. To remedy this problem, you should first train with low postures, which will give you a root even without qi and simultaneously develop your qi circulation. Only when you have accomplished grand circulation and the qi can reach the bubbling well can you use it to build the internal root. This is done by visualizing the qi flowing through your feet and extending into the ground like the roots of a tree. At this time you may start using higher postures and relaxing your leg muscles. This will facilitate the qi flow, which in turn will help you to relax even more. In the higher levels of taijiquan, muscle usage is reduced to the minimum, and all the muscles are soft and relaxed. When this stage is reached, qi is being used efficiently and is the predominant factor in the jin. Usually it takes more than thirty years of correct training to reach this level. Train according to your level of skill, starting with the larger and lower postures and only move to the smaller and higher postures as your skill increases.

To summarize: build your qi both externally and internally, and circulate it through the entire body. After the internal qi can reach the limbs, use this qi to support your jin. Gradually de-emphasize the use of the muscles, and rely more and more on using the mind to guide the qi. Train the postures from large to small, low to high, and slow to fast. First build the defensive circle large, and then make it smaller. For maximum jin, strengthen the root, develop power in the legs, balance your yi "mind" and qi, exercise control through the waist, and express your will through your hands. It is said in the Zhang, San-feng classic:

> *The root is at the feet, [jin is] generated from the legs, controlled by the waist, and expressed by the fingers. From the feet to the legs to the waist must be integrated and one unified qi. When moving forward or backward, you can then catch the opportunity and gain the superior position.*

> 其根在腳，發于腿，主宰于腰，形于手指。由腳而腿而腰，總須完整一氣。向前退后，乃能得機得勢。

Now, let us discuss the general rules of posture:

Hands and Wrists. The most common hand forms used in Yang style bare hand practice are the taiji palm and the taiji fist. The open-palm hand form can be done in various ways, depending on the style you are practicing. In the traditional Yang style we introduce here, the little finger is pulled slightly back while the thumb is pressed forward (Figure 4-2). The hand should be cupped and the middle finger should press down lightly. Here, the hands should be shaped as if you were holding a basketball with the palms, without the thumbs and little fingers touching the ball. In Yang Style Taijiquan this hand form is called "tile hand" (*wa shou,* 瓦手), because it is curved like a Chinese roof tile. In this hand

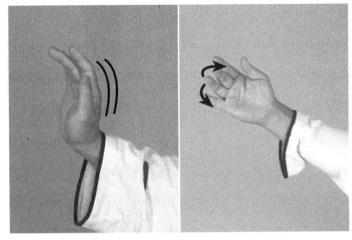

Figure 4-2

form, the thumbs and little fingers are very slightly tensed due to the hand's posture. This will slightly restrict the qi flow to these fingers and increase the flow to the middle finger and the laogong cavity (P-8, 勞宮) at the center of each palm.

The open-palm hand form is classified as a yang hand (*yang shou,* 陽手) in taijiquan. When palms are used to attack, the fingers are loosely extended and the wrists settled (dropped slightly) in order to allow the jin to reach the palms and exit easily. It is said: "Settle the wrists, extend the fingers" (坐腕 伸指).[3]

The taijiquan fist should be formed as if you were holding a ping-pong ball lightly in the center of the hand (Figure 4-3). When

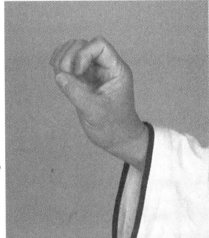

Figure 4-3

striking, the fist closes momentarily, but the fingers and palms are kept relaxed to allow the qi to circulate. The fist-hand form guides the energy back to the palm and is classi-fied as a yin hand (*yin shou,* 陰手) in taijiquan.

Elbows and Shoulders. The taiji classics say: "Sink the shoulders, drop the elbows" (沈肩垂肘).[3] There are several reasons for this. First, it allows the elbows and shoulders to be loose and the muscles relaxed. Second, dropping the elbows seals several vital cavities, such as the armpits. Third, when the elbows and shoulders are sunk, jin can be effectively stored in the postures, as well as emitted naturally from the waist without being broken. Fourth, dropped elbows and shoulders help to keep the postures stable and the mind more centered.

Head. The head should be upright. It is said: "An insubstantial energy leads the head [up-ward]" (虛領頂勁).[3] When your head is upright and feels suspended from above, your center will be firm and the spirit of vitality will be raised up. In addition, the eyes and mind should concentrate. It is said: "The eye gazes with concentrated spirit" (眼神注視).[3]

Chest. It is said: "Hold the chest in, arc the back" (含胸拔背).[3] Remember that yi leads the qi, so whenever you inhale, pull your chest in and arc your back to store jin in the posture, and visualize as vividly as possible that you are storing yi and qi. There are two large bows in the body that can store jin externally. These two bows are the spine (or torso) and the chest. If you can store jin skillfully in these two bows and maintain a strong root, the jin can be manifested powerfully.

Waist, Hips, and Thighs. The waist and hips are particularly important in taijiquan martial applications. The waist is the steering wheel that is used to direct the neutralization of the enemy's attack and the emission of jin. The waist must be relaxed, and the hips should be as if sitting so that the pelvis is level and the lower back straight. This will let your movements be agile and alive. As you move, your waist should generally stay the same distance from the floor: unnecessary up and down movement will disturb your root. The lower dan tian in the abdomen is the source of qi. It must be stimulated in order to fill it up with qi so that the abdomen is full like a drum. However, the muscles in this area must be relaxed in order to pass the qi that you have generated in the lower dan tian down to the sea bottom cavity (*haidi*, 海底) and then up the spine and out to the hands. The hips and thighs connect the waist to the legs where the jin is generated. In order to pass this jin to the waist, the hips and thighs must be relaxed and stable; otherwise the jin will be broken and the qi stagnant. In addition, if the hips and thighs are tight, the qi generated in the lower dan tian will have difficulty reaching the legs. Thus, it is said: "Relax your waist and relax your thighs" (鬆腰鬆胯).[3]

Legs, Knees, and Feet. The legs and knees must be loose and alive; then you can generate jin from the tendons and sinews. The muscles should not be tensed, for this will obstruct the generation of jin. However, the legs and knees cannot be completely loose and relaxed. They must be slightly tensed in order to keep your foundation stable. You should look loose but not be loose, look relaxed but not be relaxed.

When your weight is on the front foot, the rear leg should not be straightened, but should have a slight bend, and the front knee should generally not go past the front toe. The exception to this is when you are emitting jin. In this case the knee may momentarily go past the toe, but should immediately pull back, and the rear leg may momentarily straighten, but should immediately bend again. To avoid knee injury, the knees of both your legs are always lined up with the toes. This will provide you with firm support and a strong frame for your jin manifestation.

In taijiquan practice, once you have built the strength of the legs and have learned to use the muscles and tendons correctly and naturally, then you can exchange the substantial and insubstantial as well as the soft and the hard, skillfully and easily. Consequently, you will maintain your root and will generate jin efficiently. Thus, it is said: "The knees look relaxed, but are not relaxed."[3,4]

The feet are the root of all the postures and the source of mobility. The feet must firmly stick to the ground. It is said: "Soles touch the ground" [or "Feet flat on the ground"](足掌貼地).[3] In order to do this, your yi must be directed into the ground and the qi must be able to reach the bubbling well cavity. It takes a great deal of practice to develop a good root, but gradually you will grasp the trick and your root will grow deeper and deeper.

In conclusion, the entire body must be relaxed, centered, stable, and comfortable, and should not lean forward or backward nor tilt to either side. It is said: "Postures should not be too little or too much [i.e., neither insufficient nor excessive]. They [the postures] should seek to be centered and upright."[3,5] Every form must be continuous, smooth, and uniform: then the spirit will be calm, the yi concentrated, and the qi will flow smoothly and naturally. It is said: "Every form of every posture follows smoothly; no forcing, no opposition, the entire body is comfortable. Each form smooth."[3,6] Zhang, San-feng's *Taijiquan Treatise* says: "No part should be defective, no part should be deficient or excessive, no part should be disconnected."[7,8] Yi, qi, jin, the postures, top and bottom, inside and outside, front and back: all must act as one unit. When you reach this level, you will no doubt be a real taijiquan expert.

4-4. Fundamental Eight Stances (*Ji Ben Ba Shi*, 基本八勢)

FOLLOW ALONG FUNDAMENTAL EIGHT STANCES

Before you practice traditional Yang Style Taijiquan, you should first learn some important fundamental practices. These practices will help you understand the essence and the root of taijiquan practice. We will first introduce the most basic training in taijiquan—the fundamental stances. From these stances, you will build a firm physical foundation of taijiquan postures, which are the building blocks for the movements.

After introducing the fundamental stances, the entire primary taiji qigong set will be presented. This qigong helps a taijiquan beginner grasp the keys to using the mind to lead the qi and to coordinating the mind, breathing, and movements. After this basic qigong training, we will introduce some moving taiji qigong. This moving qigong will give you the feeling of the taijiquan movements. This feeling is the harmonization of your mind, body, breathing, and qi. Because of space limitations, no detailed theoretical discussion will be offered. Moreover, the higher level, Coiling Taiji Qigong Set will not be discussed here. If you are interested in knowing more about taiji qigong practice, you should refer to the book *The Essence of Taiji Qigong*, published by YMAA.

Taijiquan, like other martial arts has its own fundamental stances that are the basis for stability, movement, and martial technique. Basically, taijiquan uses eight stances (*ba shi*, 八勢), each of which is used during the bare hand sequence. Described below are the eight stances. When you practice these stances, you may ignore the positioning of the hands until you begin the sequence.

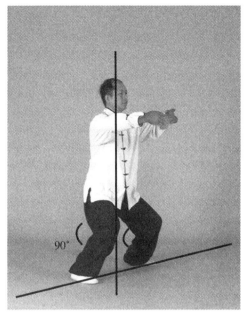

Figure 4-4

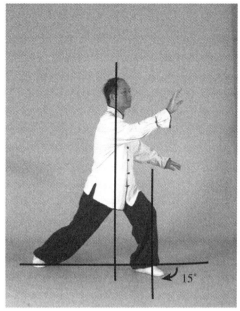

Figure 4-5

Horse Stance (*Ma Bu,* 馬步). The horse stance is commonly used as a transition between techniques and forms. To assume this stance, first place the feet parallel, slightly beyond shoulder width (Figure 4-4). Next, bend the knees until the angle between the rear thighs and calves is about 90 degrees. The torso is upright, natural, centered, and relaxed. The knees line up with the toes. Both feet must remain flat. It is important to understand that in order to avoid strain to the sides of the knees that can lead to injury, the knees must always line up with toes during your practice.

Mountain Climbing Stance or Bow-Arrow Stance (*Deng Shan Bu, Gong Jian Bu,* 蹬山步、弓箭步). This important form, the mountain climbing stance or bow-arrow stance, is the most commonly used offensive stance in taijiquan. First, place one leg forward so that the knee and toes are lined up perpendicularly and the leg as a whole supports 60 percent of the body's weight. The toe of the lead leg is pointing 15 degrees to the inside (Figure 4-5). The rear leg is firmly set down while supporting the rest of the weight. The knee of the rear leg must be slightly bent in this stance. Keep the upper body perpendicular to the ground. Again, beware of knee injury, and keep the knees lined up with the toes.

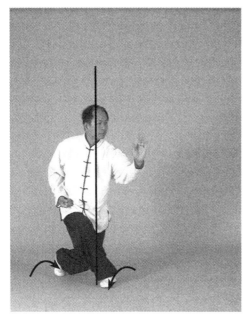

Figure 4-6

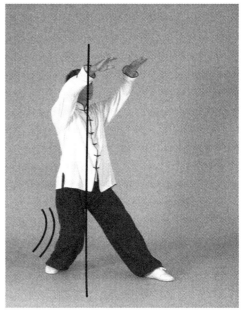

Figure 4-7

Sitting on Crossed Legs Stance (*Zuo Pan Bu,* 坐盤步). The sitting on crossed legs stance is commonly used for forward movement. First, assume ma bu (Figure 4-4). Second, turn the body and the right foot with heel 90 degrees clockwise while pivoting on the left toe (Figure 4-6). The same can be done with the left side: turn the body and the left foot with heel 90 degrees counterclockwise, and pivot on the right foot on the toes.

Four-Six Stance (*Si Liu Bu,* 四六步). The four-six stance is the most commonly used defensive stance in taijiquan. In weight distribution, it is exactly the opposite of mountain climbing stance; the front leg supports 40 percent of the weight and the rear leg supports 60 percent (Figure 4-7). The rear leg is bent, with the knee and toes turned inward, while the front leg is held loose, slightly bent, and relaxed.

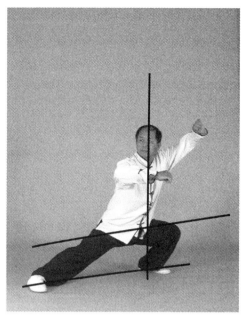

Figure 4-8

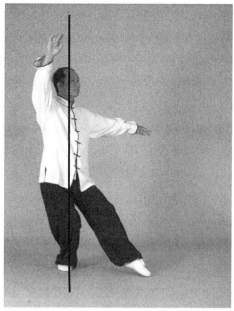

Figure 4-9

Tame the Tiger Stance (*Fu Hu Bu,* 伏虎 步). Tame the tiger stance is used for low attacks and defense. To assume this stance, stand with both feet spread. Next, squat down on one leg while keeping the other leg straight. The thigh of the squatting leg must be parallel to the ground and both feet must be flat (Figure 4-8). Again, the knee of the squatting leg should line up with the toes.

False Stance (*Xuan Ji Bu or Xu Bu,* 玄機 步、虛步). The false stance is used to set up kicks. First, place all your weight on one leg. Next, set the other leg in front of the body with only its toes lightly touching the ground (Figure 4-9). From this position the false leg can kick without hesitation.

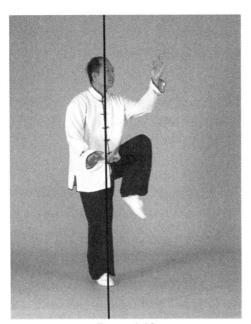

Figure 4-10

Golden Rooster Standing on One Leg Stance (*Jin Gi Du Li,* 金雞獨立). The golden rooster standing on one leg stance is similar in form to false stance and serves the same function: to set up kicks. To assume this stance lift either knee up with the toe pointing 45 degrees down (i.e., the ankle is relaxed naturally) (Figure 4-10). The raised leg can kick at any instant.

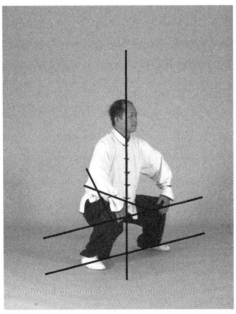

Figure 4-11

Squat Stance (*Zuo Dun,* 坐蹲). The squat stance is primarily used as a training device to build up the knees. To begin, stand with feet spread shoulder width apart. Squat down until the thighs are parallel to the ground and the back is straight (Figure 4-11). You should attempt to stay in this stance for five minutes while keeping the mind calm. In order to guard against injury, you should start at first with only one minute, and then gradually increase the time.

4-5. Taiji Qigong (太極氣功)

As with all other forms of martial qigong, taiji qigong can be categorized into both yin and yang practices (Table 4-1). The yin side of taiji qigong contains exercises that emphasize calmness without movement, and the yang side of taiji qigong has exercises that are more physically active. Moreover, the yin side of taiji qigong can again be divided into (yin) sitting relaxed meditation and (yang) standing meditation. In sitting meditation, the body is extremely relaxed, while in standing meditation the body is more tensed due to the special postures.

LECTURE
TAIJI QIGONG

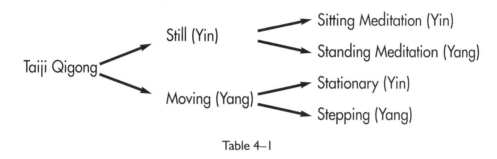

Table 4–1

Within the yang side of taiji qigong practice, stationary taiji qigong is actually considered yin, since your mind can be more concentrated by using it to lead the qi. Likewise, stepping taiji qigong is classified as yang, simply because in addition to leading the qi with the mind, you must also maintain the qi's forward and backward balance and a sense of enemy. There is essentially no difference, in terms of health goals, between the yang stepping taiji qigong and the taijiquan sequence.

When you practice taiji qigong, you must correctly coordinate your breathing to be smooth and natural. In this section, due to space limitations, we will only introduce some examples of the training. If you would like to know more about taiji qigong or general martial qigong training, both in terms of theory and practice, you should refer to these books: *The Essence of Shaolin White Crane* and *The Essence of Taiji Qigong*, published by YMAA.

On the yin side, during still taiji qigong, when you are in a sitting position, your body is in a very calm and relaxed state. However, if you are in a standing position, your legs and parts of your body will be more tensed. This does not matter for your practice goals because your physical body is not moving and your mind will be free from its obligations to direct the body's motion. Instead, you will be able to concentrate and lead the qi to circulate anywhere you desire.

Still sitting meditation is a deep and profound subject. It would take an entire volume just to explain the theory and practice of sitting meditation. Therefore, it is not possible to cover this subject completely in this book. Instead, we will provide only a summary of this practice. If you are interested in learning more about sitting meditation, please refer to the books: *Qigong Meditation—Embryonic Breathing*, and *Qigong Meditation—Small Circulation*, published by YMAA.

Still Sitting Meditation (Yin)

Sitting meditation includes a few key training practices. First, of course, is to regulate the body (*tiao shen*, 調身) until the body is in its most relaxed and natural state. That means the entire physical body is very comfortable and there is no uncomfortable feeling at all to disturb your mind.

Second, you will learn how to breathe correctly, which is considered the key to calming down or directing the qi with coordination of the mind. This is the process of regulating the breathing (*tiao xi*, 調息). In this practice, the first step is learning the normal abdominal breathing (*zheng fu hu xi* or *shun fu hu xi*, 正腹呼吸、順腹呼吸). In this step, you learn how to control the abdominal muscles smoothly and naturally. Next, you learn the reversed abdominal breathing (*fan fu hu xi* or *ni fu hu xi*, 反腹呼吸、逆腹呼吸). In this step, you are learning how to coordinate the abdominal movement with the emotional mind or wisdom mind. Reversed abdominal breathing is natural and we have used it whenever we are emotionally disturbed or we have an intention to energize our physical body to a higher level.

Once you have learned how to do the reversed abdominal breathing, then you learn the most important qigong breathing, the Embryo Breathing (*Tai Xi*, 胎息). From Embryo Breathing, you learn how to store the qi (i.e., bioelectricity) to the lower dan tian (i.e., human bioelectric battery or second human brain).[9]

Third, after you can store plenty of qi in the lower dan tian, you start to learn how to regulate your mind to a calm, peaceful, and concentrated state. This is the process of regulating the mind (*tiao xin*, 調心). That means to regulate the emotional mind (*xin*, 心) by your wisdom mind (*yi*, 意). This is the step of conquering yourself. Generally speaking, this step is the most difficult since you are dealing with your own mind. Your mind is just like a general who directs the battlefield. If this mind is not calm and wise, then the qi (soldiers) will not be led efficiently.

Fourth, after you have mastered the key to regulating your mind, you will learn how to lead the qi to circulate in two most important vessels: the conception vessel (*ren mai*,

任脈) and the governing vessel (*du mai*, 督脈) to complete the Small Circulation (*Xiao Zhou Tian*, 小周天). Moreover, you will also learn the Four Gates Breathing (*Si Xin Hu Xi*, 四心呼吸) and use the mind to lead the qi to the centers of palms and soles. Moreover, you are also learning the skin breathing or Belt Vessel Breathing (*Ti Xi, Dai Mai Hu Xi*, 体息，帶脈呼吸). These breathing techniques are considered as the foundation of the Grand Circulation (*Da Zhou Tian*, 大周天). All of the above practices are included in the step of regulating the qi (*tiao qi*, 調氣).

The fifth step or the final goal of still sitting meditation is learning how to use the mind to lead the qi from lower dan tian through thrusting vessel (*chong mai*, 衝脈) or spinal cord to the brain to energize the brain to a higher enlightened level until the third eye is opened. This is the step of regulating the spirit (*tiao shen*, 調神). It is believed that when the third eye is opened, you can feel and communicate with the natural universal energy more directly. This is the stage of unification of heaven and human (*tian ren he yi*, 天人合一).

From above very brief summary, you can see that this is a huge subject, which all of the Western and Eastern religions have been aiming for since ancient time. If you are interested in these trainings, you may refer to the future books mentioned earlier or simply participate in the related seminars and join the discussion.

Still Standing Meditation (Yang)

As mentioned, relatively speaking, still standing meditation is more yang than that of still sitting meditation. The reason of this is simply when you are in the standing posture, parts of your body are tensed. That means the physical body is more energized than in still sitting meditation.

There are many different postures of standing meditation in taijiquan or any other internal martial styles. In this place, we will only introduce two common taiji standing meditation postures for your reference and practice.

Arcing the Arms or Embracing the Moon on the Chest (*Gong Shou,* 拱手 **or *Hui Zhong Bao Yue,* 懷中抱月)**

Stand with one leg rooted on the ground, and the other in front of it with only the toes touching the ground. Both arms are held in front of the chest, forming a horizontal circle, with the fingertips almost touching (Figure 4-12). The tongue should touch the roof of the mouth to connect the yin and yang qi vessels (conception and governing vessels respectively). The mind should be calm and relaxed and concentrated on the shoulders; breathing should be deep and regular.

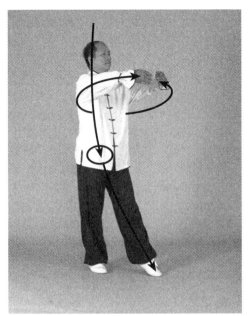

Figure 4-12

When you stand in this posture for about three minutes, your arms and one side of your back should feel sore and warm. Because the arms are held extended, the muscles and nerves are stressed. Qi will build up in this area and heat will be generated. Also, because one leg carries all the weight, the muscles and nerves in that leg and in one side of the back will be tense and will thereby build up qi. Because this qi is built up in the shoulders and legs rather than in the dan tian, it is considered "local qi" or "wai dan qi." In order to keep the qi build-up and the flow in the back balanced, after three minutes change your legs without moving your arms and stand this way for another three minutes. After the six minutes, face forward, put both feet flat on the floor, shoulder-width apart, and slowly lower your arms. The accumulated qi will then flow naturally and strongly into your arms. It is like a dam, which after accumulating a large amount of water, releases it and lets it flow out. At this time, concentrate and calm the mind and look for the feeling of qi flowing from the shoulders to the palms and fingertips. Beginners can usually sense this qi flow, which is typically felt as warmth or a slight numbness.

Naturally, when you hold your arms out you are also slowing the blood circulation, and when you lower your arms the blood will rush down into them. This may confuse you as to whether what you feel is due to qi or blood. You need to understand several things. First, every living blood cell has to have qi to keep living (each blood cell can be thought of as a dipole or small battery, which contains the "charge" of bioelectricity). Thus, when you relax after the arcing hands practice, both blood and qi will come down to the hands. Second, since blood is material and qi is energy, qi can flow beyond your body but your blood cannot. Therefore, it is possible for you to test whether the exercise has brought extra qi to your hands. Place your hands right in front of your face. You should be able to feel a slight sensation on your face, which comes from the qi. You can also hold your palms close to each other, or move one hand near the other arm. In addition to a slight feeling of warmth, you may also sense a kind of electric charge that may make the hairs on your arm move. Blood cannot cause these feelings, so they have to be symptoms of qi.

Sometimes qi is felt on the upper lip. This is because there is a channel (hand yangming large intestine, 手陽明大腸) that runs over the top of the shoulder to the upper lip (Figure 4-13). However, the qi feeling is usually stronger in the palms and fingers than in the lip, because there are six qi channels that pass through the shoulder to end in the hand, but there is only one channel connecting the lip and shoulder. Once you experience qi flowing in your arms and shoulders during this exercise, you may also find that you can sense it in your back.

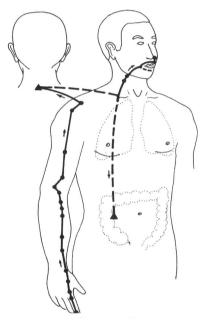

Figure 4-13

Many advanced taijiquan practitioners practice this standing, still meditation to develop their qi circulation to a higher level. It was originally called three power posture (*san cai shi*, 三才勢). "Three power" means the heaven power, the earth power, and the human power. In the posture itself, you lean, in order to lead the qi from the crown of the head (*baihui*, Gv-20, 百會), through the spinal cord (*chong mai*, 衝脈) to the lower dan tian, and then from the lower dan tian to the earth through the front leg (*yongquan*, K-1, 湧泉).

In this advanced training, in addition to building up qi in the shoulders, you are training the mind to lead the qi, in coordination with your breathing, to complete two qi circuits. The first qi circuit is a horizontal one, through your arms and chest. On the exhalation, you lead the qi to the fingertips of both hands, and then across the gap from each hand to the other. On the inhalation, you lead the qi from the fingertips to the center of your chest. It is important to realize that the qi pathway leads the qi in both directions simultaneously, so that at both the space between the fingertips and the center of the chest, the qi is actually passing through itself. Instead of clashing and creating turbulence, the qi is so smooth and uniform that it can do this effortlessly. It is important to understand this infinite smoothness of the qi. The second circuit is a vertical one that connects heaven, man, and earth. As mentioned, on the inhalation you take in qi from nature, through your baihui on the top of your head, and lead the qi downward to the lower dan tian. On the exhalation you lead the qi further downward and out of your body, through the bubbling well (*yongquan*) cavities. When you practice, circulation in the two circuits should occur simultaneuously. If you are a beginner, this is not easy to do. However, if you persevere, you can use this exercise as part of your advanced practice. The final goal of qi circulation is using the mind to lead the dan tian qi to the arms and back again; this is called grand circulation.

This exercise is one of the most common practices for leading the beginner to experience the flow of qi, and some taijiquan styles place great emphasis on it. Similar exercises are also practiced by other styles, such as Emei Da Peng Gong (峨嵋大鵬功). There is another standing still meditation called holding up the heaven posture (*tuo tian shi*, 托天勢). This is a very strenuous exercise. It is not recommended to taijiquan beginners. However, if you are interested in this training, you may refer to *The Essence of Taiji Qigong*, published by YMAA.

Moving (Yang)

Before introducing moving taiji qigong, you should first learn how to stretch and warm up. If you have done these correctly, you will have provided the best condition for you to regulate your body, breathing, and mind.

Loosening up the Joints

For stretching, the first step is loosening up the joint areas. The common joints that should be loosened are the wrists, elbows, shoulders, spine, hips, knees, and ankles.

When you loosen your wrist joints, shake your elbow sideways while letting the hands swing from side to side (Figure 4-14). This will loosen up the wrist effectively. If you use the muscles near the wrist area to move the hands from side to side, the muscles near the wrist area will be tensed, and the loosening efficiency will be low.

In the same way, when you loosen up your elbow area, you should move your shoulders and allow your arms to swing around (Figure 4-15). This will loosen up the entire arm area. Next, bounce your body up and down (Figure 4-16). When you do this, you start to loosen your torso. This up and down bouncing motion will also make the joints in the arms reach a deeper loose and relaxed state. This bouncing motion of the body is used to

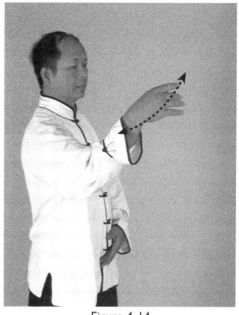

FOLLOW ALONG
STRETCHING/ WARMING UP

Figure 4-14

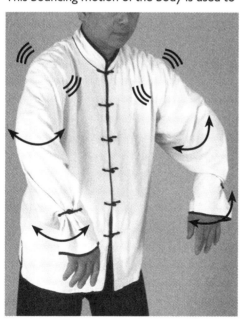

Figure 4-15

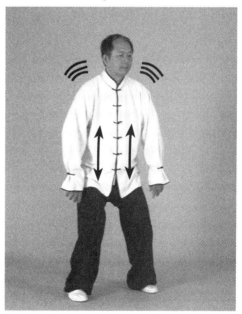

Figure 4-16

loosen up the joints. It is the most basic qigong exercise. In fact, we can still see these kinds of up and down body bouncing exercises in various ethnic dances around the world.

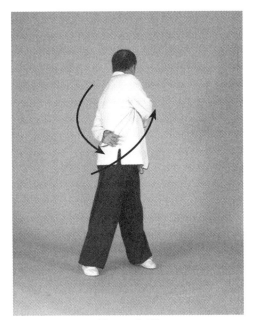

Figure 4-17

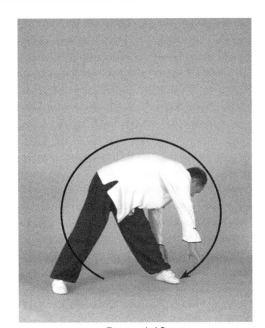

Figure 4-18

Next, twist your torso from side to side while swinging both of your arms naturally (Figure 4-17). This twisting and swinging exercise will enhance the torso's loosening, especially in the waist area. Then, circle your upper body down, up and around in each direction an equal number of times (Figure 4-18). This will help to stretch and loosen the torso.

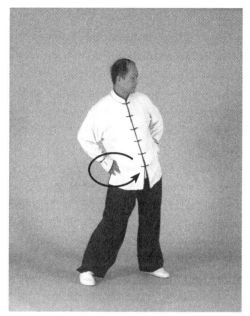

Figure 4-19

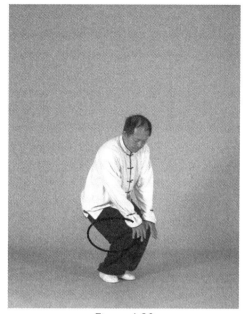

Figure 4-20

Next, circle your waist horizontally, first to one side and then to the other (Figure 4-19). This will loosen the lower back area and the hip joints. Then, squat down slightly and circle both of your knees horizontally in each direction a few times to loosen up the knee joints (Figure 4-20). Finally, circle the ankles of each leg a few times each direction (Figure 4-21). This concludes the loosening and warming up exercises. The number of repetitions for each exercise is up to you. Sometimes, when your body is tenser, you might want to move more. Other times, you may wish to do less.

Stretching

After you have loosened up your joints and warmed up, you should start to stretch your physical body. If you stretch your body correctly, you can stimulate the cells into an excited state, and this will improve qi and blood circulation. This is the key to maintaining the health

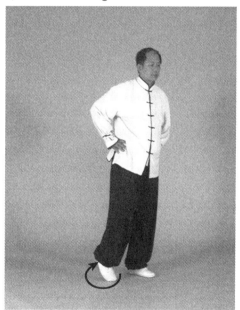

Figure 4-21

of the physical body. However, when you stretch you should treat your muscles, tendons, and ligaments like a rubber band. If you stretch too much too soon, you will break the rubber band. For muscles, tendons, and ligaments, that means the tearing off of fibers. However, if you under stretch, it will not be effective. A good stretch should feel comfortable and stimulating.

Stretching the Torso (*Shuang Shou Tuo Tian,* 雙手托天)

Theoretically, the first place that should be stretched and loosened is the trunk muscles, rather than the limbs. The trunk is at the center of the whole body, and it contains the major muscles that control the trunk and also surround the internal organs. When the trunk muscles are tense, the whole body will be tense and the internal organs will be compressed. This causes stagnation of the qi circulation in the body, and especially in the organs. For this reason, the trunk muscles should be stretched and loosened up before the limbs prior to any qigong practice. Remember, people die from failure of the internal organs, rather than problems in the limbs. The best qigong practice is to remove qi stagnation and maintain smooth qi circulation in the internal organs.

For these reasons, many qigong practices start out with movements that stretch the trunk muscles. For example, in the Standing Eight Pieces of Brocade (*Ba Duan Jin,* 八段錦), the first piece stretches the trunk to loosen up the chest, stomach, and lower abdomen (which are the triple burners in Chinese medicine). In fact, the following exercise is adapted from the Standing Eight Pieces of Brocade exercises.

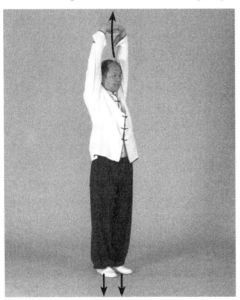

Figure 4-22

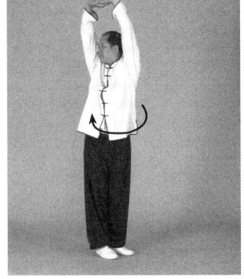

Figure 4-23

First, interlock your fingers and lift your hands up over your head while imagining that you are pushing upward with your hands and pushing downward with your feet (Figure 4-22). Do not hold your breath nor tense your muscles, because these things will constrict your body and prevent you from stretching. If you do this stretch correctly, you will feel the muscles in your waist area tensing slightly because they are being pulled simultaneously from the top and the bottom. Next, inhale and use your mind to relax and stretch out a little bit more. Remember to continue breathing deeply. After you have stretched for several breaths, on an exhalation, twist your upper body to one side to twist the trunk muscles (Figure 4-23). Stay to the side for several breaths, lengthening the body on the inhalations, and twisting on the exhalations. On an inhalation, turn your body to face forward, then exhale and turn to the other side. Stay there for several breaths. Repeat the upper body twisting three times, come back to the center, and tilt your upper body to the side and stay there for several breaths (Figure 4-24), then tilt to the other side. Next, bend forward from the waist, touch your hands to the ground and use your pelvis to wave the hips from side to

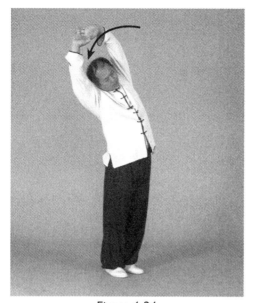

Figure 4-24

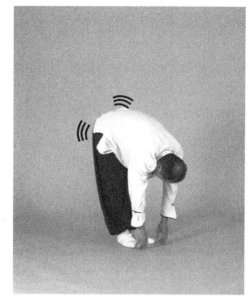

Figure 4-25

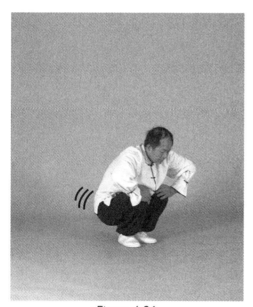

Figure 4-26

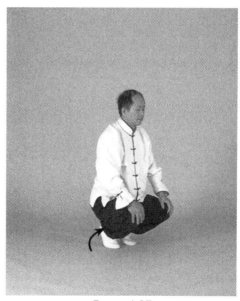

Figure 4-27

side to loosen up the lower spine (Figure 4-25). Be careful not to round the upper spine, but instead think of lengthening the back of the legs and lifting the sitting bones. Let the upper spine and the neck hang loosely. Stay there for several breaths. Finally, squat down with your feet flat on the ground to stretch your ankles (Figure 4-26) and then lift your heels up to stretch the toes (Figure 4-27). Repeat the entire process at least three times. After you finish, the inside of your body should feel very comfortable and warm. It is essential that you do not rush through these stretches. Hold each posture for between three to five seconds at a minimum. The breathing should be slow and deep, and can help you achieve a deeper stretch.

Loosening Up the Torso and Internal Organs

The torso is supported by the spine and the trunk muscles. Once you have stretched your trunk muscles, you can loosen up the torso. This also moves the muscles inside your body around, which moves and relaxes your internal organs. This, in turn, makes it possible for the qi to circulate smoothly inside your body. Next, we will introduce a few torso movements that should be performed as a warm up before you practice either taiji qigong or the taijiquan sequence.

Circle the Waist Horizontally (*Pin Yuan Niu Yao,* 平圓扭腰)

This exercise helps you to regain conscious control of the muscles in your abdomen. The lower dan tian is the main residence of your original qi. The qi in your lower dan tian can be led easily only when your abdomen is loose and relaxed. These abdominal exercises are probably the most important of all the internal qigong practices.

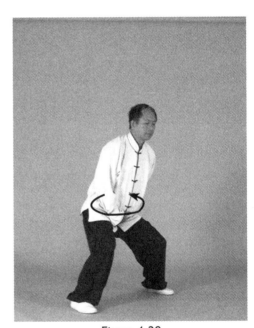

To practice this exercise, squat down slightly in the horse stance. Without moving your thighs or upper body, use the waist muscles to move the abdomen around in a horizontal circle (Figure 4-28). Circle in one direction about ten times and then in the other direction about ten times. If you hold one hand over your lower dan tian and the other on your sacrum, you may be able to focus your attention better on the area you want to control.

Figure 4-28

In the beginning, you may have difficulty making your body move the way you want. But if you keep practicing, you will quickly learn how to do it. Once you can do the movement comfortably, make the circles larger and larger. Naturally, this will cause the muscles to tense somewhat and inhibit the qi flow, but the more you practice the sooner you will again be able to relax. After you have practiced for a while and can control your waist muscles easily, start making the circles smaller and also start using your yi to lead the qi from lower dan tian to move in these circles. The final goal is to have only a slight physical movement, but a strong movement of qi.

There are four major benefits to this abdominal exercise. First, when your lower dan tian area is loose, the qi can flow in and out easily. This is especially important for martial arts qigong practitioners who use the lower dan tian as their main source of qi. Second, when the abdominal area is loose, the qi circulation in the large and small intestines will be smooth and they can absorb nutrients and eliminate waste. If your body does not eliminate effectively, the absorption of nutrients will be hindered and you may become sick. Third, when the abdominal area is loose, the qi in the kidneys will circulate smoothly and the original essence stored in the kidneys can be converted more efficiently into qi. In addition, when the kidney area is loosened, the kidney qi can be led downward and upward to nourish the entire body. Fourth, these exercises eliminate qi stagnation in the lower back, healing and preventing lower back pain. Furthermore, this exercise can also help you rebuild the strength of the muscles in the waist area.

Waving the Spine and Massaging the Internal Organs (*Ji Zhui Bo Dong, Nei Zang An Mo,* 脊椎波動，內臟按摩)

Beneath your diaphragm is your stomach, on its right is your liver and on its left is your spleen. Once you can comfortably do the movement in your lower abdomen, change the movement from horizontal to vertical and extend it up to your diaphragm. The easiest way to loosen the area around the diaphragm is to use a wave-like motion between the perineum and the diaphragm (Figure 4-29). You may find it helpful when you practice this to place one hand on your lower dan tian and your other hand above it with the thumb on the solar plexus. Use a forward and backward wave-like motion, flowing up to the diaphragm and down to the perineum and back. Repeat ten times.

Next, continue the movement while turning your body slowly to one side and then to the other (Figure 4-30). This will slightly tense the muscles on one side and loosen them on the other, which will massage the internal organs. Repeat ten times.

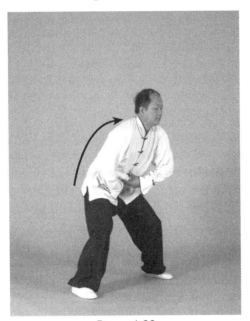 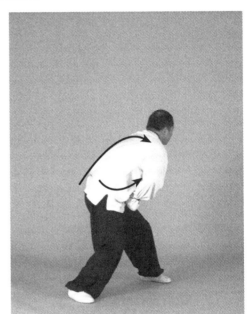

Figure 4-29 Figure 4-30

This exercise loosens the muscles around the stomach, liver, gall bladder and spleen, and therefore improves the qi circulation in these areas. It also trains you to use your mind to lead qi from your lower dan tian upward to the solar plexus area.

Thrust the Chest and Arc the Chest (*Tan Xiong Gong Bei,* 袒胸拱背)

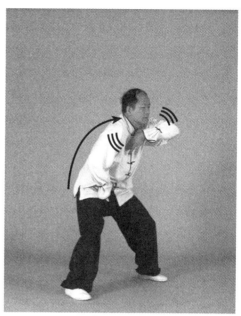

After loosening up the center portion of your body, extend the movement up to your chest. The wave-like movement starts in the abdomen, moves through the stomach and then up to the chest. You may find it easier to feel the movement if you hold one hand on your abdomen and the other lightly on your chest. You should also coordinate with the shoulders' movement. Inhale when you move your shoulders backward and exhale when you move them forward (Figure 4-31). The inhalation and exhalation should be as deep as possible and the entire chest should be very loose. When you move your spine, you should be able to feel the vertebrae move section by section. Repeat the motion ten times.

Figure 4-31

This exercise loosens up the chest and helps to regulate and improve the qi circulation in the lungs. It also teaches martial arts qigong practitioners to lead qi to the shoulders in coordination with the body's movements. In taijiquan martial applications, jin (power) is generated by the legs, directed by the waist (i.e., pelvis) and manifested by the hands. In order to do this, your body from the legs to the hands must be soft and connected like a whip. Only then will there be no stagnation to hold back the power.

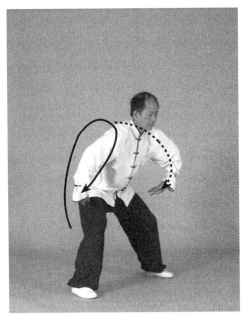

Figure 4-32

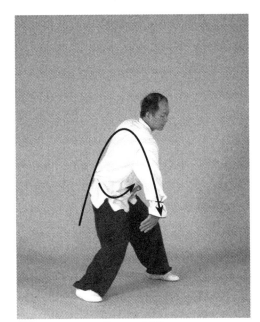

Figure 4-33

White Crane Waves Its Wings (*Bai He Dou Chi,* 白鶴抖翅)

Once you have completed the loosening up of the chest area, extend the motion to your arms and fingers. First, practice the motion with both arms ten times and then do each arm individually ten times. When you extend the movement to the arms, you first generate the motion from the legs or the waist and direct this power upward. It passes through the chest and shoulders and finally reaches the arms (Figure 4-32). When you practice with one arm, you also twist your body slightly to direct the movement (Figure 4-33).

These exercises will loosen up every joint in your body from the waist to the fingers. These exercises are in fact the fundamental practice of jin manifestation in the soft styles of Chinese martial arts.

Stationary (Yin)

There are two stationary taiji qigong sets, which I have synthesized from four different sources. These two stationary sets are identified as the primary set for taijiquan beginners, and the coiling set for advanced taijiquan practitioners who have completed the barehand solo sequence and started taiji pushing hands practice. Due to space limitations, only the primary set will be introduced in this sub-section If you are interested in learning the coiling set, please refer to the book and video, *The Essence of Taiji Qigong*, published by YMAA.

Primary Set

This set of qigong exercises has several purposes:

1. To help the taiji beginner understand and feel qi. The sooner a beginner is able to understand what qi is and to feel it, the sooner and more easily he or she can understand the internal energy of the body. This set is simple and very easy to remember, so after a short time you can do it comfortably and automatically, and can then devote your concentration to your breathing and qi.

2. To learn how to lead qi to the limbs. When you have regulated your body, breathing, and mind, you then learn how to lead qi from the limbs to the lower dan tian when you inhale, and from the lower dan tian to the limbs when you exhale. This trains you in using your yi to lead the qi (*yi yi yin qi*, 以意引氣), which is very critical in taijiquan training.

3. To gradually open up the twelve primary qi channels. After you have practiced this set for a long time, you will find that the qi is flowing more and more strongly. This stronger qi circulation will gradually open the twelve qi channels, and let the qi circulate more smoothly in your twelve internal organs. This is the key to maintaining good health

4. To loosen up the internal muscles, especially those around the internal organs. This loosening removes any qi stagnation near the internal organs, which lets them relax and receive the proper qi nourishment.

When you practice this set, in order to strongly gather the qi at the center of your palms, you should use the taiji hand form explained at the beginning of this chapter (Figure 4-2). You can relax this hand form when you complete the entire set, releasing the qi to the fingers.

FOLLOW ALONG
PRIMARY QIGONG SET

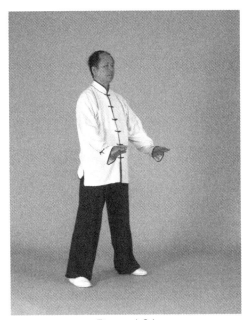

Figure 4-34

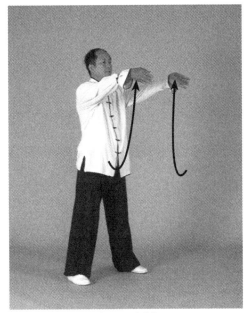

Figure 4-35

I. The Qi is Sunk to the Dan Tian
(*Qi Chen Dan Tian*, 氣沉丹田)

In this exercise you are using your mind to lead the qi to sink to the lower dan tian in coordination with the movements. First, stand still with the palms facing down right in front of your waist area (Figure 4-34). Bring your mind to the center of gravity (i.e., body's physical center)(wuji state). Inhale and exhale deeply for a few times until your mind is calm and peaceful. Next, inhale and turn your palms toward each other and lift them to shoulder height while gently and slightly arcing your back backward (Figure 4-35). Then turn both palms downward and lower them to waist level while exhaling and straightening your torso (Figure 4-36). Do ten repetitions, and each time you lower your hands imagine that you are pressing something down, and use the mind to lead the qi to the lower dan tian. Remember, even though it looks like you are moving only your hands, with practice you can generate the movement from your legs or waist through the spine, finally reaching the

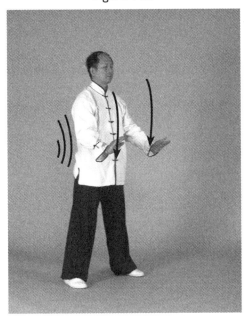

Figure 4-36

hands. The entire body moves like a soft whip. It is said in the *Taijiquan Classic*: "Once in motion, every part of the body is light and agile, and must be threaded together."[10]

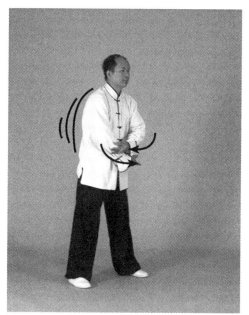

Figure 4-37

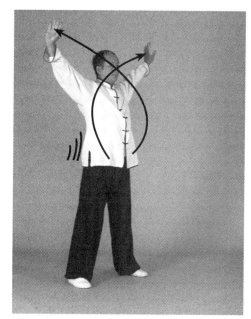

Figure 4-38

2. Expand the Chest to Cleanse the Body (*Zhan Xiong Jing Shen,* 展胸淨身)

After you have completed the last exercise, start circling your arms up in front of you and out to the sides. As they rise in front of your chest they cross while also arcing your back backward gently (Figure 4-37), then separate up and out to the sides and gently thrust your chest out (Figure 4-38). Inhale deeply as they rise, and exhale as they sink out and to the sides. The yi and the movement start at the waist, through the spine, and are passed to the limbs. The chest area is especially important in this exercise. The deep breathing and the movement of the arms loosen the muscles around the lungs. While doing this exercise you should also visualize that you are expelling the dirty qi and air from your body and lungs, and pushing them away from your body. Repeat the movements ten times.

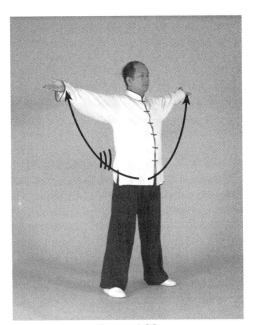

Figure 4-39

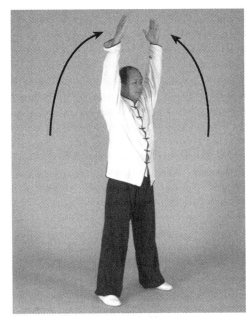

Figure 4-40

3. Pour the Qi into the Baihui
(*Baihui Guan Qi*, 百會貫氣)

After you have cleaned your body, you now visualize that you are taking in qi from the heavens through your baihui and pushing it down through your chest to the lower dan tian and finally through the bottoms of your feet into the ground. The motion of this exercise is simply the reverse of the previous one. Again, the relaxation of the chest is very important. When you inhale, open your arms out in front of your abdomen and thrust your chest out gently (Figure 4-39), and circle them up until they are above your head (Figure 4-40). As you exhale, lower your hands, palms down, in front of your body, arc your spine backward, and bring your chest in while visualizing that you are pushing the qi downward until it is below your feet (Figure 4-41). Repeat the movement ten times.

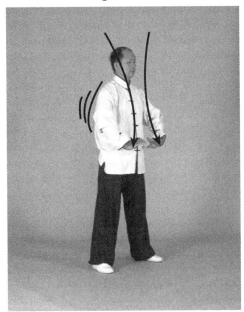

Figure 4-41

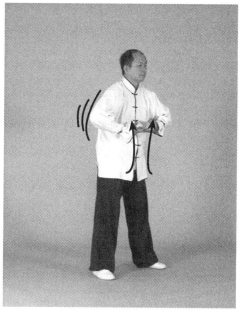

Figure 4-42

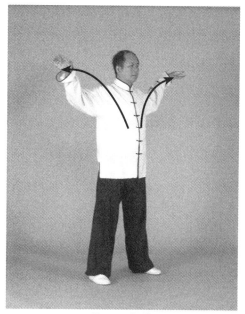

Figure 4-43

4. Left and Right to Push the Mountains (*Zuo You Tui Shan*, 左右推山)

After you have cleaned your body and absorbed qi from heaven, you start building qi internally and using it for training. As you inhale, raise your hands to chest height with the palms facing upward, while slightly and gently arcing your spine backward (Figure 4-42). Lower your elbows and turn your hands until the fingers are pointing to the sides and the palms are facing down, start to straighten your torso (Figure 4-43). Keep your wrists loose. As you exhale, extend your arms to the sides. When the arms are halfway extended, settle (lower) your wrists and push sideways with the palms as if you were pushing two mountains away, torso is straightened and spirit is raised (Figure 4-44). Inhale and bring

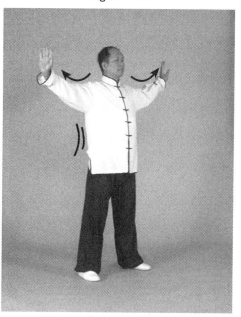

Figure 4-44

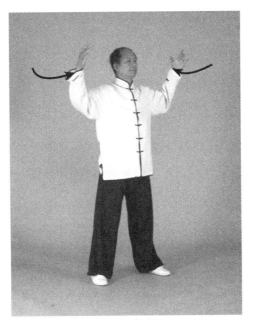

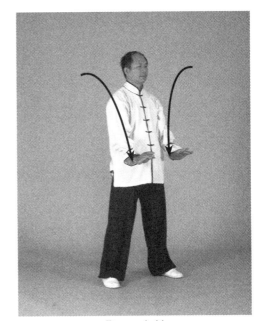

Figure 4-45   Figure 4-46

your hands back with the palms facing inward while arcing your spine gently backward (Figure 4-45), then exhale and lower the hands in front of you with the palms down and the fingers pointing forward (Figure 4-46). Resume your normal relaxed standing position. The muscles should remain relaxed throughout the exercise. Do not extend your arms to the sides as far as they can go, because this causes muscle tension and qi stagnation. Repeat the movement ten times.

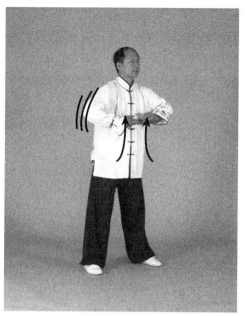

Figure 4-47

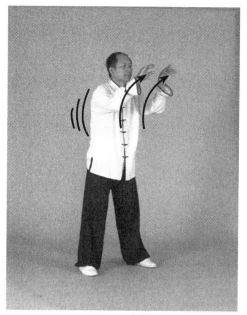

Figure 4-48

5. Settle the Wrists and Push the Palms (*Zuo Wan Tui Zhang*, 坐腕推掌)

This exercise continues the training of using your yi to lead your qi, only now you are pushing forward instead of to the sides. In order to lead the qi forward to your palms, pretend that you are pushing a car or some other heavy object. Start by raising your arms in front of you, with the palms facing upward, while inhaling and arcing your back backward gently, as you did in the previous exercise (Figure 4-47). Then lower your elbows and turn your palms forward and downward while starting to straighten the torso (Figure 4-48). The wrists are relaxed and the fingers are pointing forward. Exhale and extend your arms. When they are more than halfway out, settle (lower) the wrists and push the palms forward (Figure 4-49). Straighten your torso. Do not extend your arms all the way, because that would tense the muscles and cause stagnation of the qi circulation. Next, inhale

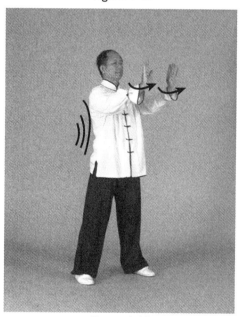

Figure 4-49

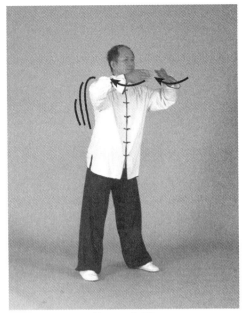

Figure 4-50

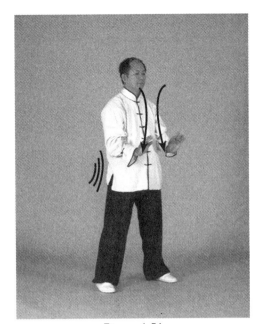

Figure 4-51

and draw your hands back, with the palms facing your chest and back arcing backward slightly (Figure 4-50), and then exhale and lower your hands to your abdomen while you straighten your torso (Figure 4-51). Repeat the movement ten times.

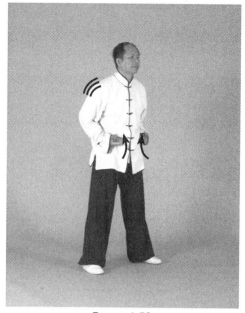

Figure 4-52

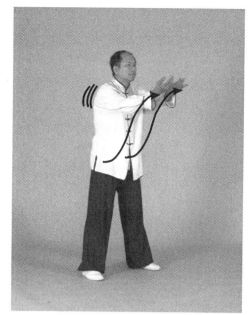

Figure 4-53

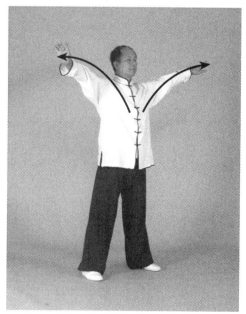

Figure 4-54

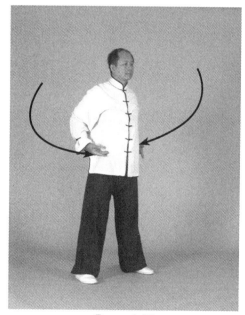

Figure 4-55

6. The Large Bear Swims in the Water (*Da Xiong You Shui*, 大熊游水)

When you have finished the last exercise and your hands are in front of your abdomen, raise them again, with the palms facing up, while inhaling (Figure 4-52). Then exhale and extend your arms forward with the palms up (Figure 4-53). Inhale and move your arms out and to the sides, turning the palms down, and then circle the hands to your waist as you rotate the palms upward (Figures 4-54 and 4-55). Continue by exhaling and extending your arms forward. The motion is similar to the breaststroke in swimming. As always in taiji, the movement is generated from the legs and directed upward to the hands. Repeat the movement ten times.

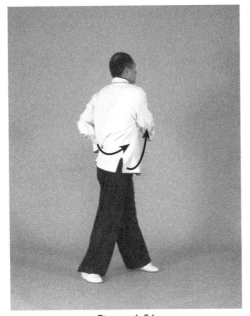

Figure 4-56

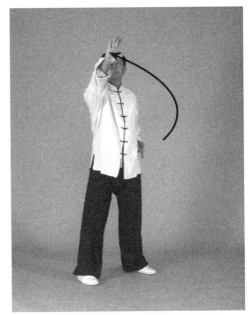

Figure 4-57

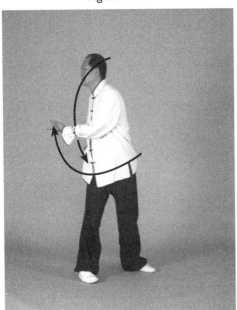

Figure 4-58

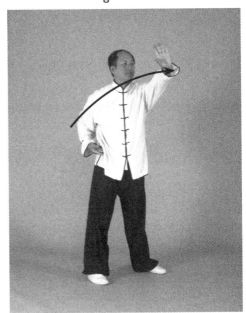

Figure 4-59

7. Left and Right to Open the Mountain (*Zuo You Kai Shan*, 左右開山)

This is similar to the last exercise, but you use only one arm at a time. From the previous movement, continue your inhalation while turning your body to the left and extending your right hand to the left (Figure 4-56); then exhale and turn the palm forward as you turn your body to your right, while sweeping your right palm in front of your chest (Figure 4-57). When the right hand reaches your waist, do the same movement with the left hand (Figures 4-58 and 4-59). Do ten repetitions of the complete movement. Let your chest open and close in coordination with the arm movement, and also turn your body slightly.

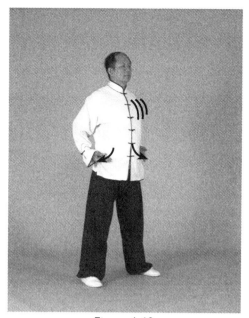

Figure 4-60

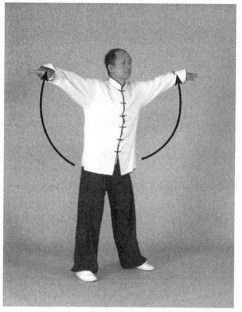

Figure 4-61

8. The Eagle Attacks Its Prey (*Lao Ying Pu Shi*, 老鷹撲食)

This exercise uses the reverse of the movement of the sixth exercise. Starting with your hands at your waist, with the palms facing up, inhale and spread your arms out to the sides, while thrusting your chest out (Figure 4-60), and then exhale as your arms circle out and forward with the palms facing down (Figure 4-61). Finally, pull your hands back to your waist as the palms rotate upward and arc your back backward (Figure 4-62). Exhale as your arms move forward, and inhale as they move back. Again, the motion originates with the legs. Repeat ten times.

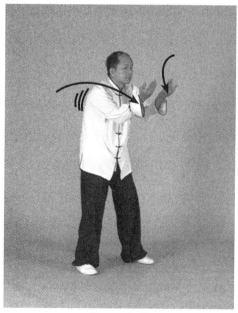

Figure 4-62

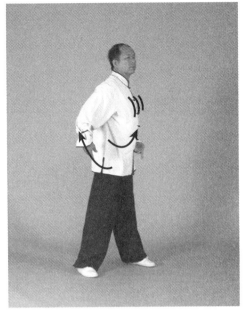

Figure 4-63

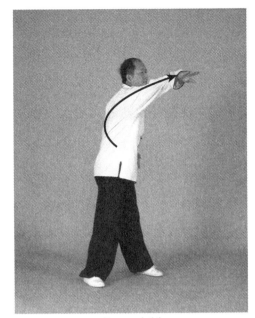

Figure 4-64

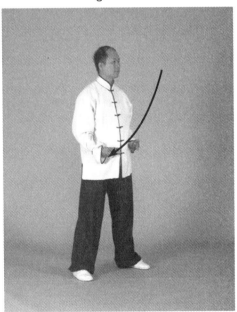

Figure 4-65

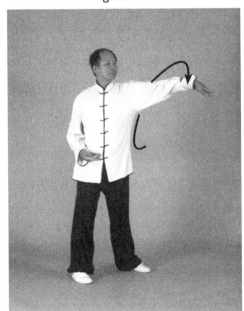

Figure 4-66

9. The Lion Rotates the Ball (*Shi Zi Gong Qiu*, 獅子拱球)

This exercise is similar to the preceding one, except that you use only one arm at a time. Starting with your hands at your waist, with the palms facing up (Figure 4-63), extend your right arm to the side and then forward in a counterclockwise movement, turning the palm down as it moves (Figure 4-64). Then inhale and draw your arm back to your waist, rotating the palm upward (Figure 4-65). Then repeat the same motion with the left hand, moving it in a clockwise circle (Figure 4-66). The movement is generated by the legs, and you can vary the size of the circles. The most important point of the training is feeling that your body is connected together from the bottom of your feet to the tips of your fingers. Repeat the complete movement ten times.

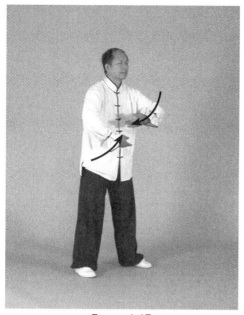

Figure 4-67

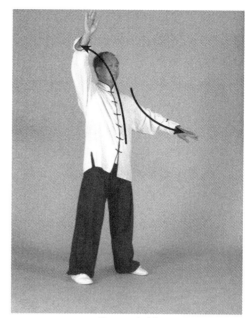

Figure 4-68

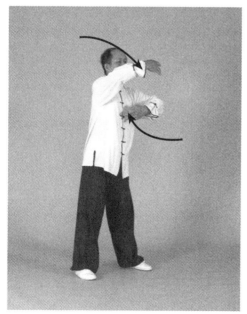

Figure 4-69

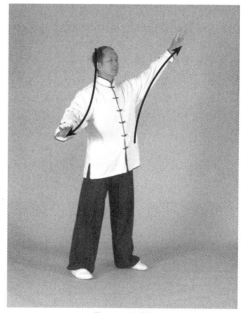

Figure 4-70

10. The White Crane Spreads Its Wing (Bai He Liang Chi, 白鶴亮翅)

This last form is used for recovery. In it the arms expand diagonally. When this motion is done in coordination with the breathing, the internal organs will relax and loosen, and any qi that may still be stagnant internally will be led to the surface of your body. Continuing from the previous exercise, cross both arms in front of your chest (Figure 4-67), then exhale and extend your arms out diagonally, with the right arm up and left arm down (Figure 4-68). Inhale as you draw both arms in and cross them in front of your chest, and then exhale and extend them out diagonally again, now with the left hand up and the right hand down (Figures 4-69 and 4-70). The mind should remain calm and the entire body should be loose. Repeat the entire movement

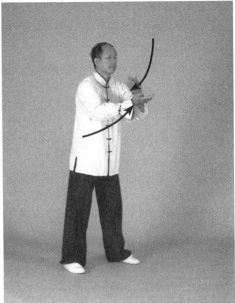

Figure 4-71

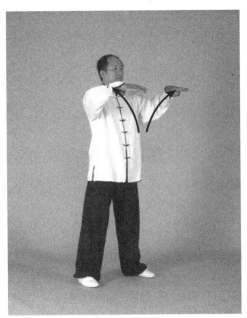

Figure 4-72

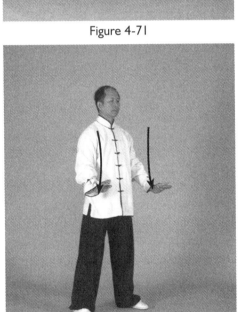

Figure 4-73

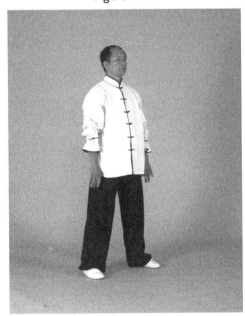

Figure 4-74

ten times. When you are finished, inhale and move both hands to in front of your chest (Figure 4-71), and then turn both palms down (Figure 4-72). Exhale and lower your hands with the feeling that you are pushing something down, and lead the qi back to your lower dan tian (Figure 4-73). Finally, drop both hands naturally to your sides (Figure 4-74). Inhale and exhale naturally ten times and feel the qi distributing itself in your body, especially in your hands.

Because you have been standing still for a while, your circulation may have become stagnant and qi and blood may have accumulated in your feet. You will notice this as a sensation of heat in your feet. To remove this qi accumulation, raise up on your toes, and then rock back on your heels several times. Alternatively, you can simply walk around for a few minutes.

Rocking Set

The rocking set was originally designed to teach the martial taijiquan practitioner to balance his qi when doing jin. It says in Zhang, San-feng's *Treatise*: "If there is a top, there is a bottom; if there is a front, there is a back; if there is a left, there is a right. If yi wants to go upward, this implies considering downward."[3] From this saying it is very clear that the secret of effective jin manifestation is balanced yi and qi.

FOLLOW ALONG
ROCKING QIGONG SET

To analyze this subject further, jin balance includes first balancing the posture, which comes from firm rooting and centering. Only then will the body be comfortable and stable, and the judgment of the yi accurate. When this yi is used to lead the qi to energize the muscles, you can manifest your strongest jin.

The motion of the rocking is very simple. You simply shift your weight from leg to leg in coordination with the arm movements. When you move forward, the rear leg balances the action of the arms, and when you shift your weight to the rear leg and withdraw your arms, the front leg balances the movement. The repeated rocking movement helps you to develop a feeling for centering and balancing, and to build the root from which power can be grown. Although this set was originally created for jin training, many taijiquan practitioners have found that it can significantly improve leg strength and also train both physical and mental centering and balance. This also contributes to good health.

We will introduce only three exercises, but after you have practiced them for a while and understand the theory, you should be able to find or create others.

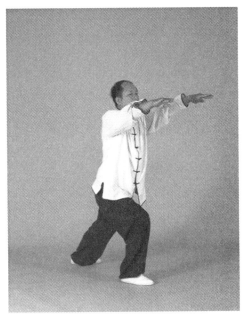

Figure 4-75

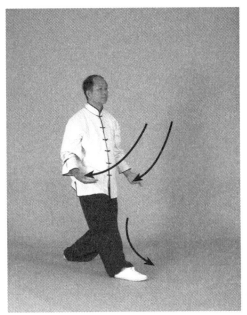

Figure 4-76

1. Embracing Arms (*Gong Bi*, 拱臂)

Start in the bow and arrow stance, with 60 percent of your weight on your front foot and both arms stretched out in front of you (Figure 4-75). Inhale and shift your weight slowly back to your rear foot until it carries 60 percent of the weight (four-six stance). As you shift back, lower and draw in your arms while rotating them so that the palms are facing up (Figure 4-76). Continue to circle both arms sideward and up to shoulder height. As you raise your arms, rotate them so that the palms are facing down when they reach shoulder height. Then exhale and move both hands forward while once again shifting 60 percent of the body's weight to the front leg (Figure 4-77). Repeat ten times, then switch your legs and repeat the same movement another ten times.

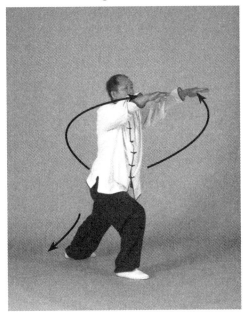

Figure 4-77

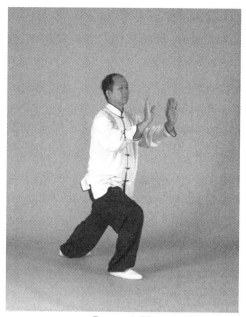

Figure 4-78

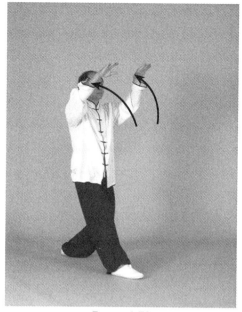

Figure 4-79

2. Press Forward (*An*, 按)

This form is adapted from the taijiquan sequence. Start by pushing forward with both hands while in the bow and arrow stance (Figure 4-78). As you inhale, shift your weight to your rear leg to take the four-six stance. Gently sink your chest, and simultaneously raise your hands up and slightly to the sides (Figure 4-79). Continue your inhalation as you draw both hands back to your chest. Finally, exhale, push your hands forward, and release your chest outward, while shifting your weight forward into the bow and arrow stance (Figure 4-80). When you push forward, you should keep your fingers pointing forward until they almost reach the imaginary target, and then settle down your wrist (i.e., fingers are pointing upward). This hand movement is called "zuo wan," (坐腕) which traslates as "sitting the wrist." As you push, you should remain relaxed, but you should also feel that you are pushing a heavy object. Always remember: you must push your rear leg backward and into the ground to produce forward pushing power. Repeat ten times on each leg.

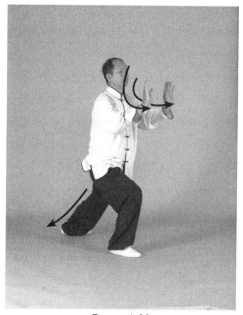

Figure 4-80

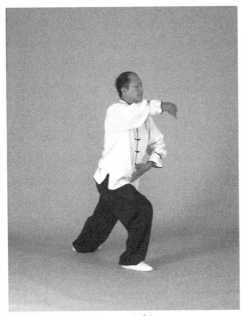

Figure 4-81

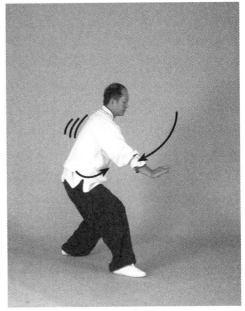

Figure 4-82

3. Wardoff (*Peng*, 掤)

This movement is also adapted from the taiji sequence. Start with your right leg forward, your right arm in front of your chest horizontally, with the palm facing in, and your left hand touching the lower abdomen (Figure 4-81). Next, inhale, arc your back, shift your weight to your rear leg, and turn your body to your left slightly. At the same time, draw down your right arm (Figure 4-82). Continuing the motion, exhale, straigthen your torso, and shift your weight to the front leg while raising your right arm in a wardoff movement (Figure 4-83). The motion is generated from the legs and is directed by the waist out to the right arm. Repeat the motion ten times, and then switch legs for another ten repetitions.

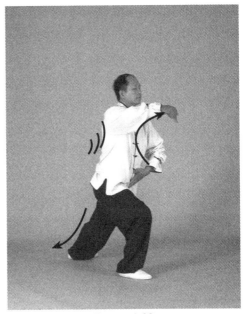

Figure 4-83

Stepping (Yang)

Stepping or walking taiji qigong is essentially taijiquan itself. Most of the walking movements are adapted from the taijiquan sequence, the only difference being that a single movement is repeated continuously until you can feel the movement of qi. Since you are only doing one basic movement it is easy to remember and master, and you can put all your attention on being relaxed, centered, and balanced, and thereby regulate your body. Then you can start regulating your breathing and mind, which is the key to leading your qi. Walking taiji qigong should be trained before the beginner starts learning the taijiquan sequence. Experienced practitioners often practice walking taiji qigong to penetrate to a deeper understanding of qi, the mind, and the body.

FOLLOW ALONG STEPPING QIGONG SET

1. Wave Hands in the Clouds (*Yun Shou*, 雲手)

Squat down into the horse stance, turn your body to your left, inhale and circle your right hand in front of your left hand, which is on the left of your waist, and upward, with the palm facing in, to chest level (Figure 4-84). Keeping your weight in the center, exhale and turn your body to the right. The hands naturally follow the turn of the body (Figure 4-85). Once your body is turned,

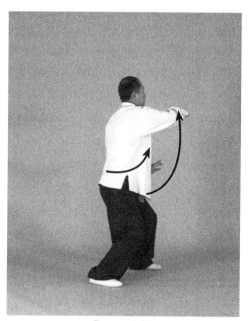

Figure 4-84

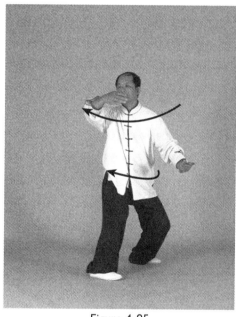

Figure 4-85

inhale and press your right hand down and lift your left arm up to chest height while moving your left leg to the side of the right leg (Figure 4-86). Then exhale and turn your body to the left, letting your hands follow naturally along (Figure 4-87). Continue by stepping your right leg to the right as you switch your hands (Figure 4-88), and then turn to the right as you start shifting your weight to the right leg. Repeat as many times as you wish. The arms should be very light, and should float around like clouds. The main purpose of this exercise is to loosen the waist and spine, and also to learn how to direct the power from the legs to the hands with a rotating motion.

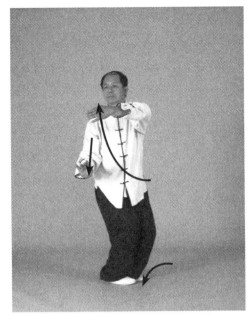

Figure 4-86

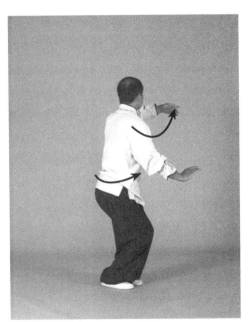

Figure 4-87

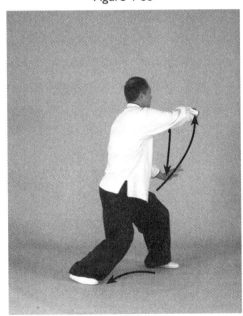

Figure 4-88

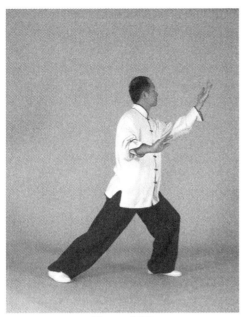

Figure 4-89

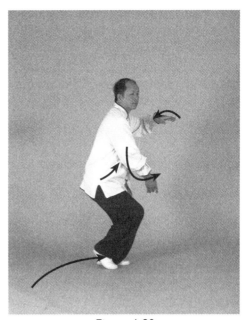

Figure 4-90

2. Diagonal Flying (*Xie Fei Shi*, 斜飛勢)

Start in the bow and arrow stance with your left hand in front of your face, palm facing in and fingers pointing up, and your right hand out to your side at lower chest height (Figure 4-89). As you inhale, rotate your body slightly to the left. As you turn, rotate your left arm so that the palm is facing down, pull your right arm in and rotate it so that the hand is palm up under the left hand, and also pull in your right leg next to your left leg (Figure 4-90). Step your right leg out to the right front (Figure 4-91). As you exhale, shift 60 percent

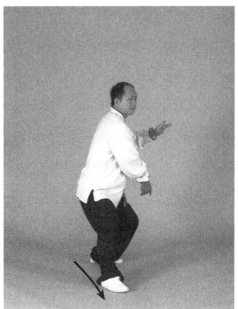

Figure 4-91

of your weight forward onto your right leg, rotate your body toward the right leg, and separate your arms (Figure 4-92). The movement of the right arm is powered by the rotation of the body. The right arm should not go out past the side of the body. Next, inhale and rotate your body slightly to your right. At the same time, rotate your right arm so the palm faces down, draw in the left arm and rotate it so that the hand is palm up under the right hand, and draw in your left leg (Figure 4-93). Step your left leg out to your left front, then exhale and shift your body forward. At the same time, rotate your body toward the left leg and separate your arms so that you end up in the position you started from (Figure 4-94). While practicing this movement you should arc in your chest as you inhale, and expand it as you exhale. This exercise is very useful for regulating the qi in the lungs and kidneys.

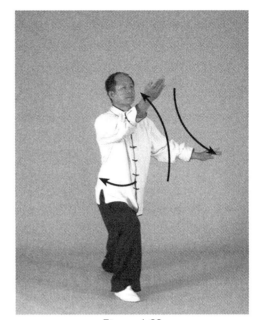

Figure 4-92

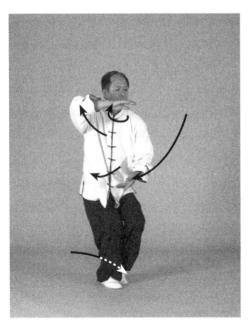

Figure 4-93

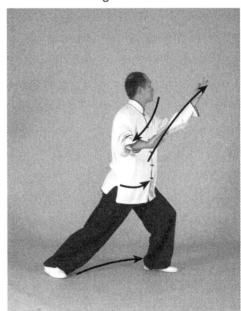

Figure 4-94

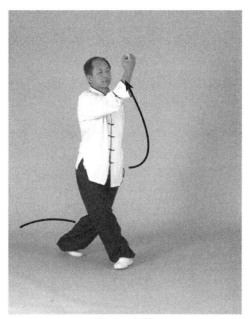

Figure 4-95

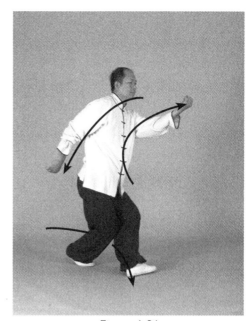

Figure 4-96

3. Twist Body and Circle the Fist (*Pie Shen Chui,* 撇身捶)

Step your right leg forward and touch the heel down. As you exhale, shift your weight forward and twist your body so that your right foot turns, on its heel, to the right front at an angle of forty-five degrees, and your right arm circles clockwise in front of your chest (Figure 4-95). Your left arm moves with your body. Inhale and step your left leg forward and touch the heel down, and at the same time start lowering your right arm and moving your left arm across your body. Then exhale and rotate your body to the left so that your left foot turns to the left front and your left arm circles counterclockwise up and to your left (Figure 4-96). Your right arm moves with your body. Remember that the waist always directs the movement of the arms. Practice at least ten times.

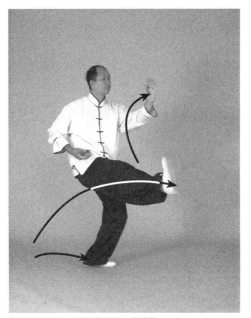

Figure 4-97

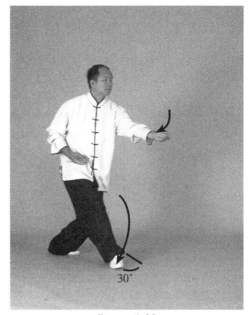

Figure 4-98

4. Stepping Leg (*Cai Tui*, 踩腿)

Stepping leg is used to train balance and also to strengthen the knees. Inhale and step your left leg forward with the toes facing about 30 degrees to the left. Shift your weight to the left leg and at the same time slowly kick out with your right heel while pushing your left hand forward and exhaling (Figure 4-97). Inhale and step your right leg forward with the toes pointing about 30 degrees to the right (Figure 4-98), and then exhale and slowly kick the left leg out while pushing the right hand forward (Figure 4-99). While you are pushing one hand out, the other should pull back to your waist with the palm facing upward. Practice ten times.

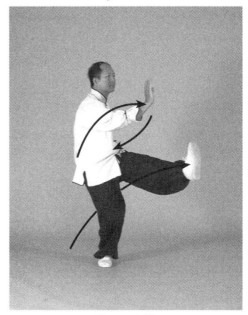

Figure 4-99

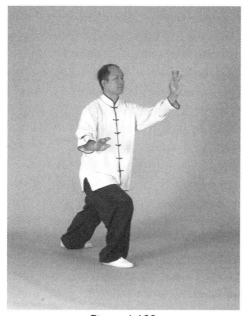

Figure 4-100

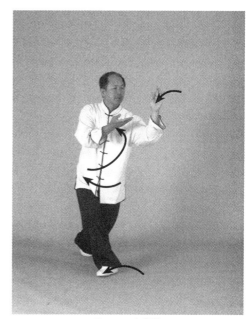

Figure 4-101

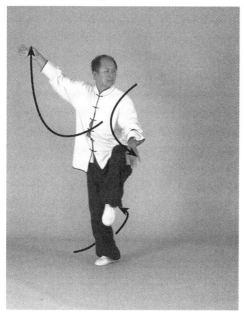

Figure 4-102

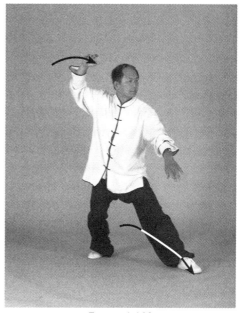

Figure 4-103

5. Brush Knee and Twist Step (*Lou Xi Ao Bu*, 摟膝拗步)

Stand in the bow and arrow stance with the right leg forward, your right hand at your waist, and your left hand pushing forward (Figure 4-100). Inhale and start to circle your right arm clockwise across your chest, rotate your body to the right, pivot your right foot to the right front corner, and push your left hand to your right. As you do this you are also shifting your weight to your front leg, and your right hand continues to circle down and to your right (Figure 4-101). Exhale and lift your left knee to waist height, circle your left arm down to brush past your knee, and circle your right arm back and up to by your right ear (Figure 4-102). Inhale and step your left leg forward (Figure 4-103).

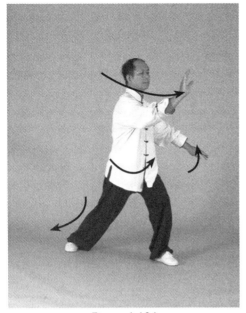

Figure 4-104

Figure 4-105

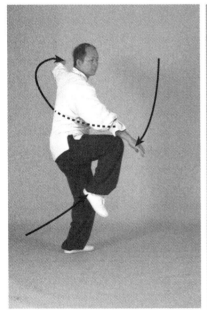

Figure 4-106

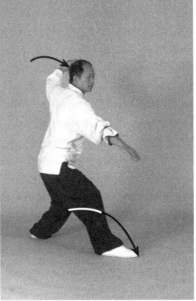

Figure 4-107

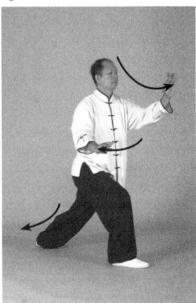

Figure 4-108

As you exhale, shift your weight forward, rotate your body to the front, push forward with your right hand, and draw your left arm back and down (Figure 4-104). Then repeat the entire sequence to the other side (Figures 4-105 to 4-108). Practice ten repetitions

4-6. Traditional Yang Style Taijiquan

In the traditional barehand sequence, the apparent number of techniques vary between 81 and 150, depending on the method used to count and group the forms. Some instructors and writers, for example, will not count repeated forms. But basically, you may judge whether a taijiquan sequence is complete by comparing the arrangement of the names given to the techniques. While the methods of counting the techniques vary, the names and their arrangement do not.

FOLLOW ALONG
TAIJIQUAN SEQUENCE (CONTINUOUS)

If your instructor has taken out techniques to shorten the sequence, you should practice the sequence several times to receive the health benefits of taijiquan. As was stated earlier, the original sequence was constructed to have enough forms to achieve results beneficial to health; shortening the sequence shortens the time of exercise.

However, if you are interested in developing the martial aspect of taijiquan, you should do the entire sequence three continuous times each morning. But if you are only interested in the health aspect of taijiquan, then the sequence can be performed once each morning.

During the morning itself, the best time to practice is before sunrise so that you can take advantage of the change in the yin and yang energies of the body and the nature around us, which is influenced by the sun. Because the sequence should take at least 20 minutes to perform, it must be done 20 minutes before the sun comes up.

By doing the sequence in a minimum of 20 minutes, the inhalations and exhalations will be relatively equal. Therefore, as beginner, you should aim for your sequence to be completed in no less than 20 minutes. Later, as you become more proficient, you can extend the time. A time of 30 minutes for one sequence is very good. The ultimate goal is to perform one complete set in 60 minutes. To achieve a time of 60 minutes requires slow, but consistent breathing, and a highly concentrated, yet relaxed, profound mind: the practitioner is in a semiconscious state while the body moves slowly.

If you practice taijiquan for improving health only, performing the taijiquan sequence with the proper series of deep breaths while maintaining a relaxed body will have the desired results. In this state, the qi will naturally circulate.

However, if you practice taijiquan as a martial art, once you achieved fluid qi circulation during the bare hand sequence, you should perform the sequence with speed and power. The fast sequence should be practiced at least once during the day. Without performing the barehand techniques with speed and power, the techniques cannot be made effective.

In terms of the practical aspects of bare hand taijiquan, listed below are major areas which the student should be aware of.

Breathing. As explained in section 2-5, if you are practicing taijiquan for relaxation and health only, you may use normal abdominal breathing, which is a better breathing method for relaxation. However, if you practice taijiquan for martial arts, you must use reversed abdominal breathing, since you need to manifest your qi into the physical form. This martial breathing training includes Four Gates Breathing and Skin/Marrow Breathing.

Be careful when you use reversed abdominal breathing. Take your time and above all, try to move slowly, in coordination with the breathing. The breathing should be deep yet smooth and light, instead of heavy and shallow. The stomach area should be relaxed, and the abdominal movement should be natural and smooth. If you cannot satisfy all of these requirements at first, you should proceed gradually and deliberately. First, practice the abdominal movements on a small scale, until it feels natural and smooth. Then, gradually increase the scale of abdominal movement. Normally, this will take about six months to one year of correct practice. If you train incorrectly, you will feel tightness in the stomach area, and may possibly experience pain and an upset stomach. Therefore, you should be very careful when you practice reversed abdominal breathing.

Warm Up. For a description of warm up exercises, please refer to the warm up qigong exercises introduced earlier. This includes: loosening up the joints, torso stretching, and the spine movements. You can also stretch your legs out, and then calm your mind by doing fundamental breathing drills. Because there are kicks in the sequence, the muscles must be properly loosened to avoid injury. To fully receive the benefits of the sequence, the mind must conduct the performance in a tranquil state. Otherwise, too much time will be spent calming the mind during the sequence. The best way to accomplish this is to practice the taiji qigong, introduced earlier, for twenty minutes before doing the form.

Movement. All the movements in the sequence are done lightly and without heavy steps. Each step is done as if the person were on ice: gently and softly. In the sequence there are many moves in which the practitioner must turn his body to an opposite direction without lifting the legs. In these particular instances, turning should be done on the heels, one at a time, in a smooth manner.

Yelling. In the taijiquan sequence there are a few places that contain fast motion and will require that the performer yell "ha." The yell should come from deep in the lungs, not from the throat. While yelling, the lower dan tian must expand. The yell will clear out the dirty air in the lungs. The times at which to yell will be stated in the description of the sequence.

External Movements. There are eight traits that you should keep in mind while performing bare hand taijiquan. These points are smoothness, natural feeling, relaxation, balance, centering, rooting, continuity, and coordination of mind, body, and breath. By noting these points while practicing the taijiquan sequence, you will soon become proficient in taijiquan.

Internal Feeling. Once you have learned the entire taijiquan sequence, you should concentrate on becoming more sensitive to the internal feelings generated during the sequence. Feeling is the language between your body and your mind. The deeper and more clearly you can sense the changes in your body, the better your mind will be at interpreting you inner state and its relationship to your circumstances. This is the key to achieving deeper relaxation, and therefore to leading the qi to circulate through the deep place in your body. This brings health. Furthermore, through this process you can learn to store the qi in the bone marrow, which is essential to storing jin (martial power).

Normally, in order to achieve a deep feeling for each form, you must understand the root and the meaning of each movement. Once you have done this, you can manifest your qi efficiently and powerfully. If you fail to grasp the essence of the taijiquan movements, it is like you are travelling without any destination. This is very similar to the practice of playing the piano. The same song, played by a beginner, will be very different from the same song played by an experienced performer. The difference is practice and experience. Each additional year of practice is an accumulation of gongfu. It is this gongfu that makes the difference. From long practice, you can grasp the deep feeling of any art or subject.

There is a very well known story, about Confucius learning how to play a piece of music on an ancient musical instrument, the gu-zheng (古箏). Confucius' music teacher at this time was Shi Xiang Zu (師襄子). After he finished learning, Confucius practiced for only ten days, yet he was able to perform the music skillfully. His teacher was very happy, and asked him: "Are you ready for the second piece?" To Shi Xiang Zi's surprise, Confucius replied: "No!" When Shi Xiang Zi asked him why not, Confucius answered: "Though I am able to play this piece skillfully, I still cannot put my whole feeling into this music and manifest my feeling in it. Therefore, I prefer to practice for a longer period of time." Confucius then practiced this piece of music for three years, until he could infuse his deepest feelings into the tones of the music. His teacher was very happy when he saw this. Again, he asked Confucius: "Now, are you ready for the second pieces?" Again, the answer was no. His teacher then asked: "Why still no, since you can already manifest your feelings into the music?" Confucius replied: "Though I am able to play this music with feeling, I still don't know the feelings of the composer. When the composer wrote this piece, he put his emotional feelings deeply into it. I must continue my practice until I am able to comprehend the composer's feelings." Again, Confucius' teacher left him alone to practice.

Three years later, Confucius came to see Shi Xiang Zi and said: "Dear teacher, now, I am ready for the new piece." His teacher was very curious and asked: "Does this mean you have figured out the feelings of the composer?" Confucius said: "From this music, I can see he is a six foot tall man. Moreover, he is a person possessing such a wide open mind and generous nature that he is able to ponder both heaven and earth in his head." Shi Xiang Zi was shocked, and said: "Amazing that you can figure these out from the music. You are completely correct. This piece is called 'Wen Wang Cao,' (文王操) and was composed by King Wen of Zhou (周文王), whose mind was wide and profound. He was also six feet tall."[11] According to Chinese history, King Wen of Zhou was six feet tall, and it was he who interpreted the *Book of Changes* (易經).

From this story, you can see that when you perform taijiquan, you must continue to search for the original motivations of its creator, and you must try to achieve the same feelings as its creator. Only then will you discover the root of the forms. When you learn taijiquan, since you are only a beginner in the art, you must learn from the experiences accumulated by your artistic ancestors. Only after you have mastered all of the forms and techniques passed down to us, which may take you more than ten years of practice, should you start to blend your own concepts and understanding into the art. When this happens, you create a new style, derived from an understanding of the past and the principles contained in the form. Therefore, this creative art can be alive, and develop from a deep and profound internal feeling, instead of being merely superficial.

Imagined Opponent. If you practice taijiquan for martial arts, then you must gradually build up a sense of enemy. This is done by imagining you are fighting with an opponent. Such practice will also help you understand the root of every movement. If done correctly, it will make each technique more accurate, and will promote the circulation of qi more abundantly. While imagining your opponent, you must regard your waist as the first master (because it directs the action), your throat as the second master (because it controls the yell, which enhances the manifestation of jin), and your heart as the third master (because it guides the mind).

Direction for the Taijiquan Sequence. For the purposes of indicating the direction of movement, Chinese martial books use a compass system. The original direction which a person faces is immediately and permanently designated (N) or North for the duration of the sequence. It does not matter which actual geographic direction the individual faces, the front will always be (N). From this designation, the right side becomes (E) or East, the left side (W) or West, and the back side (S) or South.

Finally, as a last reminder, the breathing during the sequence must be smooth and fluid. Never hold the breath. Every inhalation and exhalation should last the length of the form for which it was indicated. The breathing controls the speed of the movements, rather than the movements controlling the breathing. This is extremely important to always keep in mind.

Yang Style Taijiquan Sequence (Traditional Long Form)
傳統楊氏太極拳

I. Beginning (*Taiji Qi Shi*, 太極起勢)

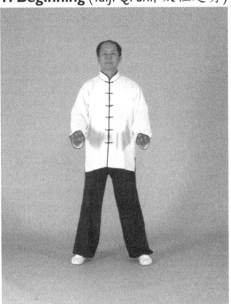

Figure 4-109: (N) Feet are slightly spread beyond shoulder width. Hands are at the waist, palms down. Wrists must be loose. Inhale and exhale naturally and comfortably. Pay attention to your lower dan tian. This is a wuji (無極) state. Remember to keep the middle finger and the thumb slightly forward while gently pushing the pinkie backward (taiji hand form).

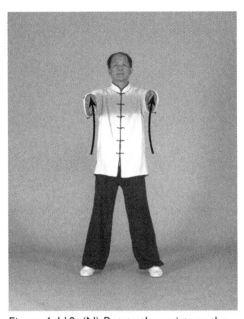

Figure 4-110: (N) Rotate the wrists so the palms face each other. Lift the arms up to shoulder height. Do not raise or make the shoulders tight. Inhale. From this movement, the yin and yang are discriminated. When you do this, imagine that you are picking up an object between your palms. One flow of qi goes to the arms and the other flow to the bottom of the feet. You should always remember that the motion of every form is directed by the waist area at the center of gravity (the real *dan tian*, 真丹田). The motion then passes through the spine and chest, finally reaching to the arms. It is said in the *Taijiquan Classic:* "The root is at the feet, [jin or the movement is] generated from the legs, controlled by the waist, and expressed by the fingers."[12] In order to reach this goal, your waist must be relaxed and loose, since it is like the steering wheel of a car. When this place is stagnant, the entire body will be stiff.

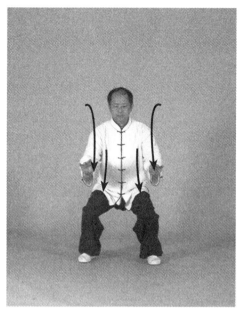

Figure 4-111: (N) Point the palms down. Move down slowly into horse stance (*ma bu*, 馬步). Lower the arms to the lower abdomen level. Exhale. When you do this, imagine that you are pushing some object downward. That means your mind is about six inches in front of the palms. In this case, the qi will be led outward through the center of the palm (*laogong* cavity, P-8, 勞宮).

Analysis

This beginning action is also called "sunken qi to the lower dan tian" (氣沉丹田). This means that you are leading the qi to the lower dan tian to build your root and firm your center. In order to accomplish this, your torso is upright, your head is suspended, and your elbows and shoulders are sunk.

2. Grasp the Sparrow's Tail: Right (*You Lan Que Wei,* 右攬雀尾)

Grasp sparrow's tail in Chinese is "lan que wei." Lan means grasp or seize. This implies that when you apply this technique you not only intercept your opponent's strike, but also grasp him. A sparrow's tail is very light and fragile, and also sensitive and mobile. Therefore, when you grasp the sparrow's tail you must be cautious and sensitive, and you cannot use muscular strength. You must lead your enemy's attack lightly and skillfully into a bad position where you can do the technique. In the taijiquan sequence there are two forms of grasp sparrow's tail: right and left. However, the left form should be the follow-up to the right form, and so some taijiquan masters would prefer to refer to the left grasp sparrow's tail as diagonal flying (left).

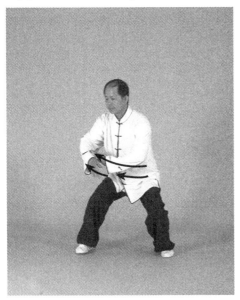

Figure 4-112: (N) Raise both arms up with right palm facing in and left hand supporting the right forearm and start to turn the body to your right. Start to inhale.

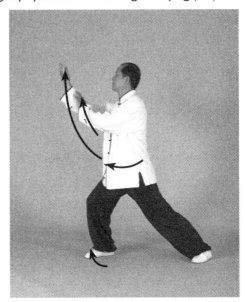

Figure 4-113: (E) Continue turning your body to your right and change your stance into mountain climbing stance (*deng shan bu,* 蹬山步) while moving both of your arms up until the right hand is on the height of the eyebrow, with the elbow down, fingers pointing up. Your right toes should be slightly inward and your left toes should be lined up with your left knee.

Analysis

Your right hand moves up to intercept the opponent's punch and lift it upward, exposing his chest to attack. Your left hand is ready to protect your chest or control his elbow. Move the left leg close to the right leg immediately after the deflection to close your groin area and prevent your opponent from kicking you. Only the toes of the left foot touch the ground, and there is no weight on it, which allows you to kick or step any way you like. Grasp sparrow's tail (right) deflects the opponent's punch and also sets him up for your attack.

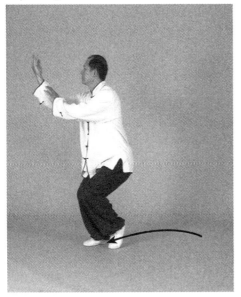

Figure 4-114: (E) Next, bring your left leg next to the right leg. Left leg is on its toes. Complete the inhalation.

3. Grasp the Sparrow's Tail: Left (*Zuo Lan Que Wei*, 左攬雀尾)

This posture is a follow-up to the previous one. While the previous posture is used for defense, this posture is used as a follow-up attack. Sometimes, this form is called diagonal flying (*xie fei shi*, 斜飛勢) instead of grasp the sparrow's tail.

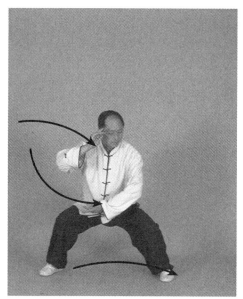

Figure 4-115: (N) Step back with your left leg. Begin to exhale. Turn on the heels into horse stance (*ma bu*, 馬步). Turn your left palm in, brushing by the face. Your right palm turns down and left palm faces up.

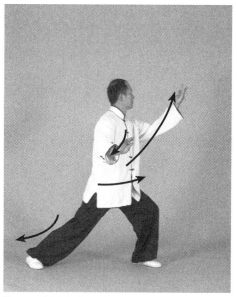

Figure 4-116: (W) Continue to exhale. Turn your body to your left and change your stance into mountain climbing stance (*deng shan bu*, 蹬山步). Swing your left arm to the front and the right hand to the side, with the left palm facing in and the right palm facing down. Complete your exhalation.

Analysis

This posture is used for attack. The right hand's downward motion generates leverage for the left hand's upward attack. Moreover, the right leg is also used to support the left hand's offensive action.

4. Wardoff (*Peng,* 掤)

The Chinese word for wardoff is "peng." Peng means to arc your arms and use them to push or bounce something away. It is used in expressions like "peng kai" (掤開) (push open or push away), which refers to the motion you wish you could use to wade through a crowd and bounce people out of your way.

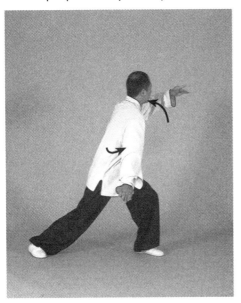

Figure 4-117: (W) Turn the body slightly to your left and rotate your left palm until it is facing downward. Inhale, cave in your chest, and arc your back.

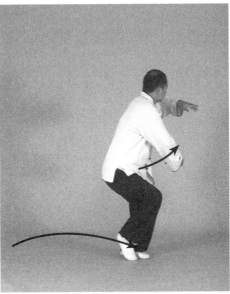

Figure 4-118: (W) Bring the right foot to the side of left foot. Continue inhaling. Swing the right hand to the front of the body, and turn the palm up to face the left palm.

Figure 4-119: (E) Step back with the right leg. Turn on the heels to (E) while shifting into mountain climbing stance (*deng shan bu,* 蹬山步) and swinging the right arm to your right with the arm horizontal, palms facing in and your left palm under the right forearm with palm facing forward and slightly down. Exhale.

Analysis
When your right leg moves close to your left leg, it protects the groin from attack, and is also set up for kicking. When you use peng to bounce your enemy, treat yourself like a beach ball bouncing an outside pressure away. Also, when you bounce, your direction should be forward and slightly upward to pull the enemy's root up so that he will move more easily.

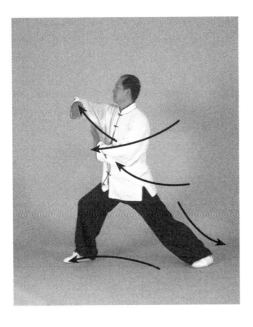

5. Rollback (*Lu*, 擺)

Rollback in Chinese is called "lu." Lu means to lead or neutralize the coming power to the side.

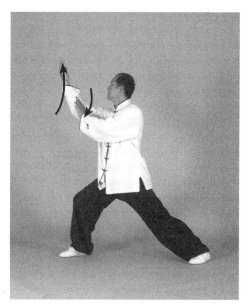

Figure 4-120: (E) Extend the right hand upward while sinking your right elbow. Continue your exhalation from last posture.

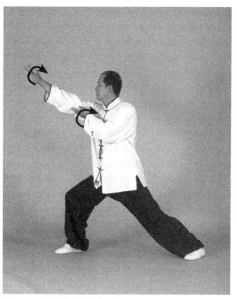

Figure 4-121: (E) Coil your right hand clockwise and forward until the palm is facing forward while turning your left palm to face upward. Begin to inhale.

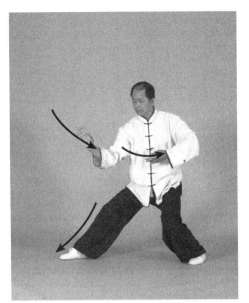

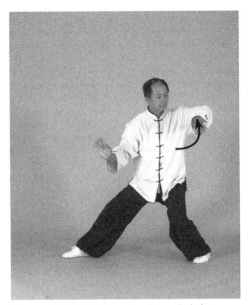

Figure 4-122: (E) Sit back into four-six stance (*si liu bu*, 四六步). Move the right arm down to the front and left hand to your left chest area. Complete your inhalation.

Figure 4-123: (E) Turn the hips slightly to your left. Make a gentle small clockwise circle with your left hand on the left side of the body. This movement does not have a practical application; instead, it is the signature of Yang Style Taijiquan. Exhale.

Analysis

The first part of this form is used to intercept and connect to the opponent's arm. Once you have connected you then rollback to lead his force sideward and past you. When you do small rollback, the movements are small and quick with the intent of exposing your opponent's vital cavities to attack. Large rollback is a larger move that is commonly used to pull the opponent's center and make him lose balance so that you can attack. It is frequently used with a step backward. In order for your rollback to be effective, you must have a firm root and good listening, understanding, adhering and sticking, and leading jins.

6. Press (*Ji*, 擠)

The Chinese word for this form is "ji," and it means to squeeze or press against. Both hands are used to press against your opponent or to squeeze part of his body.

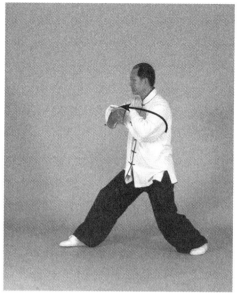

Figure 4-124: (E) Bring the left hand to the inner wrist of the right hand while inhaling. Face turn to the (E).

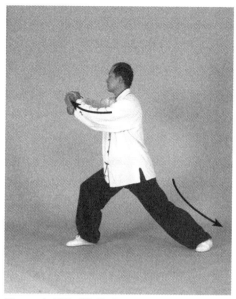

Figure 4-125: (E) Shift into mountain climbing stance (*deng shan bu*, 蹬山步) and extend both hands forward while still touching. Exhale as the arms are extended.

Analysis

The main purpose of this form is to make the opponent fall or bounce away, although it is also used to strike areas such as the solar plexus to seal the breath, or the shoulder blade to numb the shoulder.

7. Push Forward (*An*, 按)

This form is called "an" in Chinese. The Chinese character for the word is made up of two figures meaning "hand" and "peace," and has the meaning of using your hands to hold someone down and inhibit his motion. In everyday speech "an" means to press or push down. In taijiquan, "an" can be used for either offense or defense. When it is used for offense, it is used to push and bounce the opponent away or to push-strike the vital cavities. When it is used for defense, it is used to stick to the opponent's arm and immobilize it, preventing further action. When it is applied onto your enemy, he should feel that his arms have been pressed down and he can neither lift them up nor get away. In offense, "push" can be used in any direction. When it is applied to the enemy for defense, it is usually directed downward.

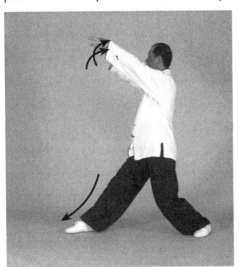

Figure 4-126: (E) Slide the left hand over the right hand. Open the arms to the width of the shoulder. Palms face down. Sit back in four-six stance (*si liu bu*, 四六步) while raising the arms up and back in a circular motion. Start to inhale.

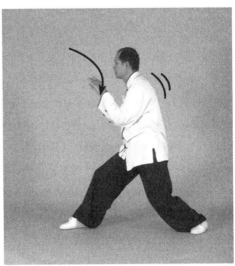

Figure 4-127: (E) Lower the arms to the chest in a circular motion. Fingers point forward. Complete your inhalation.

Analysis

Like "press," push is mainly used as a long jin, although it is sometimes used with short jin for cavity strikes. To understand how to use push jin (or press jin) to bounce the opponent, imagine that you are pushing a large beach ball and trying to bounce it away. If your jin is too short, the ball will bounce you away. However, if your jin is long and you have a good root, then the energy that the ball accumulates will bounce your opponent away.

In taijiquan, when you want to uproot the opponent and bounce him away, you should push forward and upward. When you want to make your opponent lose his stability and fall, you should push to the side or downward. To strike the opponent in the stomach or immobilize his arms, push downward. You can use a single hand push to strike the opponent's solar plexus and bounce him away by using the same principle that was explained in the discussion of press. Naturally, in order to generate enough power to bounce or uproot your opponent you must have a firm root first and then you must have strong push jin.

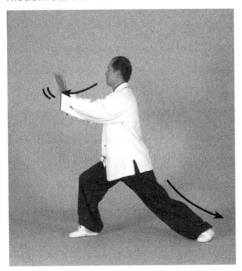

Figure 4-128: (E) Shift to mountain climbing stance (*deng shan bu*, 蹬山步) and push the hands forward while settling down your wrists. Exhale.

8. Single Whip (*Dan Bian,* 單鞭)

The name refers to the way the right hand is held in the sequence; the movement of the left hand is a follow-up movement. The Chinese name is "dan bian." Dan means single or alone. Bian is a whip that can be made of leather, rattan, or even wood. When it is made of leather it is call ruan bian (軟鞭), or soft whip. When it is made of rattan it is called ruan ying bian (軟硬鞭), which means soft-hard whip. When it is made of wood it is called ying bian (硬鞭), which means hard whip. In ancient times a whip was necessary when riding a horse, and naturally techniques were developed for using the whip in battle. Because the whip is not sharp, it is usually only used for deflecting.

In taijiquan, single whip is used to lead the opponent's hand or weapon past your body. The motion is similar to how you might use the whip when riding a horse. The deflection can be soft like a soft whip or hard like a hard whip, depending on the situation.

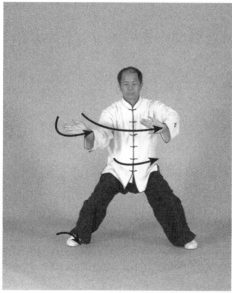

Figure 4-129: (N) Turn both hands to face forward. Keep the arms locked in the same position and turn to (N) on the right heel so the stance is horse stance (*ma bu,* 馬步). Arms swing with the body. Begin to inhale.

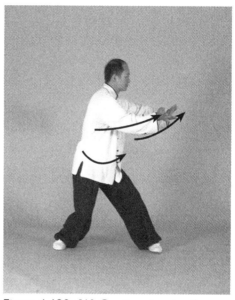

Figure 4-130: (W) Continue turning the body to your left while keeping both of your hands in the same position. Continue your inhalation.

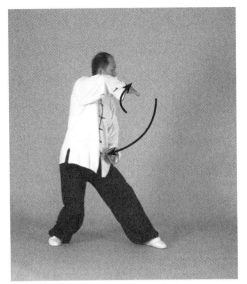

Figure 4-131: (W) Lower the left arm and turn the palm up, and turn your right palm down so that the palms face each other. Complete your inhalation.

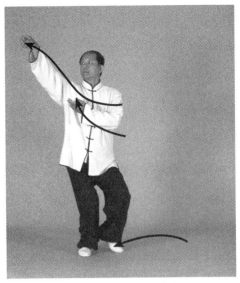

Figure 4-132: (N) Bring the left leg, on its toes, to the right leg. Swing the right arm back. All the fingertips of the right hand are touching and pointing down. Exhale.

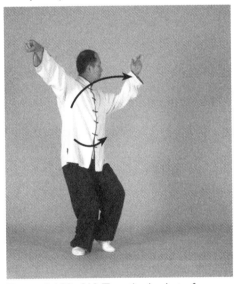

Figure 4-133: (W) Turn the body to face (W). At the same time move the left hand across the body, palm faces in. Inhale.

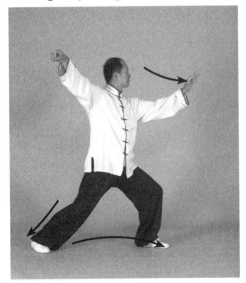

Figure 4-134: (W) Next, turn the palm out and fingers pointing forward. Step the left leg forward so the stance is mountain climbing stance (*deng shan bu*, 蹬山步), and push the left hand forward. Exhale.

Analysis

The rotation of the body to the left just before the whipping motion can be used to deflect an attack to the side. The whip-like motion of the right hand is used to lead the opponent's weapon or hand to the rear. The second half of the form is a follow-up form used for attack. Therefore, in the application you first deflect the opponent's attack with your right hand, and then immediately use your left hand to continue the deflection, if necessary, and then strike. When you deflect, your left foot touches the floor with the toes only. This allows you to kick anytime the opportunity arises.

9. Lift Hands to the Up Posture (*Ti Shou Shang Shi*, 提手上勢)

Lift hands and lean forward was translated from the Chinese name "ti shou shang shi." Ti means to raise up, pull up, or pick up. Therefore, ti shou means to raise your hands. Shang means up and shi means posture. Therefore, the entire name should be translated "raise hands to the up posture."

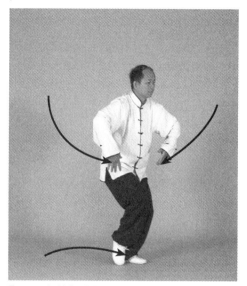

Figure 4-135: (N) Bring the right leg up to the left. Drop the hands down and arc your back. Inhale.

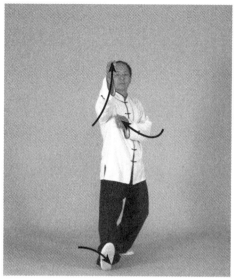

Figure 4-136: (N) Lift the right knee up at the same time as the arms. Place the right leg down on its heel. At the same time, extend the right hand forward, fingers pointing to the front. Left hand is on the right chest area. Exhale.

Analysis

When you lower both hands you protect your dan tian area from attack. Bringing your right leg near the left leg seals your groin against kicks and hand attacks. When your opponent punches your upper body, raise your hands to block his attack; since your right leg is not rooted it can be used for a quick kick.

10. The Crane Spreads Its Wings (*Bai He Liang Chi*, 白鶴亮翅)

The Chinese name of this posture is "bai he liang chi," that means white crane spreads wings. White cranes are very common in China, and are well liked by the people. When a crane fights, it usually blocks with its wings and attacks with both beak and wings. The wings derive their power from a shaking or jerking motion that starts in the body and passes to the wings. This is the same motion the crane uses to shake off water after it rains. The crane is not a muscular or strong bird, but when it strikes with its wings it can break branches and kill or injure its enemy. In order to have this kind of strong jerking power, you must have an extremely strong root. Cranes have an inborn ability to maintain balance no matter what. In China, you can often see them perched on tree branches or bamboo. No matter how strong the wind blows and the branch shakes, the crane will remain there without moving.

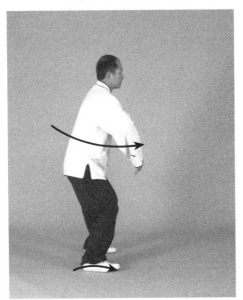

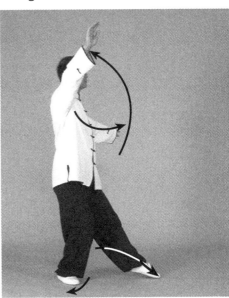

Figure 4-137: (W) Set the right foot down. Turn the body to (W) and into horse stance (*ma bu*, 馬步); simultaneously, swing the right arm down and up, making it cross the left hand that has remained stationary. Both feet are parallel. Inhale.

Figure 4-138: (W) Spread the arms, right arm higher than the left, while bringing the left leg to the right leg and then forward to form the false stance (*xu bu*, 虚步). As the arms are spread, place your weight on your right foot while pointing out 45 degrees. Exhale. The arms are the wings being spread open.

Analysis

Moving your hands to your chest seals your chest area to protect it from attack. The strongest part of the crane's body is its wings; therefore that is what it uses to block and to seal the opponent's attack. Once you have prevented the opponent from continuing his attack, you can then use your wings (hands and arms) to spread your opponent's attack to the sides. This will open the front of your opponent's body to attack.

11. Brush Knee and Step Forward: Left (*Zuo Lou Xi Ao Bu,* 左摟膝拗步)

The Chinese name of this form is "lou xi ao bu." Lou in Chinese means to embrace, to hook, or to brush, and xi means knee; therefore lou xi means to brush your knee. Yao means to twist or twist off and is commonly used in expressions such as yao zhe (拗折) or yao duan (拗斷), that means to break off by twisting. Bu means step; therefore ao bu means to step forward with a twisting motion.

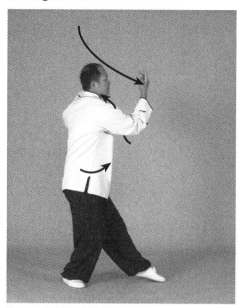

Figure 4-139: (W) Turn your body to your left slightly and swing the right arm across the body. Inhale.

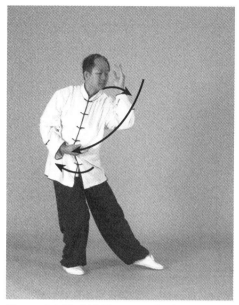

Figure 4-140: (W) Turn your body to your right. Swing the left arm across the upper body, palm facing inward, while lowering your right arm to the waist area, palm facing upward. Continue to inhale.

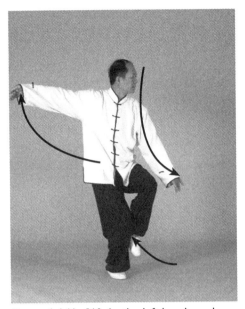

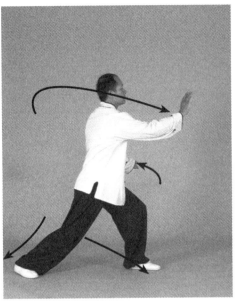

Figure 4-141: (W) As the left hand reaches the center of the body, raise the left knee, swing the left arm past it, and raise the right arm back and up to a place near the right ear. Complete your exhalation.

Figure 4-142: (W) Clear down with your left hand as you step down with the left leg into mountain climbing stance (*deng shan bu*, 蹬山步). Inhale. Push forward with the right palm with fingers pointing forward first and then settle down the wrist. Exhale.

Analysis

You pull your left knee up to seal the groin and twist your body to the right to protect your chest. Once you are in this position, your left leg is alive for kicking. Alternatively, step your left leg down behind your opponent's front leg to stop him from retreating, and at the same time use your right hand to strike.

12. Play the Guitar (*Shou Hui Pi Pa*, 手揮琵琶)

This form is called "shou hui pi pa." Shou means hands and hui means to strum on. The pi pa is a Chinese musical instrument, known as a balloon-guitar. When the pi pa is played it is held vertically in front of the chest, not against the abdomen like a Western guitar.

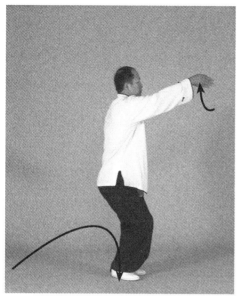

Figure 4-143: (W) Bring the right leg up with the knee lifted. Scoop your right hand clockwise and turn the right palm to the side. Step down with the right leg. Inhale.

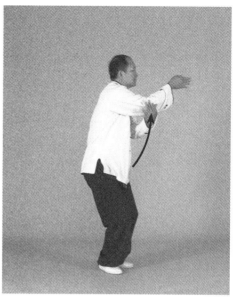

Figure 4-144: (W) Put the palm of the left hand on the outside portion of the right arm and start to lift the left knee. Begin to exhale.

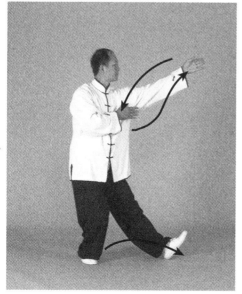

Figure 4-145: (W) Slide the left hand forward along the right arm. Put the left leg down on its heel. Extend the left hand, palm to the right side and fingers pointing forward and upward. Exhale. The left hand holds the guitar, while the right plays it. Complete your exhalation.

Analysis

When your opponent punches, first raise your right hand to lift up his punch and open his chest area to attack. Since both feet are together when you deflect, you can easily use either leg for kicking. Your left hand can either control his arm or strike.

13. Twist Body, Brush Knee and Step Forward: Left (*Zuo Lou Xi Ao Bu*, 左摟膝拗步)

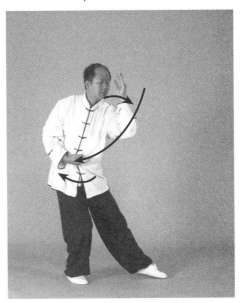

Figure 4-146: (W) Turn your body to your right. Swing the left arm across the upper body, palm facing inward, while lowering your right arm to the waist area, palm facing upward. Continue to inhale.

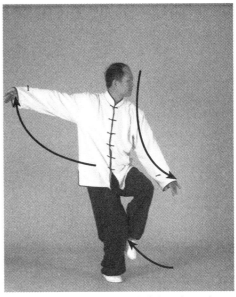

Figure 4-147: (W) As the left hand reaches the center of the body, raise the left knee, swing the left arm past it, and raise the right arm back and up to a place near the right ear. Complete your exhalation.

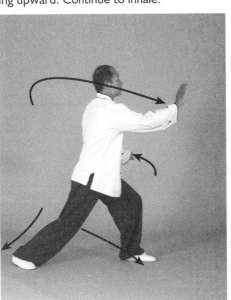

Figure 4-148: (W) Clear down with your left hand as you step down with the left leg into mountain climbing stance (*deng shan bu*, 蹬山步). Inhale. Push forward with the right palm with fingers pointing forward first and then settle down the wrist. Exhale.

14. Twist Body, Brush Knee and Step Forward: Right (*You Lou Xi Ao Bu,* 右摟膝拗步)

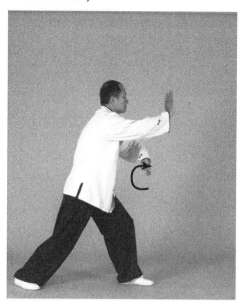

Figure 4-149: (W) Make a counterclockwise circle with the left arm. Start to inhale.

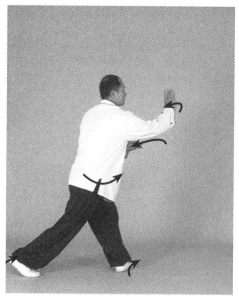

Figure 4-150: (W) Turn the left foot so the stance is sitting on crossed legs stance (*zuo pan bu,* 坐盤步). The right foot is on its toe. Complete inhale.

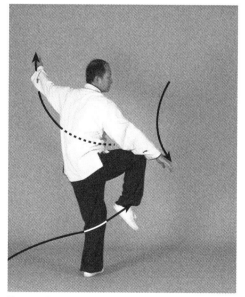

Figure 4-151: (W) Lift your right leg and brush down your right hand while circling your left hand behind you. Exhale.

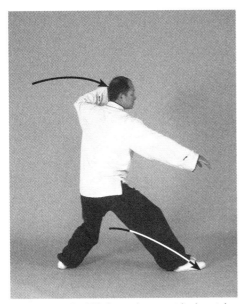

Figure 4-152: (W) Step down with the right leg. Inhale.

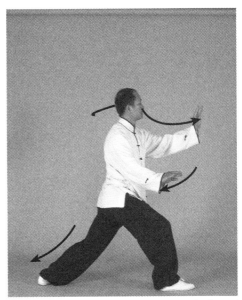

Figure 4-153: (W) Push forward with the left palm with fingers pointing forward first and then settle down the wrist. Exhale.

15. Twist Body, Brush Knee and Step Forward: Left (*Zuo Lou Xi Ao Bu,* 左搂膝拗步)

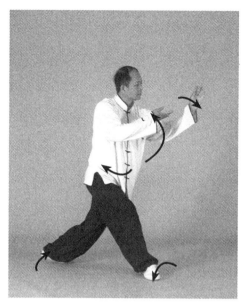

Figure 4-154: (W) Make a clockwise circle with the right hand, turn your left palm to face your right, and twist your body and shift into sitting on crossed legs stance (*zuo pan bu*, 坐盤步). Begin inhale.

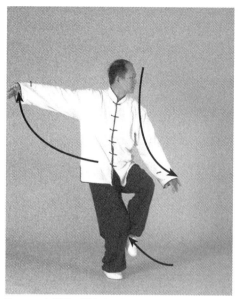

Figure 4-155: (W) As the left hand reaches the center of the body, raise the left knee, swing the left arm past it, and raise the right arm back and up to a place near the right ear. Exhale.

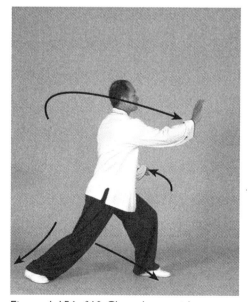

Figure 4-156: (W) Clear down with your left hand as you step down with the left leg into mountain climbing stance (*deng shan bu*, 蹬山步). Inhale. Push forward with the right palm with fingers pointing forward first and then settle down the wrist. Exhale.

16. Play the Guitar (*Shou Hui Pi Pa*, 手揮琵琶)

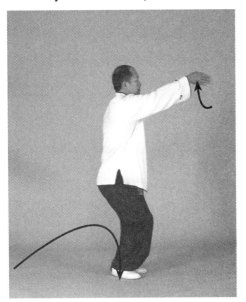

Figure 4-157: (W) Bring the right leg up with the knee lifted. Scoop your right hand clockwise and turn the right palm to the side. Step down with the right leg. Inhale.

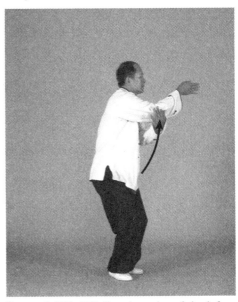

Figure 4-158: (W) Put the palm of the left hand on the outside portion of the right arm and start to lift the left knee. Begin to exhale.

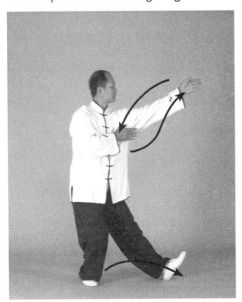

Figure 4-159: (W) Slide the left hand forward along the right arm. Put the left leg down on its heel. Extend the left hand, palm to the right side and fingers pointing forward and upward. Exhale. The left hand holds the guitar, while the right plays it. Complete your exhalation.

17. Twist Body, Brush Knee and Step Forward: Left (*Zuo Lou Xi Ao Bu,* 左摟膝拗步)

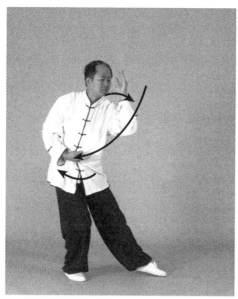

Figure 4-160: (W) Turn your body to your right. Swing the left arm across the upper body, palm facing inward, while lowering your right arm to the waist area, palm facing upward. Continue to inhale.

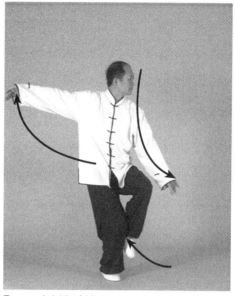

Figure 4-161: (W) As the left hand reaches the center of the body, raise the left knee, swing the left arm past it, and raise the right arm back and up to a place near the right ear. Complete your exhalation.

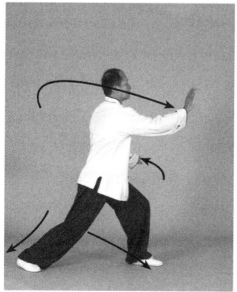

Figure 4-162: (W) Clear down with your left hand as you step down with the left leg into mountain climbing stance (*deng shan bu,* 蹬山步). Inhale. Push forward with the right palm with fingers pointing forward first and then settle down the wrist. Exhale.

18. Twist Body and Circle the Fist (*Pie Shen Chui*, 撇身捶)

This form is called "pie shen chui." Pie means to twist or swing aside. It is commonly used in expressions such as pie kai (撇開), which means to set something aside or push it away. Shen means body, and chui means to strike. Therefore, this form should be translated "twist your body and strike." This name tells you that in this form you must first turn your body to evade the opponent's attack, and then use your fist to strike the opponent. This form is generally used together with the next form: step forward, deflect downward, parry, and punch.

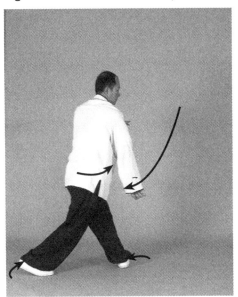

Analysis
This form is to neutralize your opponent's low attack to your left side. You are also set up for a kick with your right leg. In fact, this posture is set up for the following attack.

Figure 4-163: (W) Twist your body to your left and shift the stance to sitting on crossed legs stance (*zuo pan bu*, 坐盤步) while the right arm, in a fist, makes a big semi-circle from the front of the chest down to the thighs. Inhale.

19. Step Forward, Deflect Downward, Parry and Punch (*Jin Bu Ban Lan Chui*, 進步搬攔捶)

This form is called "jin bu ban lan chui" in Chinese. Jin bu means to move forward; ban means to remove or shift; lan means to hinder, obstruct, intercept, block, or cut off; and chui means to punch. The translation of this form should therefore be "step forward, remove, intercept, and punch." The name tells you that after doing the last form, in which you turn your body to evade your opponent's attack to the side, you continue your movements by stepping forward, moving the opponent's punch to the side and down, hindering any further action, and punching him. From this explanation you can see that from the beginning, when your hand first touches your opponent's hand, you use a few techniques to lead his punch to the side, stick with him and hinder him, and finally strike him.

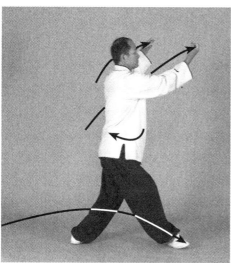

Figure 4-164: (W) Step forward with the right leg into sitting on crossed legs stance (*zuo pan bu*, 坐盤步) while circling the right arm up and forward. Start to exhale.

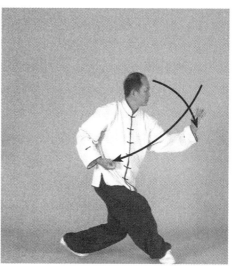

Figure 4-165: (W) Continue twisting to your right, and move your right hand to your waist while covering your left hand. Complete exhaling and then to the waist. The left arm swings across the body. Complete your inhalation.

Analysis

These forms are used to connect and then adhere and stick at close range. You first evade the opponent's attack by twisting your body to the side; your right arm moves out to seal your chest. After your opponent's punch has missed, he will immediately attempt to pull his hand back. In order to maintain the connection with your opponent, circle your right hand to your right and at the same time take two steps forward. This allows you to stick to your opponent's hand as he pulls it back, as well as lock his leg with your second step. Because your adhering and sticking have placed your opponent in a passive position, immediately use your left hand to push his arm down or to the side to allow your right hand to strike. This form is similar to brush knee and twist step, except that it is for short range while brush knee and twist step is for medium range.

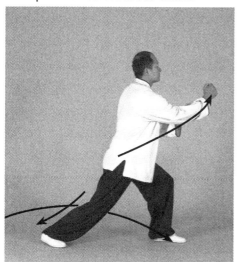

Figure 4-166: (W) Step forward with the left leg into mountain climbing stance (*deng shan bu*, 蹬山步) while punching your right fist forward and sliding your left hand to the inside of your right elbow area. When you step forward, inhale, and when you punch, exhale.

20. Seal Tightly (*Ru Feng Si Bi,* 如封似閉)

The Chinese name of this form is "ru feng si bi." Ru means like, if, or as; and feng means to seal up or blockade. Therefore ru feng means "as if sealing up." Si in Chinese means like, as, if, or seem to, and bi means close up. Therefore, si bi means, "as if closing up." Therefore, the translation of this form should be "as if sealing, as if closing up."

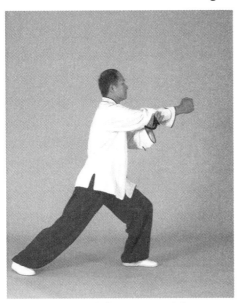

Figure 4-167: (W) Contiune to slide your left hand under the right elbow, with the palm of your left hand facing in to your right arm. Start to inhale.

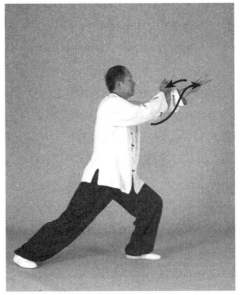

Figure 4-168: (W) Coil the left hand around the right forearm, move from the elbow to the wrist, and extend forward. When the left hand has reached its maximum extension, start to pull in the right fist. Continue to inhale.

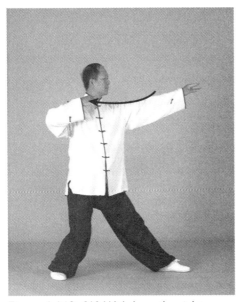

Figure 4-169: (W) Withdraw the right arm to chest area while sitting back in four-six stance (*si liu bu,* 四六步). Complete your inhalation.

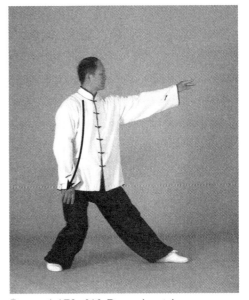

Figure 4-170: (W) Drop the right arm down. Exhale.

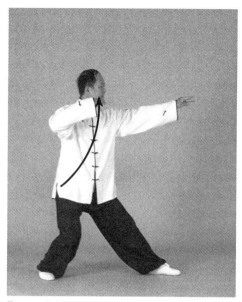

Figure 4-171: (W) Raise the right arm up so it is beside the ear. Inhale.

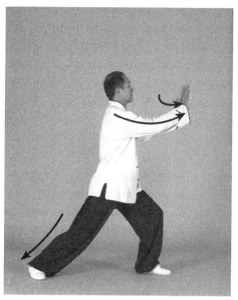

Figure 4-172: (W) Shift the stance to mountain climbing stance (*deng shan bu*, 蹬山步) and push the right palm forward. The left hand opens into a palm, pushing forward. Exhale.

Analysis
This form is commonly used to nullify the opponent's grabbing, coiling, wrapping, or drilling.

21. Embrace the Tiger and Return to the Mountain (*Bao Hu Gui Shan,* 抱虎歸山)

The Chinese name of this form is "bao hu gui shan" and means embrace tiger and return to the mountain. The tiger is a very dangerous animal, and to say that you are embracing one implies that you are embracing an enemy. In order to embrace a tiger safely, you must hold him close and tight so that he cannot claw you. You must do the same thing when you embrace an opponent—you must hold him close so that he cannot hurt you. Return to the mountain implies that it is a long way to return home and that this form is therefore a long jin. A short jin will not work. To return home with a tiger you have to carry him, which tells you that this form is meant to destroy the opponent's root.

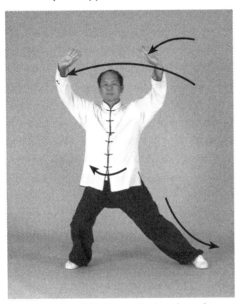

Figure 4-173: (N) Cross the hands and turn the body (N), and then open both of your arms. Lean to the right side. Inhale.

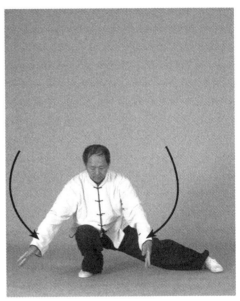

Figure 4-174: (N) Squat down into tame the tiger stance (*fu hu bu*, 伏虎步) while circling both arms out, down, and in. Weight is on the right leg. Begin to exhale.

22. **Close Taiji** (*He Taiji,* 合太極)

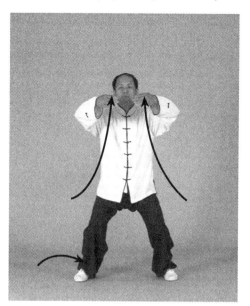

Figure 4-175: (N) Shift the weight to the left leg, raise the right knee, and step the right leg down in horse stance (*ma bu,* 馬步). Move both hands to the chest area. Arms are in a circle. Complete exhaling.

End of the First Part.

Transition Form (*Guo Du Shi*, 過渡勢)

In Yang Style Taijiquan there is no name for this transition. It is very similar to the form "white snake turns body and spits poison" in part 3 of the sequence (posture 91 in this chapter); however, there are two differences. First, in the beginning of this form only the toes of the right foot touch the floor, and there is no weight on the foot; whereas in the form white snake turns, both feet are flat on the floor. Second, the jin that is applied in this form is a long jin, while white snake turns uses short, fast jin.

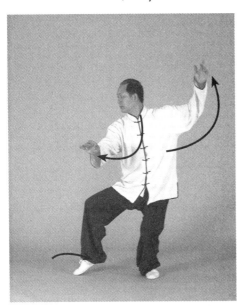 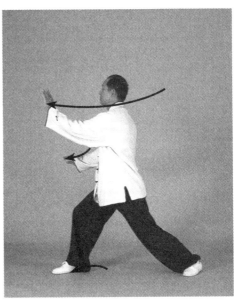

Figure 4-176: (E) Withdraw and raise the right leg on its toe. Swing the right arm down; the left arm comes up to behind the left ear. Inhale.

Figure 4-177: (E) Step right leg forward into mountain climbing stance (*deng shan bu*, 蹬山步), and push the left hand forward. Exhale.

Analysis

Your root must be solid so that you can twist your body and generate jin. This will enable you to loosen an opponent's bear hug or deflect an attack to the side. Once you have done this you will have enough time to shift your root to the left, allowing your right foot to be alive for other applications.

23. Wardoff, Rollback, Press, and Push Forward (*Peng Lu Ji An,* 掤攦擠按)

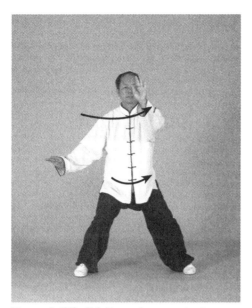

Figure 4-178: (N) Keep the arms in the same position and turn your body 90 degrees to face (N) on your right heel. Start to inhale.

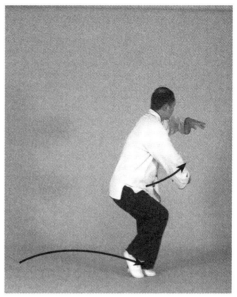

Figure 4-179: (W) Bring the right foot to the side of left foot. Continue inhaling. Swing the right hand to the front of the body, and turn the palm up to face the left palm.

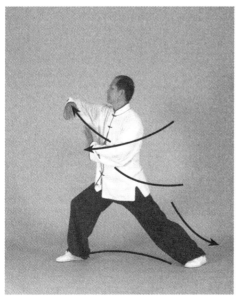

Figure 4-180: (E) Step back with the right leg. Turn on the heels to (E) while shifting into mountain climbing stance (*deng shan bu,* 蹬山步) while swinging the right arm to your right with the arm horizontal, palms facing in and your left palm under the right forearm with palm facing forward and slightly down. Exhale.

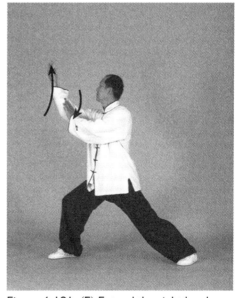

Figure 4-181: (E) Extend the right hand upward while sinking your right elbow. Continue your exhalation from last posture.

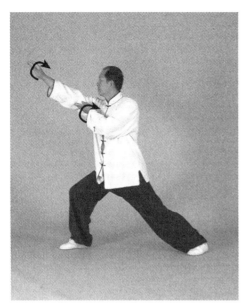

Figure 4-182: (E) Coil your right hand clockwise and forward until the palm is facing forward while turning your left palm to face upward. Begin to inhale.

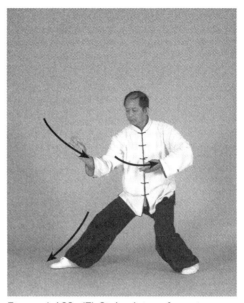

Figure 4-183: (E) Sit back into four-six stance (si liu bu, 四六步). Move the right arm down to the front and left hand to your left chest area. Complete your inhalation.

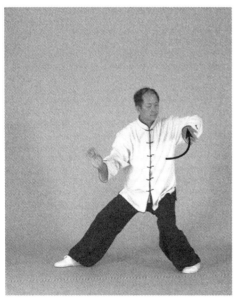

Figure 4-184: (E) Turn the hips slightly to your left. Make a gentle small clockwise circle with your left hand on the left side of the body. This movement does not have a practical application; instead, it is the signature of Yang Style Taijiquan. Exhale.

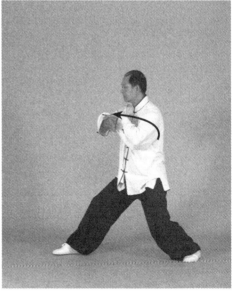

Figure 4-185: (E) Bring the left hand to the inner wrist of the right hand while inhaling. Face turn to the (E).

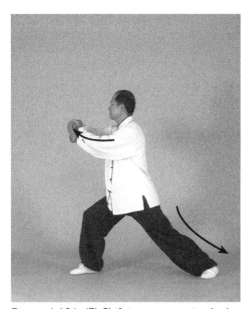

Figure 4-186: (E) Shift into mountain climbing stance (*deng shan bu*, 蹬山步) and extend both hands forward while still touching. Exhale as the arms are extended.

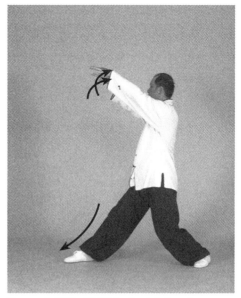

Figure 4-187: (E) Slide the left hand over the right hand. Open the arms to the width of the shoulder. Palms face down. Sit back in four-six stance (*si liu bu*, 四六步) while raising the arms up and back in a circular motion. Start to inhale.

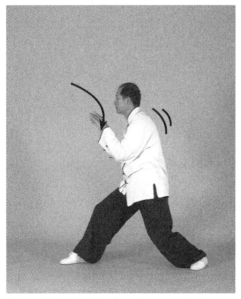

Figure 4-188: (E) Lower the arms to the chest in a circular motion. Fingers point forward. Complete your inhalation.

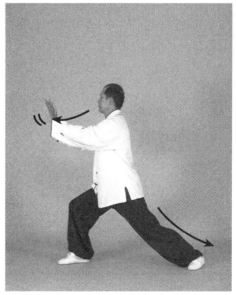

Figure 4-189: (E) Shift to mountain climbing stance (*deng shan bu*, 蹬山步) and push the hands forward while settling down your wrists. Exhale.

24. Single Whip (*Dan Bian*, 單鞭)

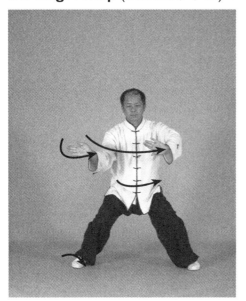

Figure 4-190: (N) Turn both hands to face forward. Keep the arms locked in the same position and turn to (N) on the right heel so the stance is horse stance (*ma bu*, 馬步). Arms swing with the body. Begin to inhale.

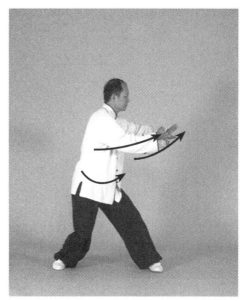

Figure 4-191: (W) Continue turning the body to your left while keeping both of your hands in the same position. Continue your inhalation.

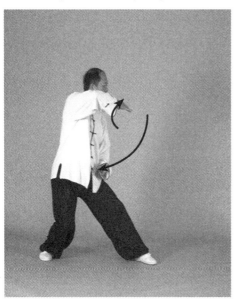

Figure 4-192: (W) Lower the left arm and turn the palm up, and turn your right palm down so that the palms face each other. Complete your inhalation.

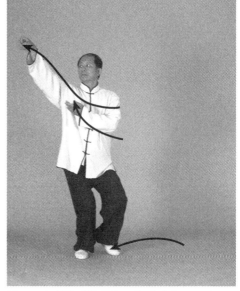

Figure 4-193: (N) Bring the left leg, on its toes, to the right leg. Swing the right arm back. All the fingertips of the right hand are touching and pointing down. Exhale.

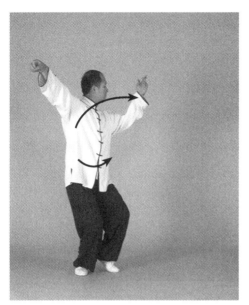 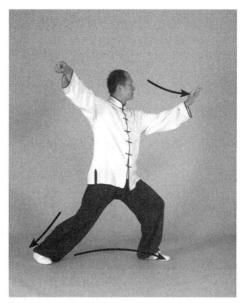

Figure 4-194: (W) Turn the body to face (W). At the same time move the left hand across the body, palm faces in. Inhale.

Figure 4-195: (W) Next, turn the palm out and fingers pointing forward. Step the left leg forward so the stance is mountain climbing stance (*deng shan bu*, 蹬山步), and push the left hand forward. Exhale.

25. Punch Under the Elbow (*Zhou Di Kan Chui*, 肘底看捶)

The Chinese name of this form is "zhou di kan chui." Zhou is "elbow," di is "bottom," kan is "look," and chui is "punch or strike." The name therefore means "look at the punch under the elbow," and implies "beware of the punch from under the elbow."

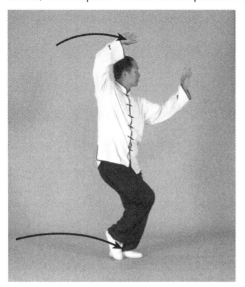

Figure 4-196: (W) Bring the right foot, on its toes, up to the left leg while moving the right hand over the head. Begin to inhale.

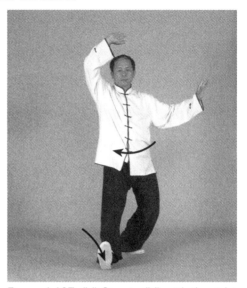

Figure 4-197: (N) Step to (N) with the right leg touching down with the heel. Complete your inhalation.

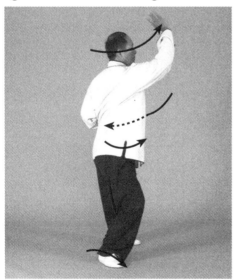

Figure 4-198: (W) Turn the body (W), raise the left leg, turn 45 degrees and touch down. At the same time, start to cover the right arm down, and move the left hand up on the inside of the right arm. Begin to exhale.

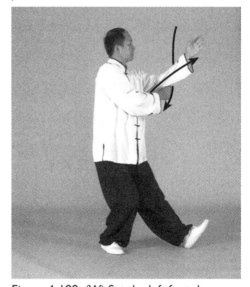

Figure 4-199: (W) Set the left foot down on the heel while bringing the left elbow up above the right fist. Complete your exhalation.

Analysis

The first step in this form is a yielding movement. Avoid the opponent's attack by stepping to the side while using your hands to neutralize the opponent's attack and trap his hands. Your left hand can attack the opponent's face and your right hand can strike his chest. Your left leg has no weight on it and can be used for kicking.

26. Step Back and Repulse the Monkey: Left (*Zuo Dao Nian Hou*, 左倒攆猴)

The Chinese name of this form is "dao nian hou." Dao means to move backward, nian means to repel or drive away, and hou is monkey. Monkeys specialize in grabbing and sticking. The name of this form tells you that it is used when someone is trying to grab your hands or arms and you are moving backward and fending him off.

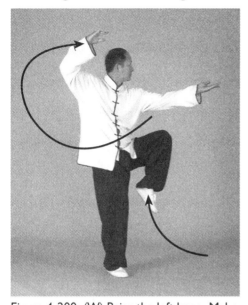

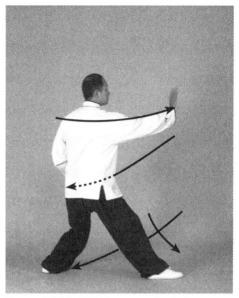

Figure 4-200: (W) Raise the left knee. Make a counterclockwise circle with the left hand so the palm ends facing up. Swing the right hand down, back, and up so the palm faces forward. Inhale.

Figure 4-201: (W) Turn your body by turning your right heel, until the toes are pointing forward. Extend the left leg back and step down. Shift into four-six stance (*si liu bu*, 四六步) while pushing forward with the right palm, withdrawing the left palm to the waist. Exhale.

Analysis

The first motion of this form is to twist your hand out of the opponent's grasp and to grasp his arm. Raising your leg prepares you for either kicking or retreating. Once you have stepped back you can control the opponent's arm and either strike him or knock him down.

27. Step Back and Repulse the Monkey: Right (*You Dao Nian Hou,* 右倒攆猴)

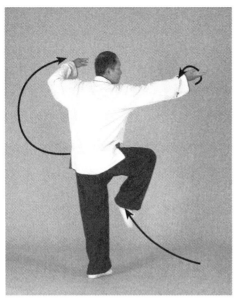

Figure 4-202: (W) Lift the right knee up. Make a clockwise circle with the right hand, palm up. Swing the left hand down, back, and up so the palm faces front. Inhale.

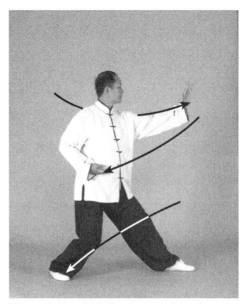

Figure 4-203: (W) Turn your left heel until the toes are pointing forward. Extend the right leg back and step down. Shift into four-six stance (*si liu bu,* 四六步) while pushing the left palm forward and retreating the right palm to the waist. Exhale.

28. Step Back and Repulse the Monkey: Left (*Zuo Dao Nian Hou,* 左倒攆猴)

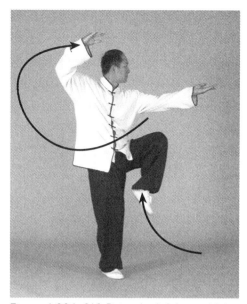

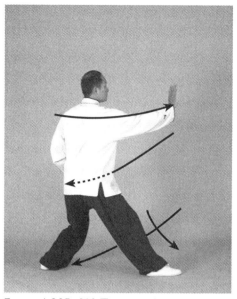

Figure 4-204: (W) Raise the left knee. Make a counterclockwise circle with the left hand so the palm ends facing up. Swing the right hand down, back, and up so the palm faces forward. Inhale.

Figure 4-205: (W) Turn your body by turning your right heel, until the toes are pointing forward. Extend the left leg back and step down. Shift into four-six stance (*si liu bu,* 四六步) while pushing forward with the right palm, withdrawing the left palm to the waist. Exhale.

29. Diagonal Flying (*Xie Fei Shi*, 斜飛勢)

The Chinese name of this form is "xie fei shi." Xie means slanted, inclined, or oblique, fei means to fly, and shi means posture. Therefore, the translation should be "oblique flying posture." The name tells you that when you use this posture your arms move out diagonally as if you were flying.

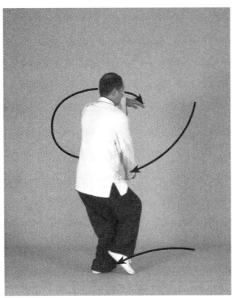

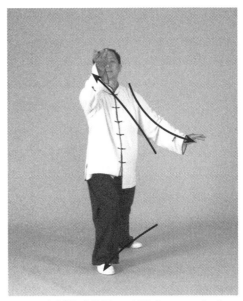

Figure 4-206: (S) Circle the left hand up, palm facing down, and the right hand down, palm facing up, while bringing your right leg in to the side of the left leg. Inhale.

Figure 4-207: (N) Turn 180 degrees clockwise on the left heel. Step the right leg down into mountain climbing stance (*deng shan bu*, 蹬山步) while spreading both of your hands apart, right palm up to the front of the face. The left hand moves, palm down, down to the side. Exhale.

Analysis

This form neutralizes an attack by deflecting with your left hand and twisting your body to the side. Your arm or shoulder is then used to push or bounce the opponent diagonally upward to uproot him and make him fall. When you defend, there is no weight on your right leg, so you can easily use it for kicking.

30. Lift Hands to the Up Posture (*Ti Shou Shang Shi,* 提手上勢)

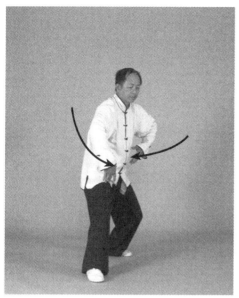

Figure 4-208: (N) Move both arms in toward your abdominal area, while shifting your weight onto your left foot. Inhale.

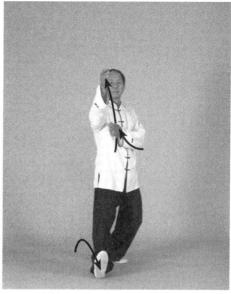

Figure 4-209: (N) Lift your right leg up, and then touch down with heel while raising both your hands up to the chest area. Exhale.

31. The Crane Spreads Its Wings (*Bai He Liang Chi,* 白鶴亮翅)

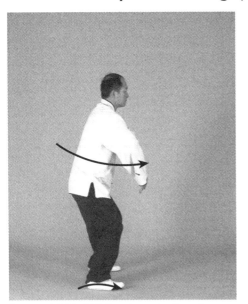 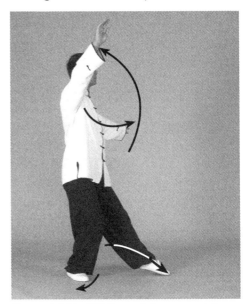

Figure 4-210: (W) Set the right foot down. Turn the body to (W) and into horse stance (*ma bu,* 馬步); simultaneously, swing the right arm down and up, making it cross the left hand that has remained stationary. Both feet are parallel. Inhale.

Figure 4-211: (W) Spread the arms, right arm higher than the left, while bringing the left leg to the right leg and then forward to form the false stance (*xu bu,* 虛步). As the arms are spread, place your weight on your right foot while pointing out 45 degrees. Exhale. The arms are the wings being spread open.

32. Brush Knee and Step Forward: Left (*Zuo Lou Xi Ao Bu,* 左摟膝拗步)

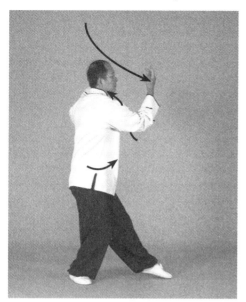

Figure 4-212: (W) Turn your body to your left slightly and swing the right arm across the body. Inhale.

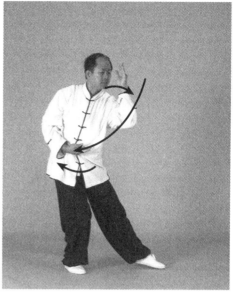

Figure 4-213: (W) Turn your body to your right. Swing the left arm across the upper body, palm facing inward, while lowering your right arm to the waist area, palm facing upward. Continue to inhale.

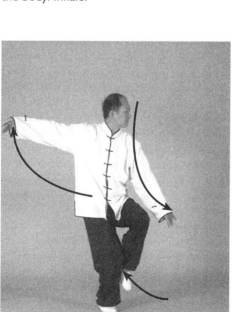

Figure 4-214: (W) As the left hand reaches the center of the body, raise the left knee, swing the left arm past it, and raise the right arm back and up to a place near the right ear. Complete your exhalation.

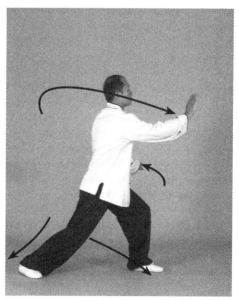

Figure 4-215: (W) Clear down with your left hand as you step down with the left leg into mountain climbing stance (*deng shan bu,* 蹬山步). Inhale. Push forward with the right palm with fingers pointing forward first and then settle down the wrist. Exhale.

33. Pick Up the Needle from the Sea Bottom (*Hai Di Lao Zhen,* 海底撈針)

The Chinese name of this form is "hai di lao zhen." Hai di means sea bottom, lao means to scoop up, and zhen means needle. Therefore, the translation of this form is "scoop up needle from the sea bottom." According to Chinese custom, the top of the head is called tian ling gai (天靈蓋) and means heaven spirit cover, and the perineum is called hai di (海底) and means sea bottom. Therefore, the name of this form indicates that you are attacking the groin from below.

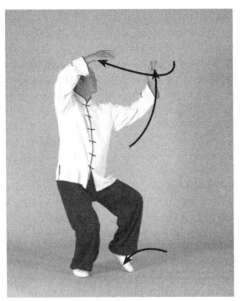

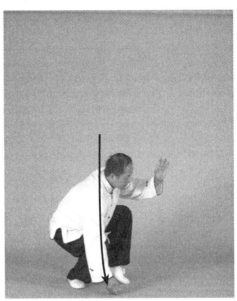

Figure 4-216: (W) Withdraw the left leg in on its toes while bringing the right hand back, palm facing in, and pushing out the left palm. Inhale.

Figure 4-217: (W) Scoop down, the right hand "picking" an object from the floor. Exhale.

Analysis
When your opponent attacks high, pull back your body and use both hands to intercept and deflect his attack. His right side is now exposed to attack. Since your left leg has no weight on it, it can be used for a quick kick. The dropping motion in this technique can also be used as a downward pluck.

34. Fan Back (*Shan Tong Bei,* 扇通背)

The Chinese name of this form is "shan tong bei." Shan means fan, tong means through or reachable, and bei means back. In China there is a kind of monkey with very long arms. Their arms are so long they can easily scratch their backs, and so they are called tong bei yuan (通背猿), which means reach the back apes, or tong bi yuan (通臂猿) that means reachable arm apes. This indicates that when you use this form your arms are long and stretched out far, and therefore the jin is a long jin. When you draw back in the first part of this form you should arc your back to accumulate as much jin as possible; then when you straighten out, you extend your arms like a Chinese fan.

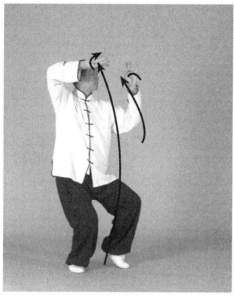

Figure 4-218: (W) Stand up into the position of 4-216 but with the right palm facing out. Inhale.

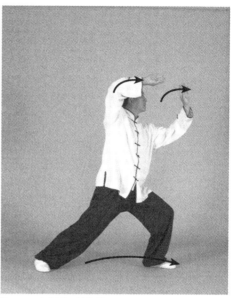

Figure 4-219: (W) Shift the stance into mountain climbing stance (*deng shan bu,* 蹬山步) while moving both arms forward. Exhale.

Analysis

This form is generally used for close range. After you neutralize the opponent's attack, use both hands to push him off balance.

35. Turn, Twist Body, and Circle the Fist (*Zhuan Shen Pie Shen Chui*, 轉身撇身捶)

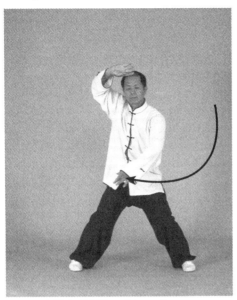

Figure 4-220: (N) Turn N into horse stance (*ma bu*, 馬步) and circumscribe a large counterclockwise circle in front of the body with the left hand. Start to inhale.

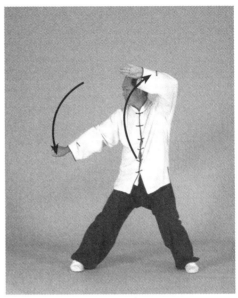

Figure 4-221: (N) Continue to circle your left hand up while circling your right hand down. Complete the inhalation.

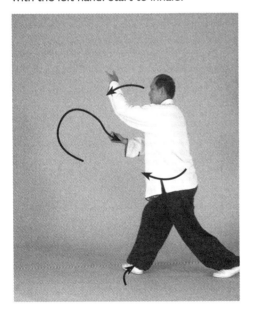

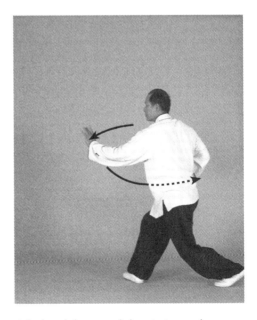

Figures 4-222 and 4-223: (E) Continue circling your right hand down and then in toward you, and finally out to strike from high to low. Then pull your right hand back to your right waist, while covering down with your left hand. While doing this, you are also turning your body to your right on the front heel and the toes of the rear foot. Exhale.

36. Step Forward, Deflect Downward, Parry and Punch (*Jin Bu Ban Lan Chui*, 進步搬攔捶)

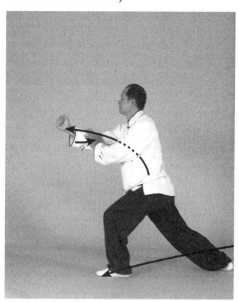

Figure 4-224: (E) Step forward with the left leg into mountain climbing stance (*deng shan bu*, 蹬山步). Inhale. Then, punch with the right fist. Exhale. Refer No. 19.

37. Step Forward, Wardoff, Rollback, Press and Push Forward (*Shang Bu Beng Lu Ji An*, 上步掤攦擠按)

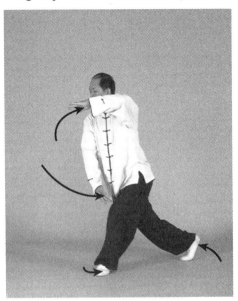

Figure 4-225: (E) Turn the legs so that you are in the sitting on crossed legs stance (*zuo pan bu*, 坐盤步) while lowering your right hand, palm up. As you do this, you also raise your left hand straight up and neutralize to your left. Inhale.

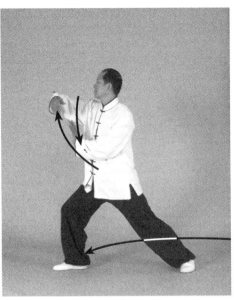

Figure 4-226: (E) Step forward with the right leg into mountain climbing stance (*deng shan bu*, 蹬山步) and swing the right arm up. Exhale.

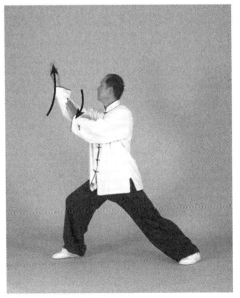

Figure 4-227: (E) Extend the right hand upward while sinking your right elbow. Continue your exhalation from last posture.

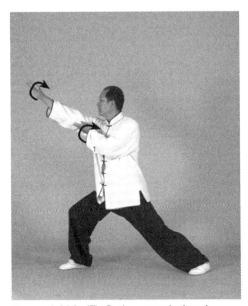

Figure 4-228: (E) Coil your right hand clockwise and forward until the palm is facing forward while turning your left palm to face upward. Begin to inhale.

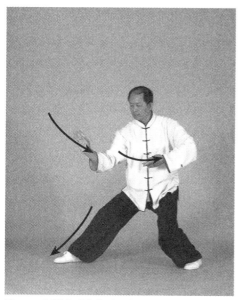

Figure 4-229: (E) Sit back into four-six stance (*si liu bu*, 四六步). Move the right arm down to the front and left hand to your left chest area. Complete your inhalation.

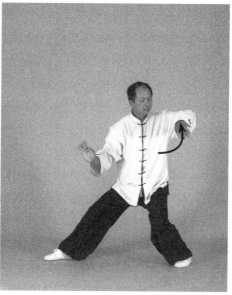

Figure 4-230: (E) Turn the hips slightly to your left. Make a gentle small clockwise circle with your left hand on the left side of the body. This movement does not have a practical application; instead, it is the signature of Yang Style Taijiquan. Exhale.

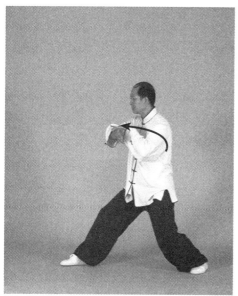

Figure 4-231: (E) Bring the left hand to the inner wrist of the right hand while inhaling. Face turn to the (E).

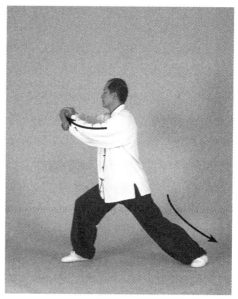

Figure 4-232: (E) Shift into mountain climbing stance (*deng shan bu*, 蹬山步) and extend both hands forward while still touching. Exhale as the arms are extended.

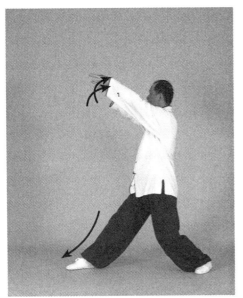

Figure 4-233: (E) Slide the left hand over the right hand. Open the arms to the width of the shoulder. Palms face down. Sit back in four-six stance (*si liu bu*, 四六步) while raising the arms up and back in a circular motion. Start to inhale.

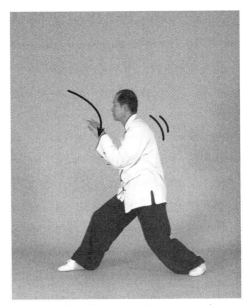

Figure 4-234: (E) Lower the arms to the chest in a circular motion. Fingers point forward. Complete your inhalation.

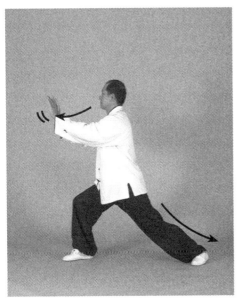

Figure 4-235: (E) Shift to mountain climbing stance (*deng shan bu*, 蹬山步) and push the hands forward while settling down your wrists. Exhale.

38. Single Whip (*Dan Bian,* 單鞭)

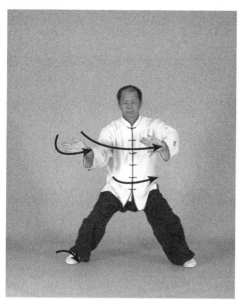

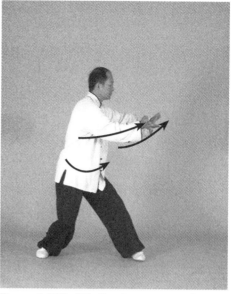

Figure 4-236: (N) Turn both hands to face forward. Keep the arms locked in the same position and turn to (N) on the right heel so the stance is horse stance (*ma bu,* 馬步). Arms swing with the body. Begin to inhale.

Figure 4-237: (W) Continue turning the body to your left while keeping both of your hands in the same position. Continue your inhalation.

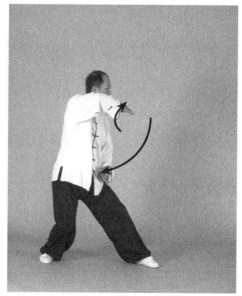

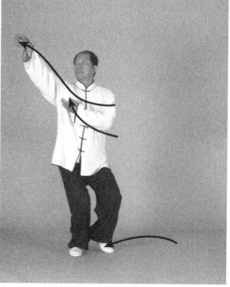

Figure 4-238: (W) Lower the left arm and turn the palm up, and turn your right palm down so that the palms face each other. Complete your inhalation.

Figure 4-239: (N) Bring the left leg, on its toes, to the right leg. Swing the right arm back. All the fingertips of the right hand are touching and pointing down. Exhale.

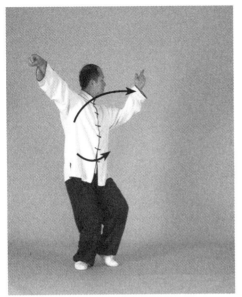

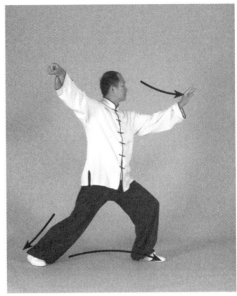

Figure 4-240: (W) Turn the body to face (W). At the same time move the left hand across the body, palm faces in. Inhale.

Figure 4-241: (W) Next, turn the palm out and fingers pointing forward. Step the left leg forward so the stance is mountain climbing stance (*deng shan bu*, 蹬山步), and push the left hand forward. Exhale.

39. Wave Hands in the Clouds: Right (*You Yun Shou,* 右雲手)

The Chinese name of this form is "yun shou" and means cloud hands, which implies waving your hands like floating clouds. The movement of clouds can be fast or slow, but it is steady and continuous. Therefore, when you perform this form you wave your hands the way clouds move. It is a long-range, continuous jin application.

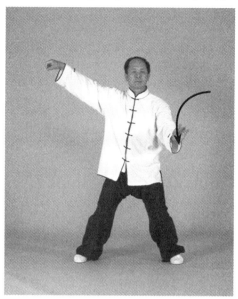

Figure 4-242: (N) Turn N into horse stance (*ma bu,* 馬步) while dropping the left hand down. Start your inhalation.

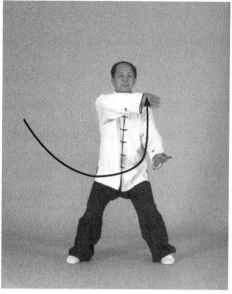

Figure 4-243: (N) Swing the right arm clockwise, with the palm facing your body, down and up so that it passes directly in front of the left hand. Move the right arm up until it is at shoulder height and above the left hand. Complete your inhalation.

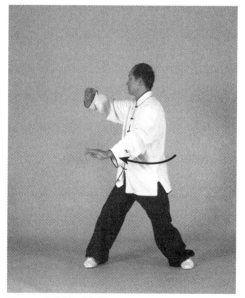

Figure 4-244: (E) Turn the upper body to the right while keeping the arms locked. The arms will turn with the body. Exhale.

Analysis

This form is designed to neutralize the opponent's grabbing. You neutralize his grab to the side and use your twisting jin to make him lose his balance. When you twist your body it must be centered and balanced.

40. Wave Hands in the Clouds: Left (*Zuo Yun Shou,* 左雲手)

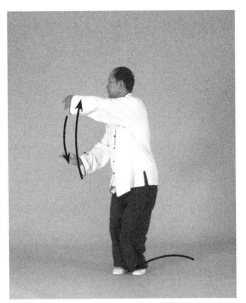

Figure 4-245: (E) Close the left leg in to the right leg. Turn the right palm to face the ground and move it down. At the same time, turn the left palm in and move it up. Inhale.

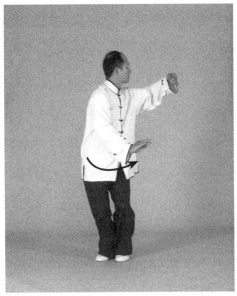

Figure 4-246: (W) Turn the upper body to the left side. Exhale.

41. Wave Hands in the Clouds: Right (*You Yun Shou,* 右雲手)

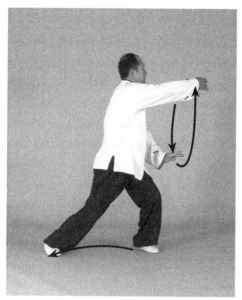 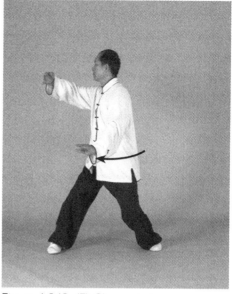

Figure 4-247: (W) Turn the left palm to face the ground while moving the left arm down; at the same time, turn the right palm in while moving the right arm up. Step to the side with the right leg. Inhale.

Figure 4-248: (E) Change to horse stance (*ma bu,* 馬步) and turn the upper body to the right. Complete your exhalation.

42. Single Whip (*Dan Bian,* 單鞭)

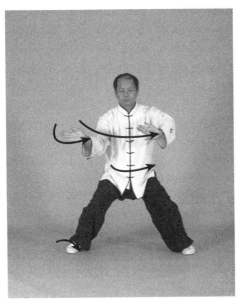

Figure 4-249: (N) Turn both hands to face forward. Keep the arms locked in the same position and turn to (N) on the right heel so the stance is horse stance (*ma bu,* 馬步). Arms swing with the body. Begin to inhale.

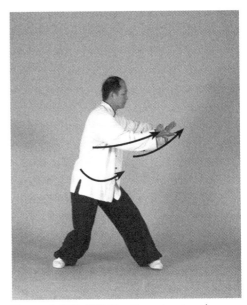

Figure 4-250: (W) Continue turning the body to your left while keeping both of your hands in the same position. Continue your inhalation.

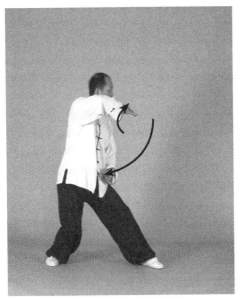

Figure 4-251: (W) Lower the left arm and turn the palm up, and turn your right palm down so that the palms face each other. Complete your inhalation.

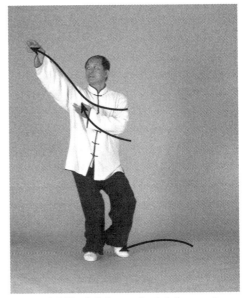

Figure 4-252: (N) Bring the left leg, on its toes, to the right leg. Swing the right arm back. All the fingertips of the right hand are touching and pointing down. Exhale.

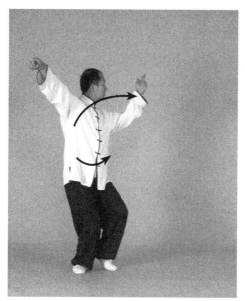

Figure 4-253: (W) Turn the body to face (W). At the same time move the left hand across the body, palm faces in. Inhale.

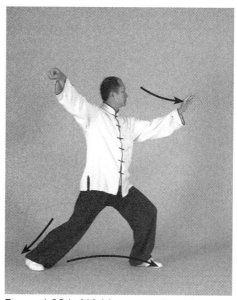

Figure 4-254: (W) Next, turn the palm out and fingers pointing forward. Step the left leg forward so the stance is mountain climbing stance (*deng shan bu*, 蹬山步), and push the left hand forward. Exhale.

43. Stand High to Search Out the Horse (*Gao Tan Ma*, 高探馬)

The Chinese name of this form is "gao tan ma." Gao means high, tan means to try or search out, and ma means horse. When you search for your horse in the field, you must use your hands to shade your eyes from the sun in order to see far and clear. This indicates that the hands are used for blocking. The horse fights mainly by kicking, so the name implies that your leg can be used for kicking and also that when you stand up high, your lower body is exposed to a kicking attack.

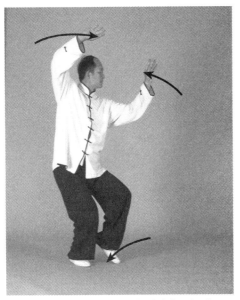

Analysis
This form is similar to the beginning of both "pick up needle from sea bottom" and "fan back." The difference is that this form is applied in a shorter and quicker manner to set up your opponent for your kick.

Figure 4-255: (W) Bring the left leg back on its toe while opening both hands and raising them up slightly. Begin to inhale.

44. Separate Right Foot (*You Fen Jiao*, 右分腳)

The Chinese name of this form is "fen jiao" and means "separate foot." It implies that the feet are separated sideward.

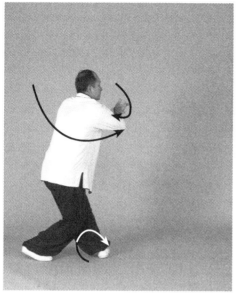

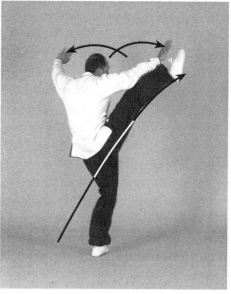

Figure 4-256: (W) Pick up the left knee and then set the left foot down into sitting on crossed legs stance (*zuo pan bu*, 坐盤步). Exhale. Cross your hands in front of your chest, palms facing inward. Inhale.

Figure 4-257: (W) Open up both arms, palms out, and snap kick the right leg so it touches the right palm. Exhale.

Analysis

In this form you must first deflect upward to protect yourself and to expose your opponent's side. If possible, grab your opponent's hand to prevent him from escaping or blocking.

45. **Separate Left Foot** (*Zuo Fen Jiao,* 左分腳)

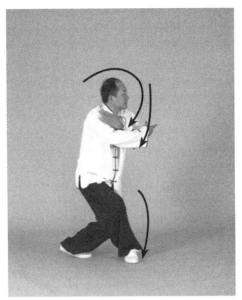

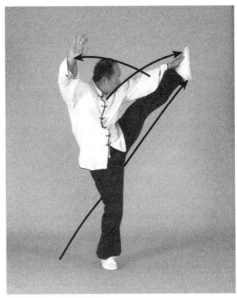

Figure 4-258: (W) Draw your right leg in and then step the right leg down, going into sitting on crossed legs stance (*zuo pan bu,* 坐盤步). Cross your arms in front of the body, palms facing inward. Inhale.

Figure 4-259: (W) Open both arms, palms out, and snap kick the left leg so it touches the left palm. Exhale.

46. Turn and Kick with the Heel: 90 degrees (*Zhuan Shen Deng Jiao,* 轉身蹬腳)

The Chinese name of this form is "deng jiao" and means to use your heel to step or kick, usually forward.

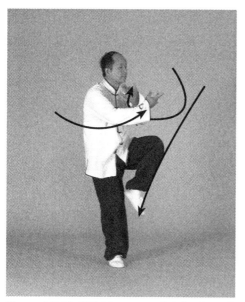

Analysis

Before you kick you must seal all your vital points from your opponent's strike. Therefore, first cross your hands in front of your chest to protect your chest area, and at the same time lift your left leg to protect your groin and dan tian. Then, if you have a suitable target, kick. When you kick, you make the shouting sound of "ha" to raise up your spirit and to release any tight or stagnant feeling in the chest area.

Figure 4-260: (W) Draw your left leg in and scoop both of your hands down and then up to cross (forming an "X") in front of your chest. Inhale

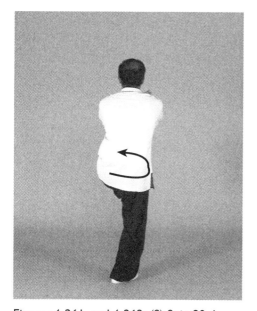

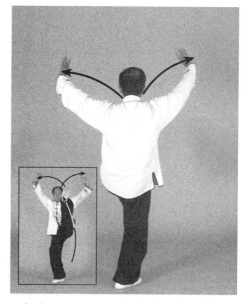

Figures 4-261, and 4-262: (S) Spin 90 degrees counterclockwise on the right heel to face (S). Open both arms and kick with the left heel (fast kick), while shouting with a sound "ha." Exhale.

47. Brush Knee and Step Forward: Left (*Zuo Lou Xi Ao Bu*, 左摟膝拗步)

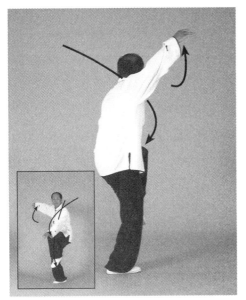

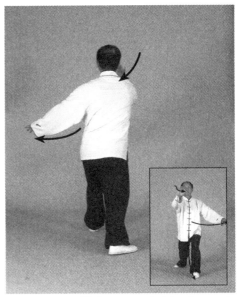

Figures 4-263: (S) Bring the left foot in, knee raised, and swing the left hand past the left knee while raising the right hand up to the area of your right ear. Inhale.

Figure 4-264: (S) Step your left leg forward and brush your left hand to your left while pushing your right palm forward. Exhale.

48. Brush Knee and Step Forward: **Right** (*You Lou Xi Ao Bu*, 右摟膝拗步)

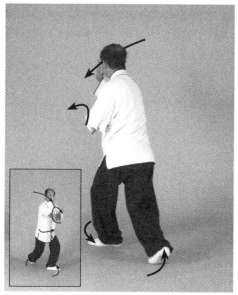

Figure 4-265: (S) Make a counterclockwise circle with the left arm. Start to inhale. Turn the left foot so the stance is sitting on crossed legs stance (*zuo pan bu*, 坐盤步). The right foot is on its toe. Complete inhale.

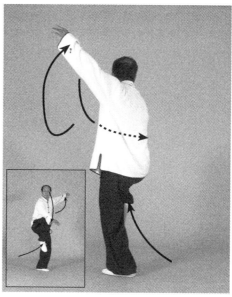

Figure 4-266: (S) Lift your right leg and brush down your right hand while circling your left hand behind you. Exhale.

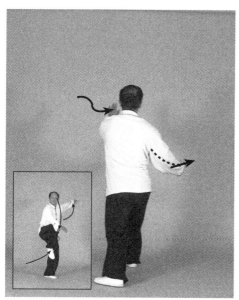

Figure 4-267: (S) Step down with the right leg. Inhale. Push forward with the left palm with fingers pointing forward first and then settle down the wrist. Exhale.

49. Step Forward and Strike Down with the Fist (*Jin Bu Zai Chui*, 進步栽捶)

The Chinese name of this form is "jin bu zai chui." Jin bu means to step forward, zai means to fall, and chui means to punch. There are not too many vital points in the lower body to strike. Common targets are the dan tian, groin, and upper thigh.

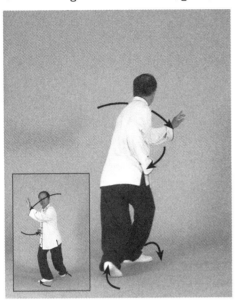

Figure 4-268: (S) Turn legs so the stance is sitting on crossed legs stance (*zuo pan bu*, 坐盤步). Swing the left arm across the body and retreat the right hand in a fist to the waist. Inhale.

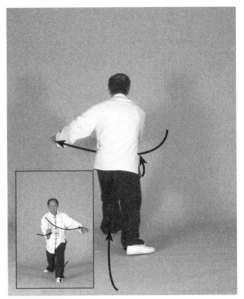

Figure 4-269: (S) Step forward with the left leg, sweep the left arm down and to the left while punching your right fist down to the groin area. Exhale.

Analysis

This form is for deflecting low punches and kicks. After you deflect, shift your body forward close to your opponent to immobilize him. This will give you a good opportunity to strike.

50. Turn, Twist Body, and Circle the Fist (*Zhuan Shen Pie Shen Chui*, 轉身撇身捶)

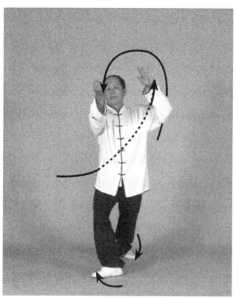

Figure 4-270: (N) Turn 180 degrees clockwise in the crossed legs stance (*zuo pan bu*, 坐盤步) to face (N) while swinging your right fist up and down and covering down with the left hand. Start to inhale.

51. Step Forward, Deflect Downward, Parry and Punch (Jin Bu Ban Lan Chui, 進步搬攔捶)

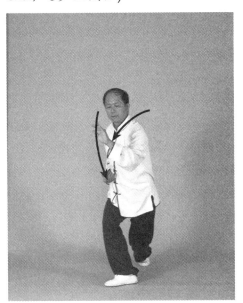

Figure 4-271: (N) Continue swinging your right fist down, and then withdraw it to the right waist area while covering down with your left hand. Complete your inhalation.

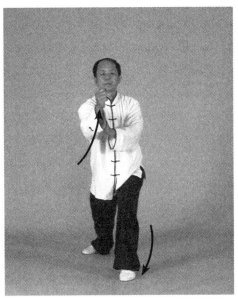

Figure 4-272: (N) Step forward with the left leg and punch your right fist forward while sliding your left hand in along the right forearm. Exhale.

52. Kick Right (*You Ti Jiao, 右踢腳*)

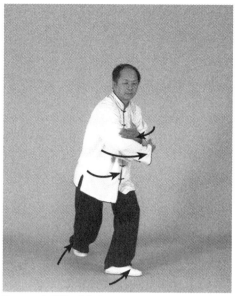

Figure 4-273: (N) Turn legs so the stance is sitting on crossed legs stance (*zuo pan bu*, 坐盤步) and cross your arms in front of your body. Inhale.

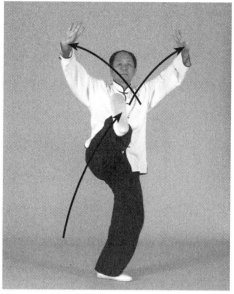

Figure 4-274: (N) Open your arms and kick with the right heel. Exhale.

53. Strike the Tiger: Right (*You Da Hu,* 右打虎)

This form is called "da hu" in Chinese and means strike the tiger. When a tiger leaps toward you, you can squat down to avoid its attack. This squatting stance can be used against an opponent who initiates a high, jumping kick toward you.

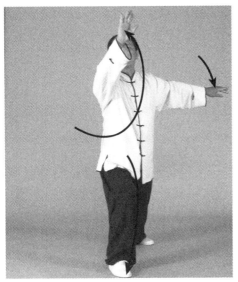

Figure 4-275: (N) Step down with the right leg into mountain climbing stance (*deng shan bu,* 蹬山步) and swing the right hand down and up. Start your inhalation.

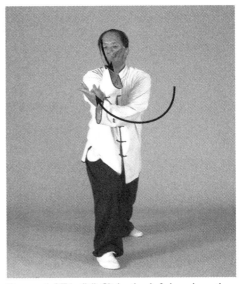

Figure 4-276: (N) Slide the left hand up the right arm, and start to bring the right hand to the waist. Continue your inhalation.

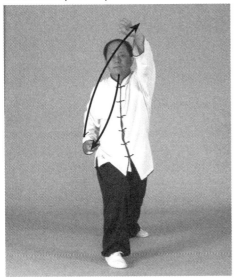

Figure 4-277: (N) Withdraw your right fist to the waist while continuing to circle your left hand up, changing it to a fist. Complete your inhalation.

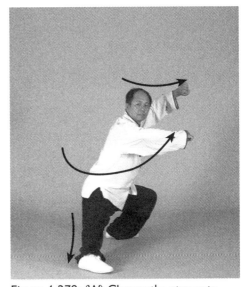

Figure 4-278: (W) Change the stance to tame the tiger stance (*fu hu bu,* 伏虎步), weight on the left leg. Hook the right fist across the body. The left arm remains up. Exhale.

Analysis

Your right hand deflects the attack and your left hand immediately takes over to put your opponent in a passive situation. Once you have the opportunity, pull him down to make him lose balance and use the right hand to strike him. Your root and your waist-twisting jin are extremely important in this application.

54. Strike the Tiger: Left (*Zuo Da Hu,* 左打虎)

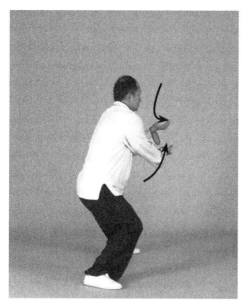

Figure 4-279: (W) Move the right hand under the left elbow. Slide the right arm up the left forearm. Begin to inhale.

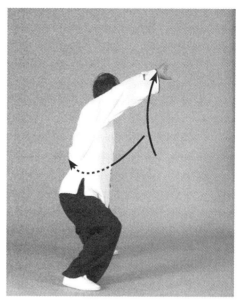

Figure 4-280: (W) Bring the left fist to the waist while the right hand swings up, palm out. Complete your inhalation.

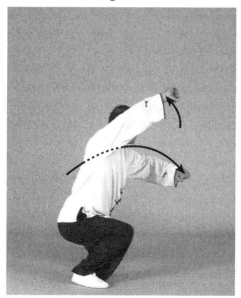

Figure 4-281: (W) Shift weight to the right leg into the tame the tiger stance (*fu hu bu,* 伏虎步) posture. Hook the left fist across the body. Exhale.

55. Kick Right (*You Ti Jiao,* 右踢腳)

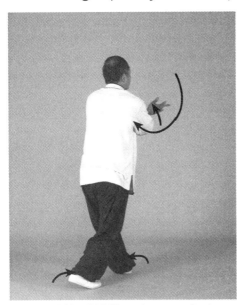 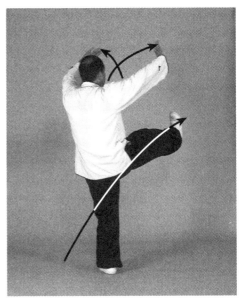

Figure 4-282: (SW) Turn the upper body to (SW) while raising your body up to sitting on crossed legs stance (*zuo pan bu,* 坐盤步), crossing your hands. Inhale.

Figure 4-283: (SW) Open your hands and heel kick with your right foot (slow kick). Exhale.

56. Attack the Ears with the Fists (*Shuang Feng Guan Er,* 雙風貫耳)

The Chinese name of this form is "shuang feng guan er." Shuang means a pair, double, or both, feng means the wind, guan means to go through or pass through, and er means ears. Therefore, the translation of this form should be "two winds pass through the ears." In this form, the fists generate the wind. The strikes must be fast and powerful to approach the targets, which are the temples or other cavities.

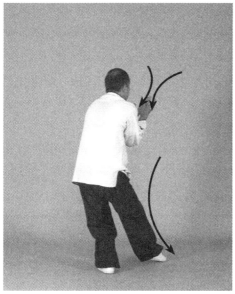 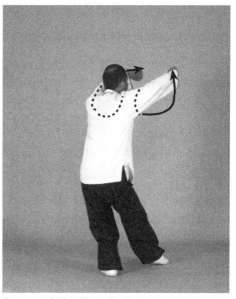

Figure 4-284: (SW) Set the right foot down on its toes and withdraw both of your hands in relaxed fists with the palms up, in to the chest area. Inhale.

Figure 4-285: (SW) Circle both of your fists down, to the sides, and then up and in, palms facing out. Exhale.

Analysis
Bringing both hands in front of your chest seals it from your opponent's attack, and emptying your right leg gives you the opportunity to kick. Once you have sealed your opponent's strike, you can follow his striking limbs to attack his body or head.

57. Kick Left (*Zuo Ti Jiao*, 左踢腳)

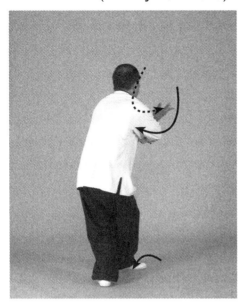

Figure 4-286: (S) Raise the right knee, and then step down into sitting on crossed legs stance (*zuo pan bu*, 坐盤步) while crossing your arms. Face (S). Inhale.

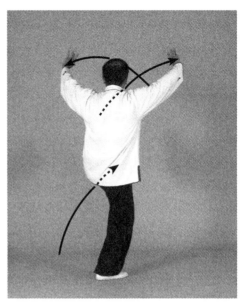

Figure 4-287: (S) Open both arms and kick with the left heel (slow kick). Exhale.

58. Turn and Kick with the Heel: 270 degrees (*Zhuan Shen Deng Jiao,* 轉身蹬腳)

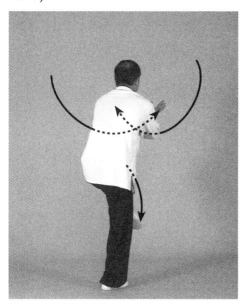

Figure 4-288: (S) Bring the left leg in, knee raised, and cross your hands in front of your chest, palms facing in. Start to inhale.

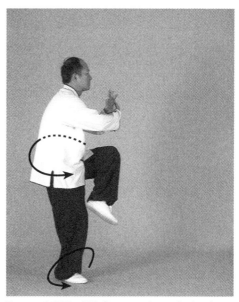

Figure 4-289: (W) Spin on the right heel 270 degrees counterclockwise to face (W). Continue your inhalation.

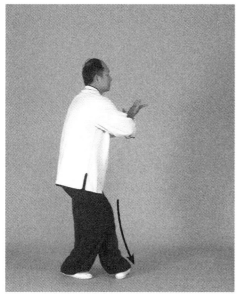

Figure 4-290: (W) Step the left leg down into sitting on crossed legs stance (*zuo pan bu,* 坐盤步). Draw both hands up to the chest, palms facing in. Complete your inhalation.

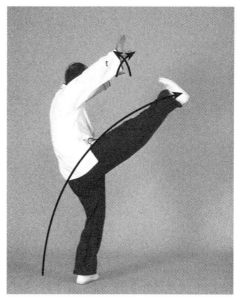

Figure 4-291: (W) Turn the palms of both hands out and clear your chest as you kick your right heel forward (fast kick) and exhale, while making the shouting sound "ha."

59. Twist the Body and Circle the Fist (*Pie Shen Chui,* 撇身捶)

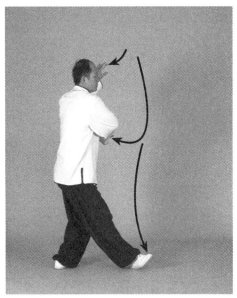

Figure 4-292: (W) Step the right leg down into sitting on crossed legs stance (*zuo pan bu,* 坐盤步) while swinging the right fist down across your body, then up across your body. Start your inhalation.

60. Step Forward, Deflect Downward, Parry, and Punch (*Jin Bu Ban Lan Chui*, 進步搬欄捶)

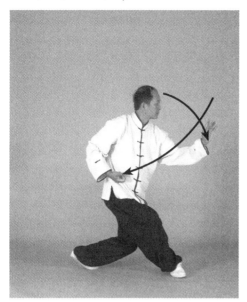

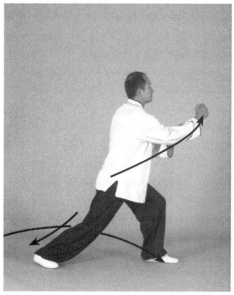

Figure 4-293: (W) Continue twisting to your right, and move your right hand to your waist while covering your left hand. The left arm swings across the body. Complete your inhalation.

Figure 4-294: (W) Step forward with the left leg into mountain climbing stance (*deng shan bu*, 蹬山步) while punching your right fist forward and sliding your left hand to the inside of your right elbow area. When you step forward, inhale, and when you punch, exhale.

61. Seal Tightly (*Ru Feng Si Bi,* 如封似閉)

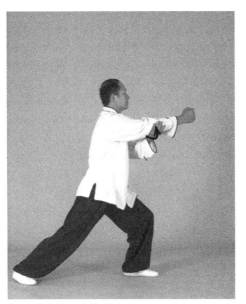

Figure 4-295: (W) Continue to slide your left hand under the right elbow, with the palm of your left hand facing in to your right arm. Start to inhale.

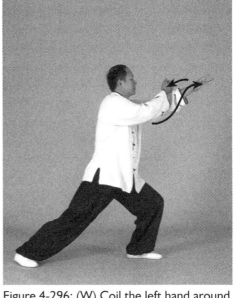

Figure 4-296: (W) Coil the left hand around the right forearm, move from the elbow to the wrist, and extend forward. When the left hand has reached its maximum extension, start to pull in the right fist. Continue to inhale.

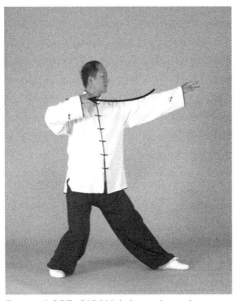

Figure 4-297: (W) Withdraw the right arm to chest area while sitting back in four-six stance (*si liu bu,* 四六步). Complete your inhalation.

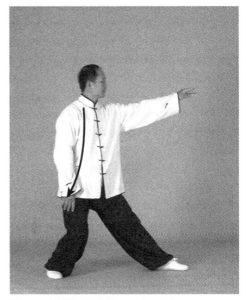

Figure 4-298: (W) Drop the right arm down. Exhale.

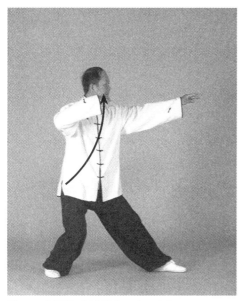

Figure 4-299: (W) Raise the right arm up so it is beside the ear. Inhale.

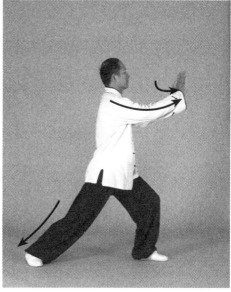

Figure 4-300: (W) Shift the stance to mountain climbing stance (*deng shan bu*, 蹬山步) and push the right palm forward. The left hand opens into a palm, pushing forward. Exhale.

62. Embrace the Tiger and Return to the Mountain (*Bao Hu Gui Shan,* 抱虎歸山)

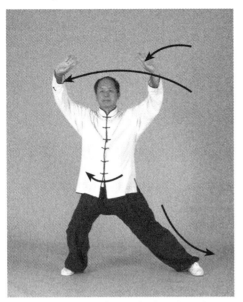

Figure 4-301: (N) Cross the hands and turn the body (N), and then open both of your arms. Lean to the right side. Inhale.

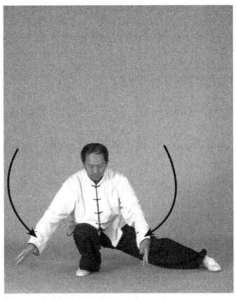

Figure 4-302: (N) Squat down into tame the tiger stance (*fu hu bu,* 伏虎步) while circling both arms out, down, and in. Weight is on the right leg. Begin to exhale.

63. Close Taiji (*He Taiji*, 合太極)

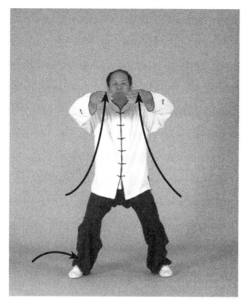

End of the Second Part.

Figure 4-303: (N) Shift the weight to the left leg, raise the right knee, and step the right leg down in horse stance (*ma bu*, 馬步). Move both hands to the chest area. Arms are in a circle. Complete exhaling.

Transition Form (*Guo Du Shi*, 過渡勢)

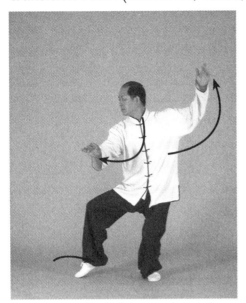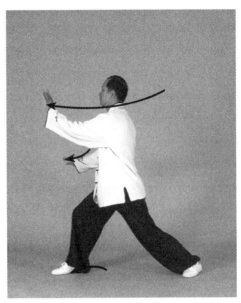

Figure 4-304: (E) Withdraw and raise the right leg on its toe. Swing the right arm down; the left arm comes up to behind the left ear. Inhale.

Figure 4-305: (E) Step right leg forward into mountain climbing stance (*deng shan bu*, 蹬山步), and push the left hand forward. Exhale.

64. Wardoff, Rollback, Press, and Push Forward (*Peng Lu Ji An,* 掤攦擠按)

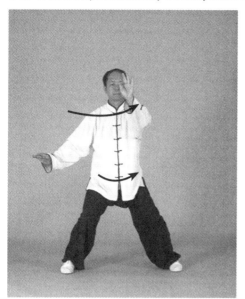

Figure 4-306: (N) Keep the arms in the same position and turn your body 90 degrees to face (N) on your right heel. Start to inhale.

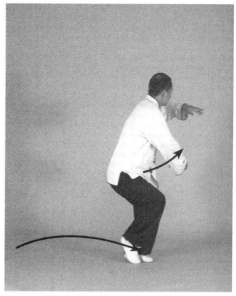

Figure 4-307: (W) Bring the right foot to the side of left foot. Continue inhaling. Swing the right hand to the front of the body, and turn the palm up to face the left palm.

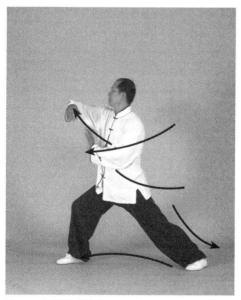

Figure 4-308: (E) Step back with the right leg. Turn on the heels to (E) while shifting into mountain climbing stance (*deng shan bu,* 蹬山步) while swinging the right arm to your right with the arm horizontal, palms facing in and your left palm under the right forearm with palm facing forward and slightly down. Exhale.

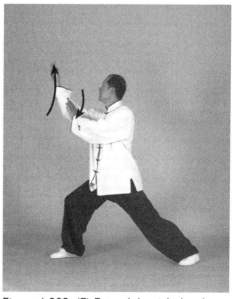

Figure 4-309: (E) Extend the right hand upward while sinking your right elbow. Continue your exhalation from last posture.

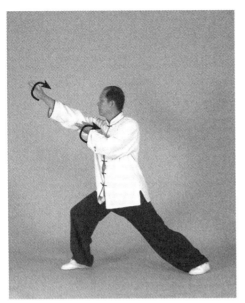

Figure 4-310: (E) Coil your right hand clockwise and forward until the palm is facing forward while turning your left palm to face upward. Begin to inhale.

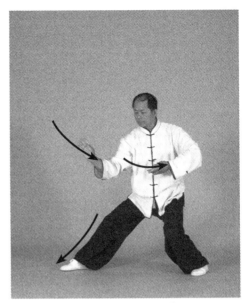

Figure 4-311: (E) Sit back into four-six stance (si liu bu, 四六步). Move the right arm down to the front and left hand to your left chest area. Complete your inhalation.

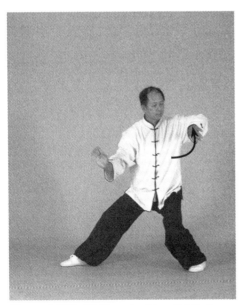

Figure 4-312: (E) Turn the hips slightly to your left. Make a gentle small clockwise circle with your left hand on the left side of the body. This movement does not have a practical application; instead, it is the signature of Yang Style Taijiquan. Exhale.

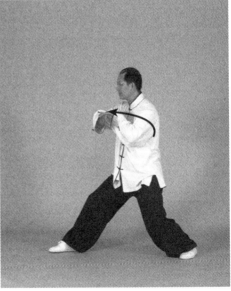

Figure 4-313: (E) Bring the left hand to the inner wrist of the right hand while inhaling. Face turn to the (E).

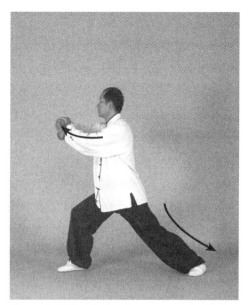

Figure 4-314: (E) Shift into mountain climbing stance (*deng shan bu*, 蹬山步) and extend both hands forward while still touching. Exhale as the arms are extended.

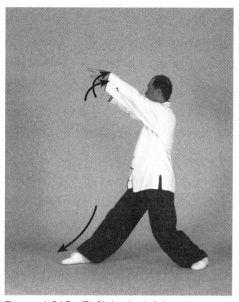

Figure 4-315: (E) Slide the left hand over the right hand. Open the arms to the width of the shoulder. Palms face down. Sit back in four-six stance (*si liu bu*, 四六步) while raising the arms up and back in a circular motion. Start to inhale.

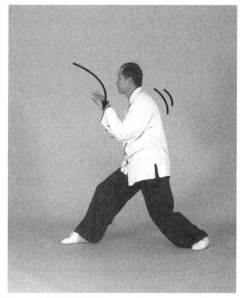

Figure 4-316: (E) Lower the arms to the chest in a circular motion. Fingers point forward. Complete your inhalation.

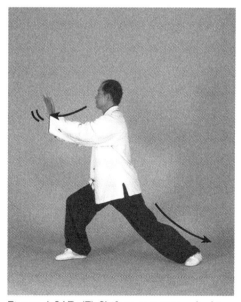

Figure 4-317: (E) Shift to mountain climbing stance (*deng shan bu*, 蹬山步) and push the hands forward while settling down your wrists. Exhale.

65. Single Whip (*Dan Bian,* 單鞭)

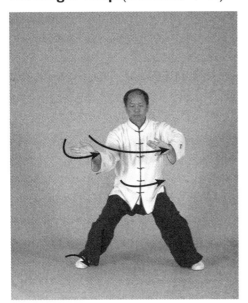

Figure 4-318: (N) Turn both hands to face forward. Keep the arms locked in the same position and turn to (N) on the right heel so the stance is horse stance (*ma bu,* 馬步). Arms swing with the body. Begin to inhale.

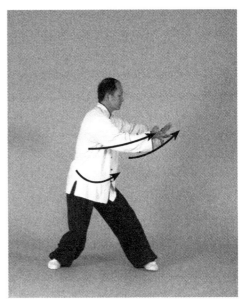

Figure 4-319: (W) Continue turning the body to your left while keeping both of your hands in the same position. Continue your inhalation.

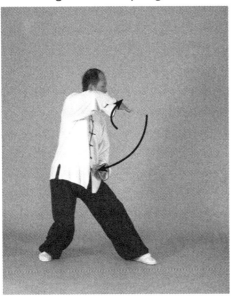

Figure 4-320: (W) Lower the left arm and turn the palm up, and turn your right palm down so that the palms face each other. Complete your inhalation.

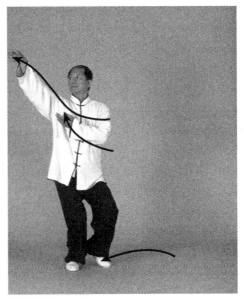

Figure 4-321: (N) Bring the left leg, on its toes, to the right leg. Swing the right arm back. All the fingertips of the right hand are touching and pointing down. Exhale.

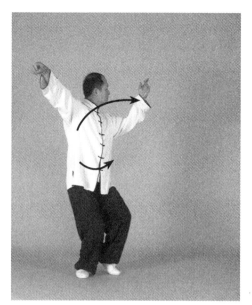

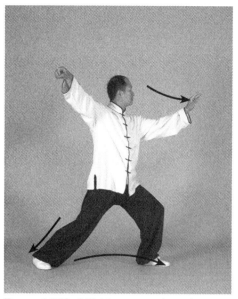

Figure 4-322: (W) Turn the body to face (W). At the same time move the left hand across the body, palm faces in. Inhale.

Figure 4-323: (W) Next, turn the palm out and fingers pointing forward. Step the left leg forward so the stance is mountain climbing stance (*deng shan bu*, 蹬山步), and push the left hand forward. Exhale.

66. The Wild Horse Parts Its Mane: Right (*You Ye Ma Fen Zong*, 右野馬分鬃)

The Chinese name of this form is "ye ma fen zong." Ye means wild, ma means horse, fen means to shear or divide, and zong means mane. The horse is a powerful animal, and a wild horse is particularly forceful and vigorous. The name of this form gives the image of a horse tossing its head vigorously and shaking its mane. The word "shear" is used because when you do this form you "tear" your hands apart as you turn your body. The motion is continuous, extended, and powerful. It is a long jin that can rend the opponent off his feet.

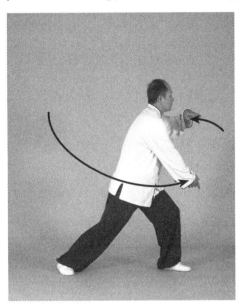

Figure 4-324: (W) Swing your right hand down and move your left hand in to your chest area. Inhale.

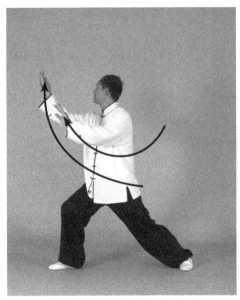

Figure 4-325: (E) Turn the body on your heels 180 degrees clockwise while swinging the right hand up. Left hand is on the left hand side of the right forearm, palm facing forward. The stance is mountain climbing stance (*deng shan bu*, 蹬山步). Exhale.

Analysis

In order to shear or divide your opponent you must grasp part of his body, usually an arm, and pull it in one direction, and at the same time use your other arm against his body to move him in the other direction. Also, your right leg should be placed so that it blocks the opponent from retreating or kicking. This is an example of rend jin because you move the opponent in two directions at once.

67. The Wild Horse Parts Its Mane: Left (*Zuo Ye Ma Fen Zong,* 左野馬分鬃)

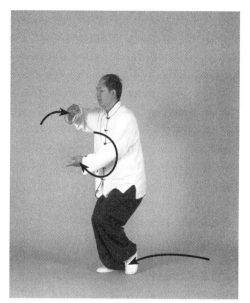

Figure 4-326: (NW) Bring the left foot up to the right leg and turn your palms in to face each other, left palm up, right palm down. Inhale.

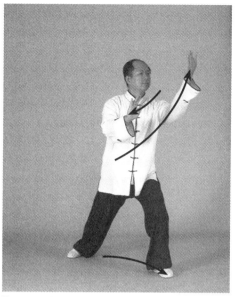

Figure 4-327: (NW) Step forward to (NW) with the left leg into mountain climbing stance (*deng shan bu,* 蹬山步) and slide the left hand up, palm facing in. Exhale.

68. The Wild Horse Parts Its Mane: Right *(You Ye Ma Fen Zong, 右野馬分鬃)*

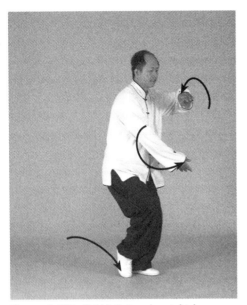 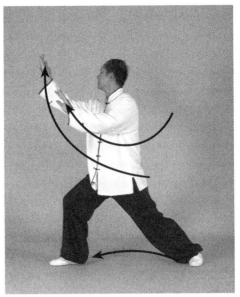

Figure 4-328: (NW) Bring the right leg up to the left leg. Turn your palms toward each other, left palm facing down, right palm facing up. Inhale.

Figure 4-329: (E) Step straight back with the right leg. Turn your body to face the (E) while sliding the right hand up. Left hand moves to the side of the right forearm. The stance is mountain climbing stance *(deng shan bu, 蹬山步)*. Exhale.

69. Grasp the Sparrow's Tail: Left (*Zuo Lan Que Wei,* 左攬雀尾)

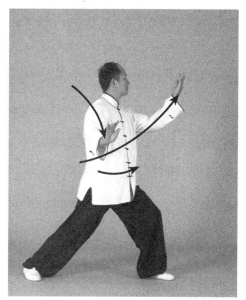

Figure 4-330: (W) Turn your body to face (W), and press the right palm down while sliding your left arm up and to the left. The stance is mountain climbing stance (*deng shan bu,* 蹬山步). When you turn your body, first you inhale until you face (N), and then exhale until you face (W).

70. Wardoff, Rollback, Press, and Push Forward (*Peng Lu Ji An*, 掤攦擠按)

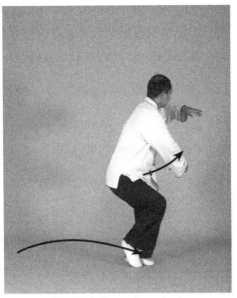

Figure 4-331: (W) Bring the right foot to the side of left foot. Inhale. Swing the right hand to the front of the body, and turn the palm up to face the left palm.

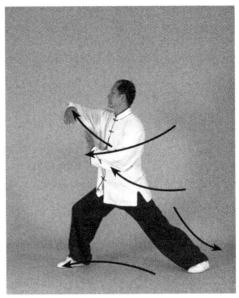

Figure 4-332: (E) Step back with the right leg. Turn on the heels to (E) while shifting into mountain climbing stance (*deng shan bu*, 蹬山步) while swinging the right arm to your right with the arm horizontal, palms facing in and your left palm under the right forearm with palm facing forward and slightly down. Exhale.

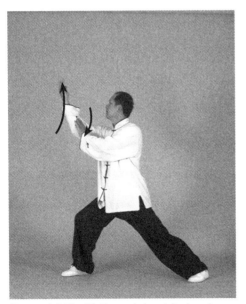

Figure 4-333: (E) Extend the right hand upward while sinking your right elbow. Continue your exhalation from last posture.

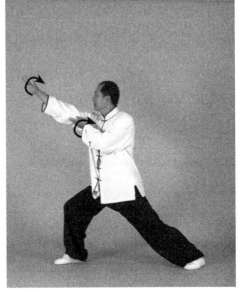

Figure 4-334: (E) Coil your right hand clockwise and forward until the palm is facing forward while turning your left palm to face upward. Begin to inhale.

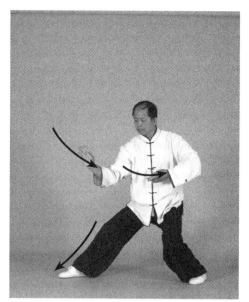

Figure 4-335: (E) Sit back into four-six stance (*si liu bu*, 四六步). Move the right arm down to the front and left hand to your left chest area. Complete your inhalation.

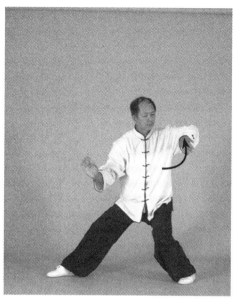

Figure 4-336: (E) Turn the hips slightly to your left. Make a gentle small clockwise circle with your left hand on the left side of the body. This movement does not have a practical application; instead, it is the signature of Yang Style Taijiquan. Exhale.

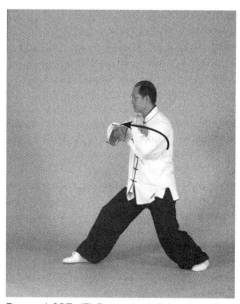

Figure 4-337: (E) Bring the left hand to the inner wrist of the right hand while inhaling. Face turn to the (E).

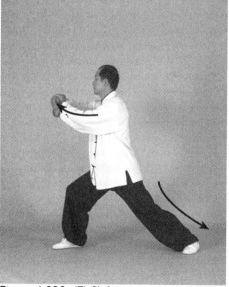

Figure 4-338: (E) Shift into mountain climbing stance (*deng shan bu*, 蹬山步) and extend both hands forward while still touching. Exhale as the arms are extended.

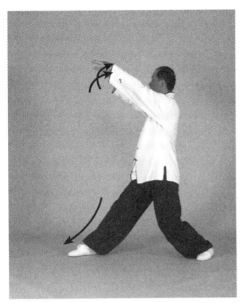

Figure 4-339: (E) Slide the left hand over the right hand. Open the arms to the width of the shoulder. Palms face down. Sit back in four-six stance (*si liu bu*, 四六步) while raising the arms up and back in a circular motion. Start to inhale.

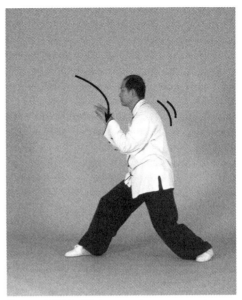

Figure 4-340: (E) Lower the arms to the chest in a circular motion. Fingers point forward. Complete your inhalation.

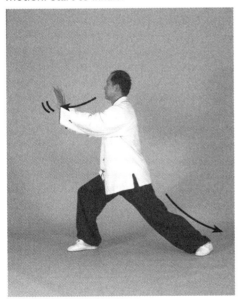

Figure 4-341: (E) Shift to mountain climbing stance (*deng shan bu*, 蹬山步) and push the hands forward while settling down your wrists. Exhale.

71. Single Whip (*Dan Bian,* 單鞭)

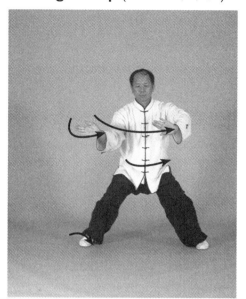

Figure 4-342: (N) Turn both hands to face forward. Keep the arms locked in the same position and turn to (N) on the right heel so the stance is horse stance (*ma bu,* 馬步). Arms swing with the body. Begin to inhale.

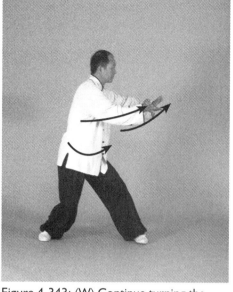

Figure 4-343: (W) Continue turning the body to your left while keeping both of your hands in the same position. Continue your inhalation.

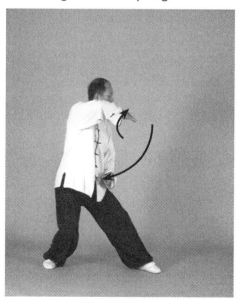

Figure 4-344: (W) Lower the left arm and turn the palm up, and turn your right palm down so that the palms face each other. Complete your inhalation.

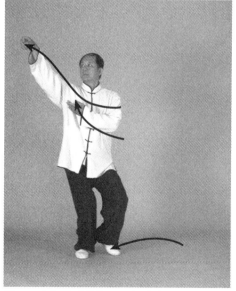

Figure 4-345: (N) Bring the left leg, on its toes, to the right leg. Swing the right arm back. All the fingertips of the right hand are touching and pointing down. Exhale.

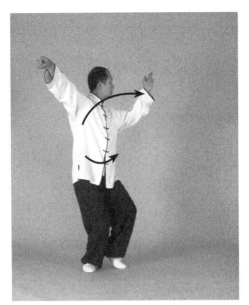

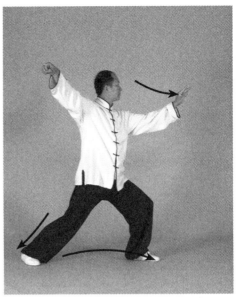

Figure 4-346: (W) Turn the body to face (W). At the same time move the left hand across the body, palm faces in. Inhale.

Figure 4-347: (W) Next, turn the palm out and fingers pointing forward. Step the left leg forward so the stance is mountain climbing stance (*deng shan bu*, 蹬山步), and push the left hand forward. Exhale.

72. The Fair Lady Weaves with Shuttle: Left (*Zuo Yu Nu Chuan Suo,* 左玉女穿梭)

The Chinese name of this form is "yu nu chuan suo." Yu is jade, nu is girl or lady; together they refer to a fair or beautiful lady. Chuan means to thread or pass through, and suo is a weaver's shuttle. In order to weave a piece of cloth, you must move the horizontal threads back and forth through the vertical threads with a shuttle. As you do the repetitions of the form, your body moves back and forth as if you were working a loom. You have to watch carefully in order to insert the shuttle accurately through the threads.

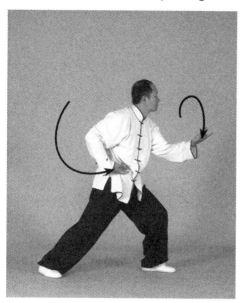

Figure 4-348: (W) Lower both arms to waist level. Inhale.

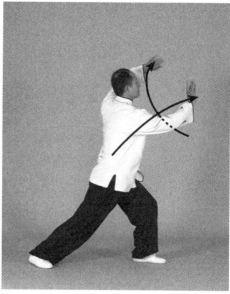

Figure 4-349: (W) Raise the left arm up and push the right palm forward. Exhale.

Analysis
This form is generally used at close range. From the movements of the form it is understood that you are attacking the vital cavity in the armpit, where a correct strike can cause a heart attack. You must first expose the target by raising his elbow, and then use the secret sword hand form (index and middle fingers) in order to reach the cavity, which is deep in the armpit.

73. The Fair Lady Weaves with Shuttle: Right (*You Yu Nu Chuan Suo,* 右玉女穿梭)

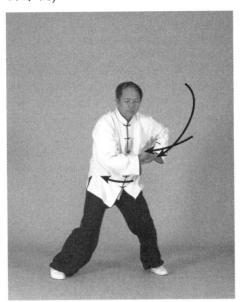

Figure 4-350: (N) Turn the body into horse stance (*ma bu,* 馬步) facing (N) while lowering both hands down to the waist area. Inhale.

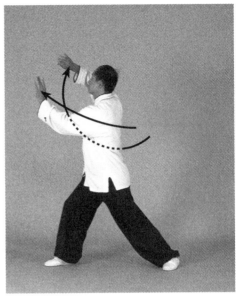

Figure 4-351: (E) Continue turning your body to face (E), and shift into mountain climbing stance (*deng shan bu,* 蹬山步). Raise the right hand while pushing the left palm forward. Exhale.

74. The Fair Lady Weaves with Shuttle: Left (*Zuo Yu Nu Chuan Suo*, 左玉女穿梭)

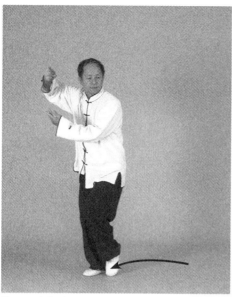

Figure 4-352: (E) Bring the left leg up to the right leg. Begin to inhale.

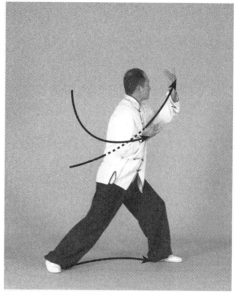

Figure 4-353: (SW) Step the left leg back to the (SW). Lower both arms to waist level, and then scoop up the left arm while preparing to push out with the right palm. Inhale.

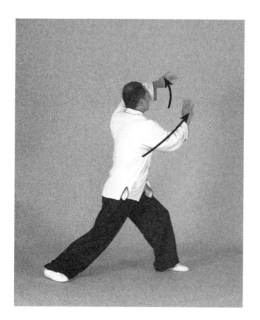

Figure 4-354: (SW) Raise your left arm while pushing out with your right palm. The stance is mountain climbing stance (*deng shan bu*, 蹬山步). Exhale.

75. The Fair Lady Weaves with Shuttle: Right (You Yu Nu Chuan Suo, 右玉女穿梭)

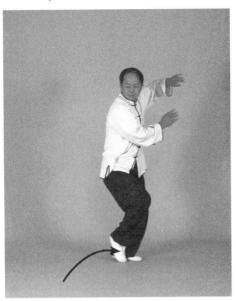

Figure 4-355: (SW) Bring the right leg to the left leg. Begin to inhale.

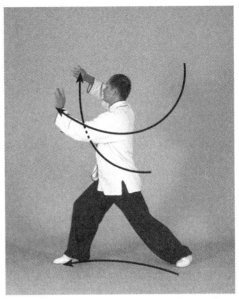

Figure 4-356: (E) Step your right leg to the (E), and shift into mountain climbing stance (*deng shan bu*, 蹬山步). Raise your right arm while pushing out with the left palm. Exhale.

76. Grasp Sparrow's Tail: Left (*Zuo Lan Que Wei*, 左攬雀尾)

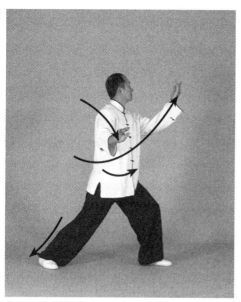

Figure 4-357: (W) Turn your body to face (W) and press the right palm down while sliding your left arm up and to the left. The stance is mountain climbing stance (*deng shan bu*, 蹬山步). When you turn your body, first inhale until you face (N), and then exhale until you face (W).

77. Wardoff, Rollback, Press, and Push Forward (*Peng Lu Ji An*, 掤攦擠按)

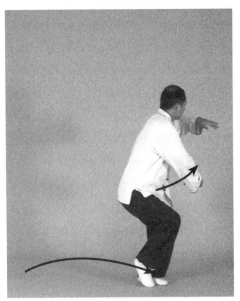

Figure 4-358: (W) Bring the right foot to the side of left foot. Inhale. Swing the right hand to the front of the body, and turn the palm up to face the left palm.

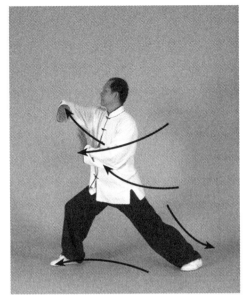

Figure 4-359: (E) Step back with the right leg. Turn on the heels to (E) while shifting into mountain climbing stance (*deng shan bu*, 蹬山步) while swinging the right arm to your right with the arm horizontal, palms facing in and your left palm under the right forearm with palm facing forward and slightly down. Exhale.

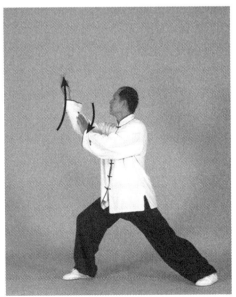

Figure 4-360: (E) Extend the right hand upward while sinking your right elbow. Continue your exhalation from last posture.

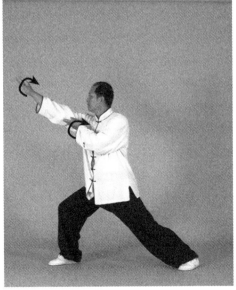

Figure 4-361: (E) Coil your right hand clockwise and forward until the palm is facing forward while turning your left palm to face upward. Begin to inhale.

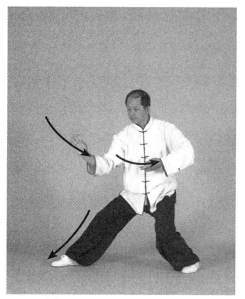

Figure 4-362: (E) Sit back into four-six stance (*si liu bu*, 四六步). Move the right arm down to the front and left hand to your left chest area. Complete your inhalation.

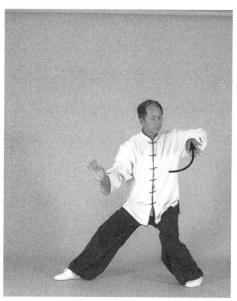

Figure 4-363: (E) Turn the hips slightly to your left. Make a gentle small clockwise circle with your left hand on the left side of the body. This movement does not have a practical application; instead, it is the signature of Yang Style Taijiquan. Exhale.

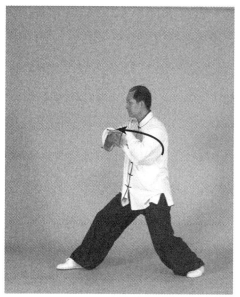

Figure 4-364: (E) Bring the left hand to the inner wrist of the right hand while inhaling. Face turn to the (E).

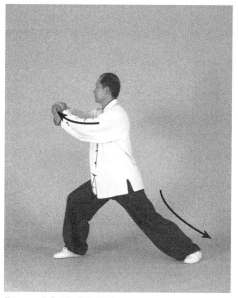

Figure 4-365: (E) Shift into mountain climbing stance (*deng shan bu*, 蹬山步) and extend both hands forward while still touching. Exhale as the arms are extended.

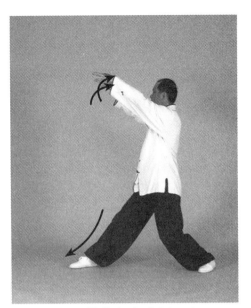

Figure 4-366: (E) Slide the left hand over the right hand. Open the arms to the width of the shoulder. Palms face down. Sit back in four-six stance (*si liu bu*, 四六步) while raising the arms up and back in a circular motion. Start to inhale.

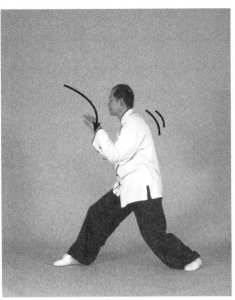

Figure 4-367: (E) Lower the arms to the chest in a circular motion. Fingers point forward. Complete your inhalation.

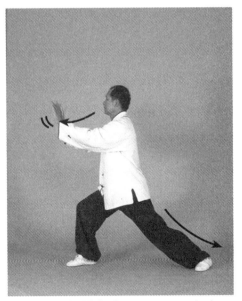

Figure 4-368: (E) Shift to mountain climbing stance (*deng shan bu*, 蹬山步) and push the hands forward while settling down your wrists. Exhale.

78. Single Whip (Dan Bian, 單鞭)

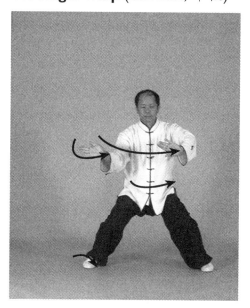

Figure 4-369: (N) Turn both hands to face forward. Keep the arms locked in the same position and turn to (N) on the right heel so the stance is horse stance (ma bu, 馬步). Arms swing with the body. Begin to inhale.

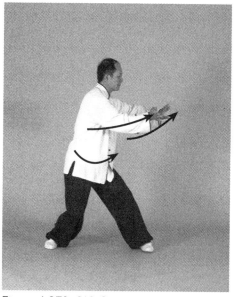

Figure 4-370: (W) Continue turning the body to your left while keeping both of your hands in the same position. Continue your inhalation.

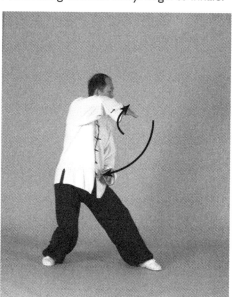

Figure 4-371: (W) Lower the left arm and turn the palm up, and turn your right palm down so that the palms face each other. Complete your inhalation.

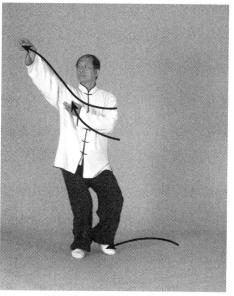

Figure 4-372: (N) Bring the left leg, on its toes, to the right leg. Swing the right arm back. All the fingertips of the right hand are touching and pointing down. Exhale.

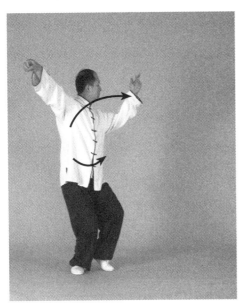

Figure 4-373: (W) Turn the body to face (W). At the same time move the left hand across the body, palm faces in. Inhale.

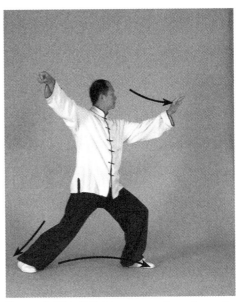

Figure 4-374: (W) Next, turn the palm out and fingers pointing forward. Step the left leg forward so the stance is mountain climbing stance (*deng shan bu*, 蹬山步), and push the left hand forward. Exhale.

79. Wave Hands in the Clouds: Right (*You Yun Shou,* 右雲手)

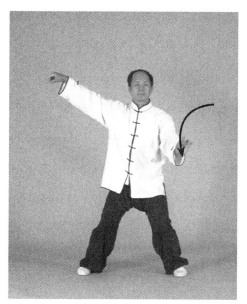

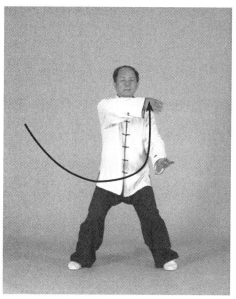

Figure 4-375: (N) Turn N into horse stance (*ma bu*, 馬步) while dropping the left hand down. Start your inhalation.

Figure 4-376: (N) Swing the right arm clockwise, with the palm facing your body, down and up so that it passes directly in front of the left hand. Move the right arm up until it is at shoulder height and above the left hand. Complete your inhalation.

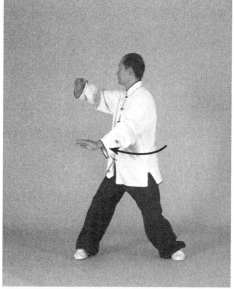

Figure 4-377: (E) Turn the upper body to the right while keeping the arms locked. The arms will turn with the body. Exhale.

80. Single Whip (*Dan Bian*, 單鞭)

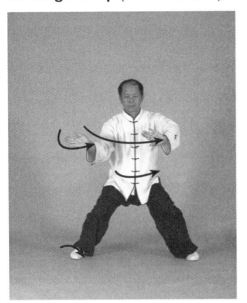

Figure 4-378: (N) Turn both hands to face forward. Keep the arms locked in the same position and turn to (N) on the right heel so the stance is horse stance (*ma bu*, 馬步). Arms swing with the body. Begin to inhale.

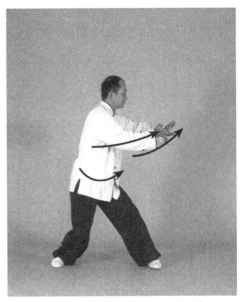

Figure 4-379: (W) Continue turning the body to your left while keeping both of your hands in the same position. Continue your inhalation.

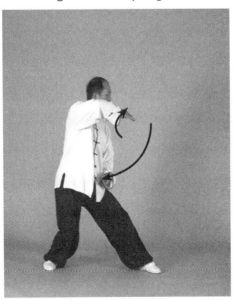

Figure 4-380: (W) Lower the left arm and turn the palm up, and turn your right palm down so that the palms face each other. Complete your inhalation.

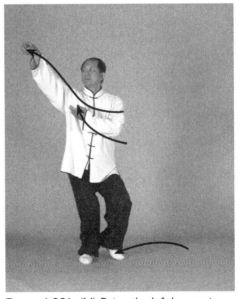

Figure 4-381: (N) Bring the left leg, on its toes, to the right leg. Swing the right arm back. All the fingertips of the right hand are touching and pointing down. Exhale.

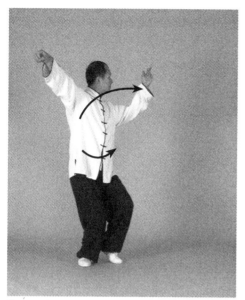

Figure 4-382: (W) Turn the body to face (W). At the same time move the left hand across the body, palm faces in. Inhale.

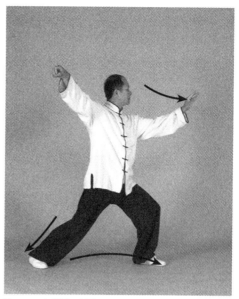

Figure 4-383: (W) Next, turn the palm out and fingers pointing forward. Step the left leg forward so the stance is mountain climbing stance (*deng shan bu*, 蹬山步), and push the left hand forward. Exhale.

81. The Snake Creeps Down (She Shen Xia Shi, 蛇身下勢)

The Chinese name of this form is "she shen xia shi." She means snake, shen means body. Xia means down or to lower, and shi means aspect or manner. The image is that of a snake wrapped around a branch, lowering its head as if about to attack. The name implies that you must first wrap, coil, stick and adhere with your opponent before you lower your body to attack. When a snake creeps down a branch, its head is lower than its body, searching the air to find and attack a target. This means that you coil and wrap on the top while you attack your opponent's lower body.

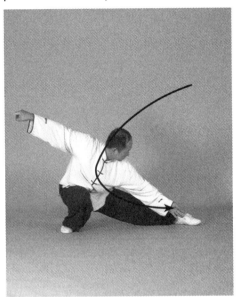

Figure 4-384: (W) Squat into tame the tiger stance (fu hu bu, 伏虎步) with weight on the right leg while swinging your left hand past your face and down to your left foot. Inhale.

Analysis

This is a defensive form that also sets up the opponent for your counterattack, for example, "rooster stands on one leg" (see next form) or "step forward to seven stars" (see No. 104). Your left hand must stick and adhere, coiling like a snake around a branch, as it leads the opponent's attacking arm into a position advantageous to you.

82. The Golden Rooster Stands on One Leg: Right (You Jin Ji Du Li, 右金雞 獨立)

The Chinese name of this form is "jin ji du li." The usual translation is correct. When a rooster stands on one leg, it is very stable and balanced. When you apply this form, you too must be balanced and stable. When you are in this stance you can kick very easily with the lifted leg.

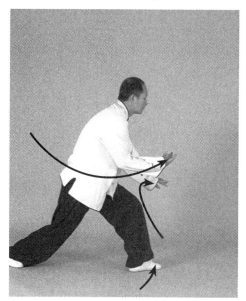 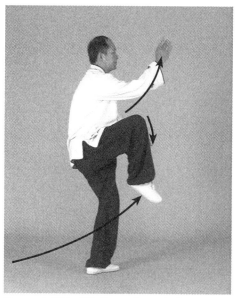

Figure 4-385: (W) Start to shift your weight forward, and turn your left foot toes 45 degrees to the side while moving your right hand to your front. Start to exhale.

Figure 4-386: (W) Bring the right leg up while moving the right hand to face height, turning the palm to the side, and pressing the left palm down. Complete your exhalation.

Analysis

Once you have sealed your opponent's attack and led his attacking hand to the side, the front of his body is exposed. You can now attack with your right hand or your right leg, or both.

83 Golden Rooster Stands on One Leg: Left (*Zuo Jin Ji Du Li,* 左金雞獨立)

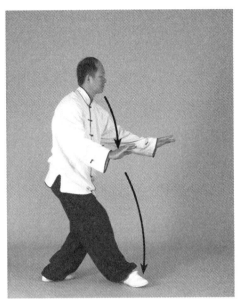

Figure 4-387: (W) Step down with the right leg and lower the right hand, palm down, to waist level. Inhale.

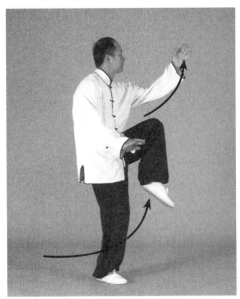

Figure 4-388: (W) Raise the left knee and hand, left elbow bent, left palm facing to the side with fingers pointing up. Exhale.

84. Step Back and Repulse the Monkey: Left (*Zuo Dao Nian Hou*, 左倒攆猴)

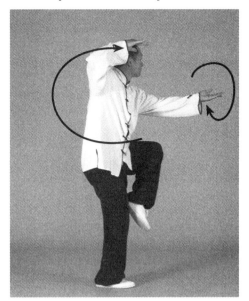

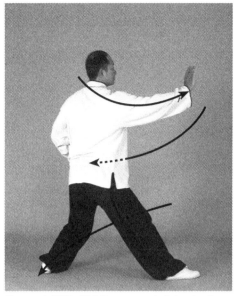

Figures 4-389: (W) Circle your right hand up to the side of your right ear while rotating your left palm counterclockwise until the palm faces up. Inhale.

Figure 4-390: (W) Step your left leg back into four-six stance (*si liu bu*, 四六步). Push your right palm forward and withdraw your left hand back to the side of the waist. Exhale.

85. Diagonal Flying (*Xie Fei Shi,* 斜飛勢)

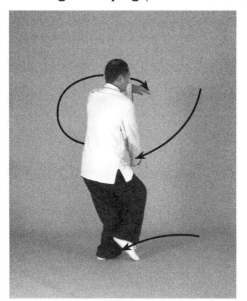

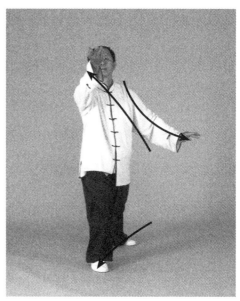

Figure 4-391: (S) Circle the left hand up, palm facing down, and the right hand down, palm facing up, while bringing your right leg in to the side of the left leg. Inhale.

Figure 4-392: (N) Turn 180 degrees clockwise on the left heel. Step the right leg down into mountain climbing stance (*deng shan bu,* 蹬山步) while spreading both of your hands apart, right palm up to the front of the face. The left hand moves, palm down, down to the side. Exhale.

86. Lift Hands to the Up Posture (*Ti Shou Shang Shi,* 提手上勢)

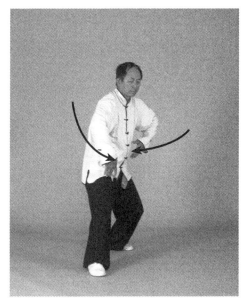

Figure 4-393: (N) Move both arms in toward your abdominal area, while shifting your weight onto your left foot. Inhale.

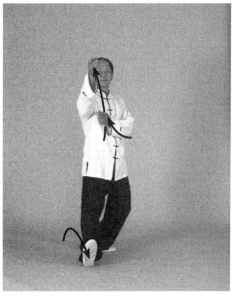

Figure 4-394: (N) Lift your right leg up, and then touch down with heel while raising both your hands up to the chest area. Exhale.

87. The White Crane Spreads Its Wings (Bai He Liang Chi, 白鶴亮翅)

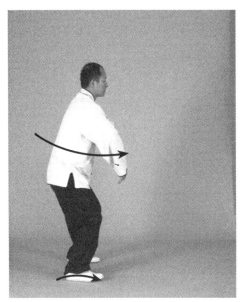

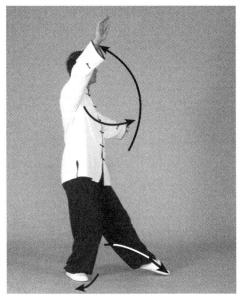

Figure 4-395: (W) Set the right foot down. Turn the body to (W) and into horse stance (ma bu, 馬步); simultaneously, swing the right arm down and up, making it cross the left hand that has remained stationary. Both feet are parallel. Inhale.

Figure 4-396: (W) Spread the arms, right arm higher than the left, while bringing the left leg to the right leg and then forward to form the false stance (xu bu, 虛步). As the arms are spread, place your weight on your right foot while pointing out 45 degrees. Exhale. The arms are the wings being spread open.

88. Brush Knee and Step Forward: Left (*Zuo Lou Xi Ao Bu,* 左摟膝拗步)

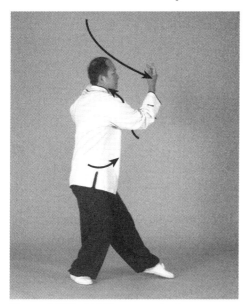

Figure 4-397: (W) Turn your body to your left slightly and swing the right arm across the body. Inhale.

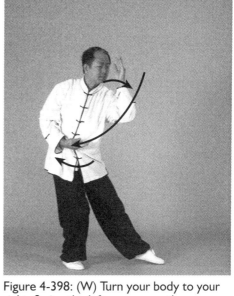

Figure 4-398: (W) Turn your body to your right. Swing the left arm across the upper body, palm facing inward, while lowering your right arm to the waist area, palm facing upward. Continue to inhale.

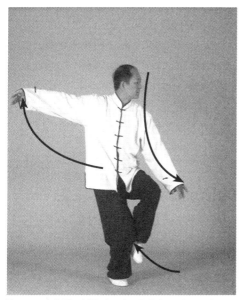

Figure 4-399: (W) As the left hand reaches the center of the body, raise the left knee, swing the left arm past it, and raise the right arm back and up to a place near the right ear. Complete your exhalation.

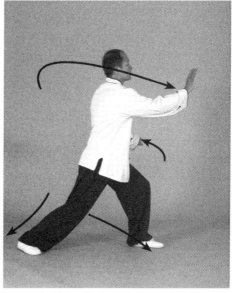

Figure 4-400: (W) Clear down with your left hand as you step down with the left leg into mountain climbing stance (*deng shan bu,* 蹬山步). Inhale. Push forward with the right palm with fingers pointing forward first and then settle down the wrist. Exhale.

89. Pick Up the Needle from the Sea Bottom (*Hai Di Lao Zhen,* 海底撈針)

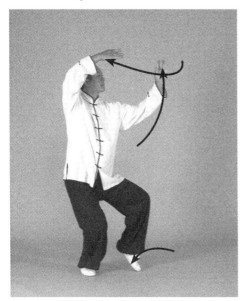

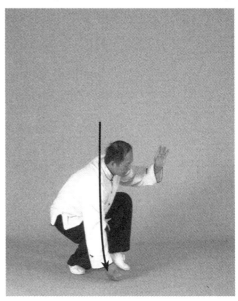

Figure 4-401: (W) Withdraw the left leg in on its toes while bringing the right hand back, palm facing in, and pushing out the left palm. Inhale.

Figure 4-402: (W) Scoop down, the right hand "picking" an object from the floor. Exhale.

90. Fan Back (*Shan Tong Bei,* 扇通背)

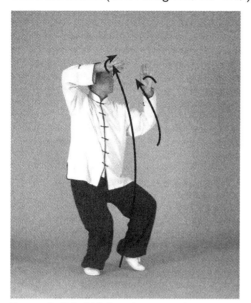 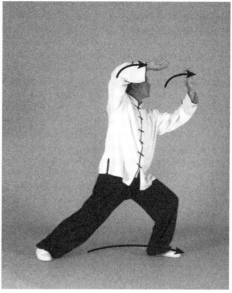

Figure 4-403: (W) Stand up into the position of Figure 4-216 but with the right palm facing out. Inhale.

Figure 4-404: (W) Shift the stance into mountain climbing stance (*deng shan bu,* 蹬山步) while moving both arms forward. Exhale.

91. The White Snake Turns Its Body and Spits Poison (*Zhuan Shen Bai She Tu Xin*, 轉身白蛇吐信)

The Chinese name of this form is "bai she tu xin." Bai she means white snake, Tu means spits and xin means truth or a pledge—here it means poison. When a snake spits poison it must use speed and surprise to hit its target.

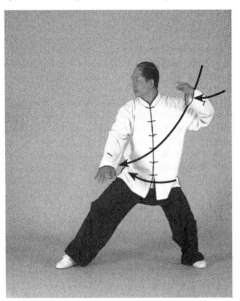 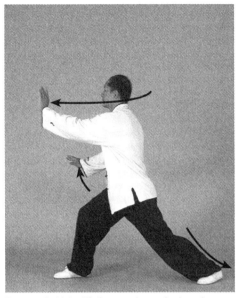

Figure 4-405: (E) Turn the upper body to (E) while sitting back in four-six stance (*si liu bu*, 四六步) and sweeping the right hand down. Inhale.

Figure 4-406: (E) Swing the right hand to the side. Shift the stance forward into mountain climbing stance (*deng shan bu*, 蹬山步) and push with the left palm. When you push your left hand forward, your fingers first extend forward, and then up. At the same time, your wrist settles downward, ending with the palm facing forward for a push. Exhale.

Analysis

When your opponent grabs or strikes your back, turn your body and sit back to evade the attack and expose his cavities. Shift your weight forward and attack. The strike must be fast for this form to be effective.

92. Step Forward, Deflect Downward, Parry, and Punch (*Jin Bu Ban Lan Chui*, 進步搬攔捶)

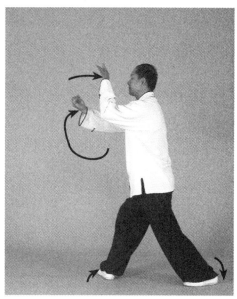

Figure 4-407: (E) Twist your body to your right and change into sitting on crossed legs stance (*zuo pan bu*, 坐盤步) while circling your right fist to the side and covering your left hand down. Start to inhale.

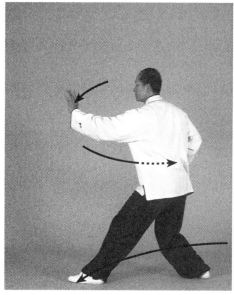

Figure 4-408: (E) Step your left leg forward into four-six stance (*si liu bu*, 四六步), and continue to cover your left hand down while pulling your right fist back to the waist. Complete your inhalation.

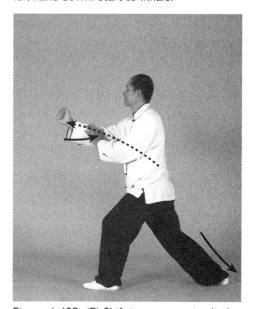

Figure 4-409: (E) Shift into mountain climbing stance (*deng shan bu*, 蹬山步), pushing your right fist forward while sliding your left hand back to the right forearm area. Exhale.

93. Step Forward, Wardoff, Rollback, Press, and Push Forward (*Shang Bu Peng Lu Ji An,* 上步掤攦擠按)

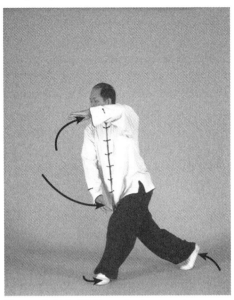

Figure 4-410: (E) Turn the legs so that you are in the sitting on crossed legs stance (*zuo pan bu,* 坐盤步) while lowering your right hand, palm up. As you do this, you also raise your left hand straight up and neutralize to your left. Inhale.

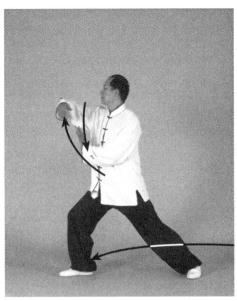

Figure 4-411: (E) Step forward with the right leg into mountain climbing stance (*deng shan bu,* 蹬山步) and swing the right arm up. Exhale.

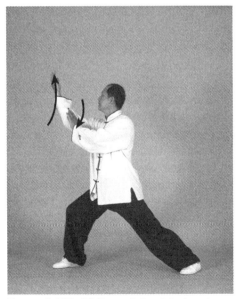

Figure 4-412: (E) Extend the right hand upward while sinking your right elbow. Continue your exhalation from last posture.

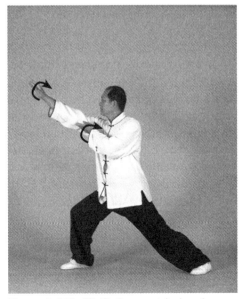

Figure 4-413: (E) Coil your right hand clockwise and forward until the palm is facing forward while turning your left palm to face upward. Begin to inhale.

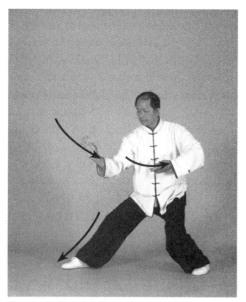

Figure 4-414: (E) Sit back into four-six stance (*si liu bu*, 四六步). Move the right arm down to the front and left hand to your left chest area. Complete your inhalation.

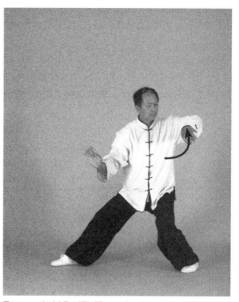

Figure 4-415: (E) Turn the hips slightly to your left. Make a gentle small clockwise circle with your left hand on the left side of the body. This movement does not have a practical application; instead, it is the signature of Yang Style Taijiquan. Exhale.

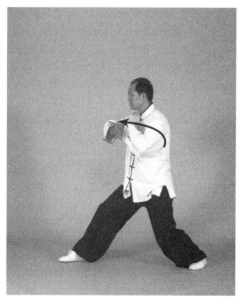

Figure 4-416: (E) Bring the left hand to the inner wrist of the right hand while inhaling. Face turn to the (E).

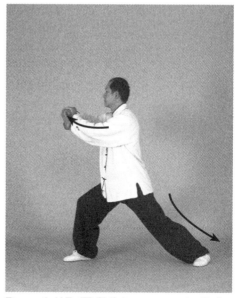

Figure 4-417: (E) Shift into mountain climbing stance (*deng shan bu*, 蹬山步) and extend both hands forward while still touching. Exhale as the arms are extended.

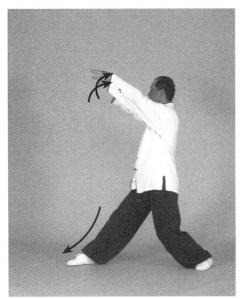

Figure 4-418: (E) Slide the left hand over the right hand. Open the arms to the width of the shoulder. Palms face down. Sit back in four-six stance (*si liu bu*, 四六步) while raising the arms up and back in a circular motion. Start to inhale.

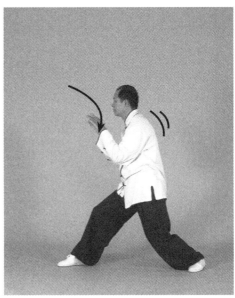

Figure 4-419: (E) Lower the arms to the chest in a circular motion. Fingers point forward. Complete your inhalation.

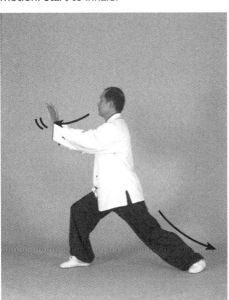

Figure 4-420: (E) Shift to mountain climbing stance (*deng shan bu*, 蹬山步) and push the hands forward while settling down your wrists. Exhale.

94. Single Whip (Dan Bian, 單鞭)

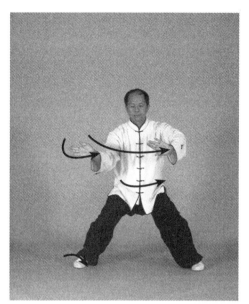

Figure 4-421: (N) Turn both hands to face forward. Keep the arms locked in the same position and turn to (N) on the right heel so the stance is horse stance (ma bu, 馬步). Arms swing with the body. Begin to inhale.

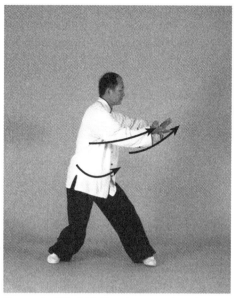

Figure 4-422: (W) Continue turning the body to your left while keeping both of your hands in the same position. Continue your inhalation.

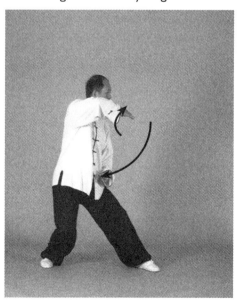

Figure 4-423: (W) Lower the left arm and turn the palm up, and turn your right palm down so that the palms face each other. Complete your inhalation.

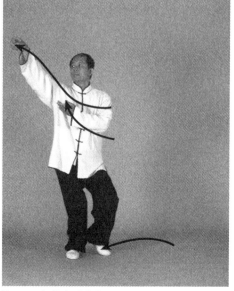

Figure 4-424: (N) Bring the left leg, on its toes, to the right leg. Swing the right arm back. All the fingertips of the right hand are touching and pointing down. Exhale.

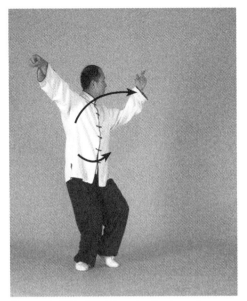

Figure 4-425: (W) Turn the body to face (W). At the same time move the left hand across the body, palm faces in. Inhale.

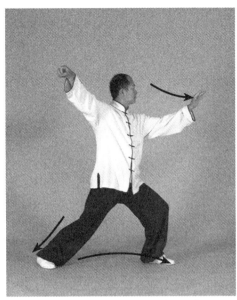

Figure 4-426: (W) Next, turn the palm out and fingers pointing forward. Step the left leg forward so the stance is mountain climbing stance (*deng shan bu*, 蹬山步), and push the left hand forward. Exhale.

95. Wave Hands in the Clouds: Right (You Yun Shou, 右雲手)

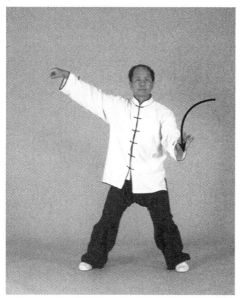

Figure 4-427: (N) Turn N into horse stance (ma bu, 馬步) while dropping the left hand down. Start your inhalation.

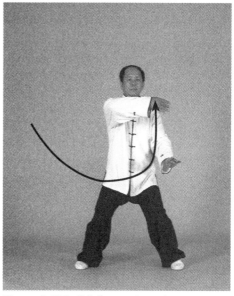

Figure 4-428: (N) Swing the right arm clockwise, with the palm facing your body, down and up so that it passes directly in front of the left hand. Move the right arm up until it is at shoulder height and above the left hand. Complete your inhalation.

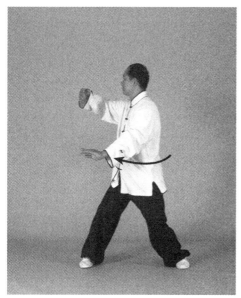

Figure 4-429: (E) Turn the upper body to the right while keeping the arms locked. The arms will turn with the body. Exhale.

96. Single Whip (Dan Bian, 單鞭)

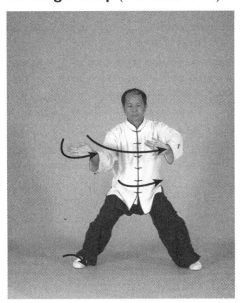

Figure 4-430: (N) Turn both hands to face forward. Keep the arms locked in the same position and turn to (N) on the right heel so the stance is horse stance (ma bu, 馬步). Arms swing with the body. Begin to inhale.

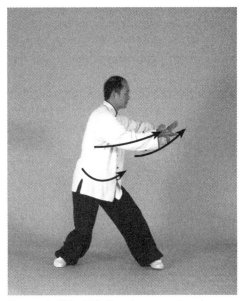

Figure 4-431: (W) Continue turning the body to your left while keeping both of your hands in the same position. Continue your inhalation.

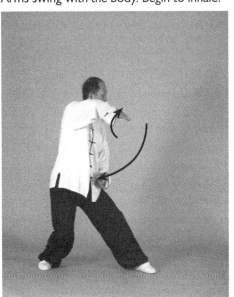

Figure 4-432: (W) Lower the left arm and turn the palm up, and turn your right palm down so that the palms face each other. Complete your inhalation.

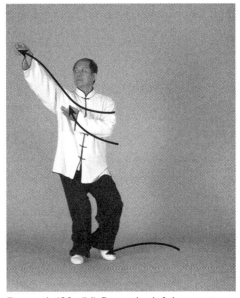

Figure 4-433: (N) Bring the left leg, on its toes, to the right leg. Swing the right arm back. All the fingertips of the right hand are touching and pointing down. Exhale.

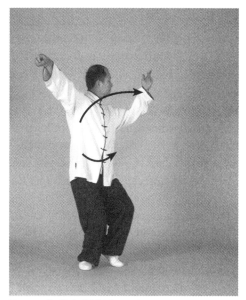

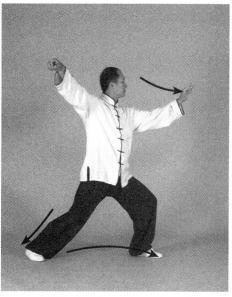

Figure 4-434: (W) Turn the body to face (W). At the same time move the left hand across the body, palm faces in. Inhale.

Figure 4-435: (W) Next, turn the palm out and fingers pointing forward. Step the left leg forward so the stance is mountain climbing stance (*deng shan bu*, 蹬山步), and push the left hand forward. Exhale.

97. Stand High to Search Out the Horse (*Gao Tan Ma,* 高探馬)

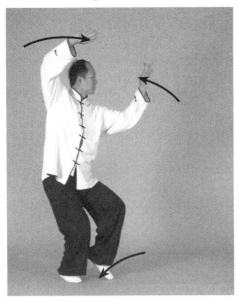

Figure 4-436: (W) Bring the left leg back on its toe while opening both hands and raising them up slightly. Begin to inhale.

98. Cross Hands (*Shi Zi Shou*, 十字手)

The Chinese name of this form is "shi zi shou." Shi means ten, zi means word, and shou means hands; therefore the accurate translation of this form would be "the word 'ten' hands." The Chinese character for ten (十) is formed by two crossed lines like a Christian cross, which reflects how your hands are held in this form.

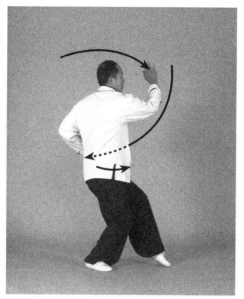

Figure 4-437: (W) Twist your body to your left while starting to cover your right hand down and pulling your left hand back to the waist. Inhale.

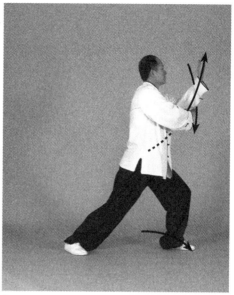

Figure 4-438: (W) Shift into mountain climbing stance (*deng shan bu*, 蹬山步). Continue to swing the right forearm down across the body. Raise the left hand up and inside the right arm while moving the right hand under the left elbow. Exhale.

Analysis

You sit back to yield, and at the same time use your right hand to neutralize the opponent's attack. After neutralizing, press his arm down further to expose his face to your attack. Your left leg should be placed in an advantageous position when you step forward. While deflecting the opponent's attack there is no weight on your left leg, and you can easily kick with it.

99. Turn and Kick (*Zhuan Shen Shi Zi Tui*, 轉身十字腿)

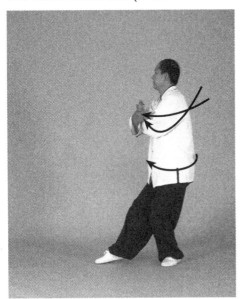 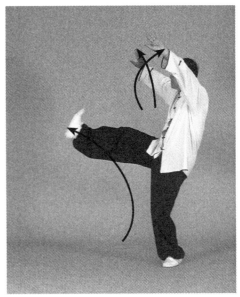

Figure 4-439: (E) Turn 180 degrees clockwise while shifting the weight onto your left leg; the right foot is on its toes. Cross your hands, right hand on the outside, both hands facing in, and inhale.

Figure 4-440: (E) Spread your arms open, turn the palms out, and kick with the right heel. Exhale.

100. Brush Knee and Punch Down (*Lou Xi Zhi Dang Chui,* 摟膝指襠捶)

This form is called "lou xi zhi dang chui" in Chinese. Lou xi means to embrace the knee. Zhi means finger or to aim, dang means the seat of a pair of trousers and actually refers to the groin area, and chui means punch. The name therefore tells you that this form is designed for brushing the opponent's kick out of the way and punching his groin. This form is very similar to No. 49: "Step Forward and Strike Down with the Fist," the difference being that this form is for long-range fighting while the other form is for shorter-range fighting.

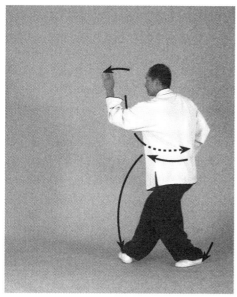 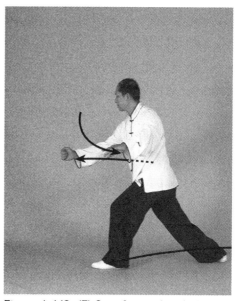

Figure 4-441: (E) Step down with the right leg into sitting on crossed legs stance (*zuo pan bu,* 坐盤步) and swing the left arm down across the body. Withdraw the right fist to the waist. Inhale.

Figure 4-442: (E) Step forward with the left leg into mountain climbing stance (*deng shan bu,* 蹬山步). Continue to swing your left arm to the side and punch down with the right fist. Exhale.

Analysis

You cannot use your hand to block a hard kick, or you might break your arm. You must sit back to yield and use your hand to gently connect to his leg and lead it to the side. This exposes your opponent's groin to your punch.

101. Step Forward, Wardoff, Rollback, Press, and Push Forward (*Shang Bu Peng Lu Ji An* 上步掤捋擠按)

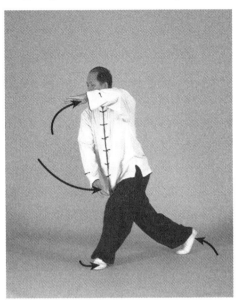

Figure 4-443: (E) Turn the legs so that you are in the sitting on crossed legs stance (*zuo pan bu*, 坐盤步) while lowering your right hand, palm up. As you do this, you also raise your left hand straight up and neutralize to your left. Inhale.

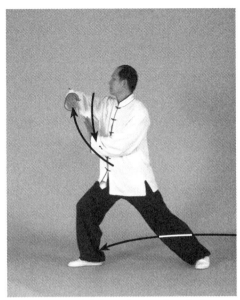

Figure 4-444: (E) Step forward with the right leg into mountain climbing stance (*deng shan bu*, 蹬山步) and swing the right arm up. Exhale.

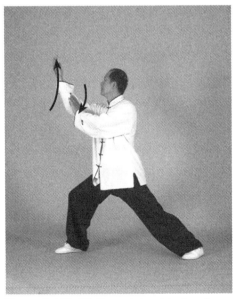

Figure 4-445: (E) Extend the right hand upward while sinking your right elbow. Continue your exhalation from last posture.

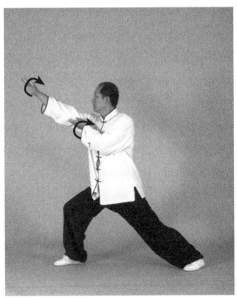

Figure 4-446: (E) Coil your right hand clockwise and forward until the palm is facing forward while turning your left palm to face upward. Begin to inhale.

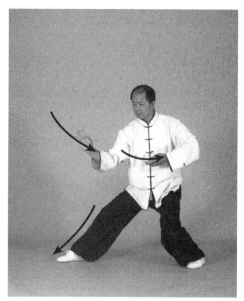

Figure 4-447: (E) Sit back into four-six stance (*si liu bu*, 四六步). Move the right arm down to the front and left hand to your left chest area. Complete your inhalation.

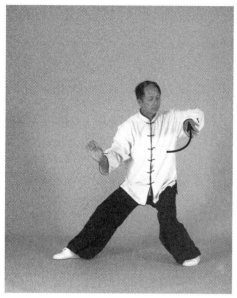

Figure 4-448: (E) Turn the hips slightly to your left. Make a gentle small clockwise circle with your left hand on the left side of the body. This movement does not have a practical application; instead, it is the signature of Yang Style Taijiquan. Exhale.

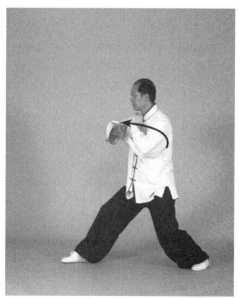

Figure 4-449: (E) Bring the left hand to the inner wrist of the right hand while inhaling. Face turn to the (E).

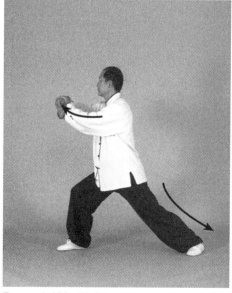

Figure 4-450: (E) Shift into mountain climbing stance (*deng shan bu*, 蹬山步) and extend both hands forward while still touching. Exhale as the arms are extended.

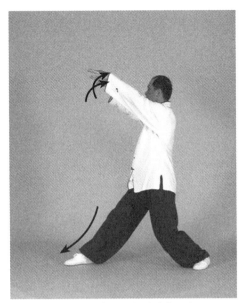

Figure 4-451: (E) Slide the left hand over the right hand. Open the arms to the width of the shoulder. Palms face down. Sit back in four-six stance (*si liu bu*, 四六步) while raising the arms up and back in a circular motion. Start to inhale.

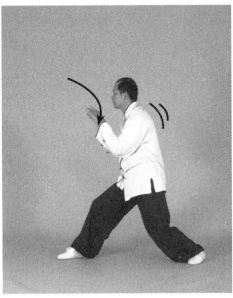

Figure 4-452: (E) Lower the arms to the chest in a circular motion. Fingers point forward. Complete your inhalation.

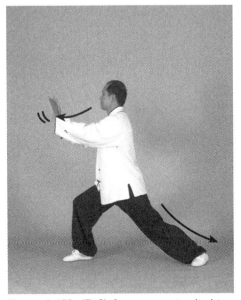

Figure 4-453: (E) Shift to mountain climbing stance (*deng shan bu*, 蹬山步) and push the hands forward while settling down your wrists. Exhale.

102. Single Whip (*Dan Bian,* 單鞭)

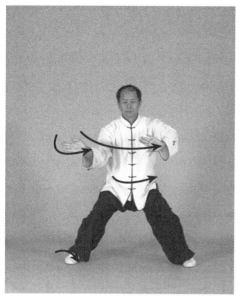

Figure 4-454: (N) Turn both hands to face forward. Keep the arms locked in the same position and turn to (N) on the right heel so the stance is horse stance (*ma bu,* 馬步). Arms swing with the body. Begin to inhale.

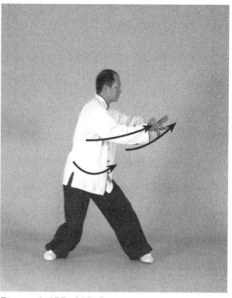

Figure 4-455: (W) Continue turning the body to your left while keeping both of your hands in the same position. Continue your inhalation.

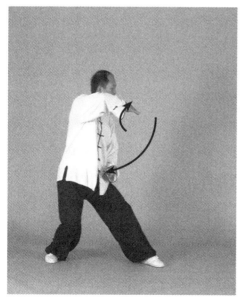

Figure 4-456: (W) Lower the left arm and turn the palm up, and turn your right palm down so that the palms face each other. Complete your inhalation.

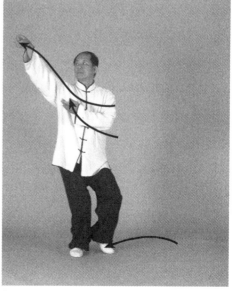

Figure 4-457: (N) Bring the left leg, on its toes, to the right leg. Swing the right arm back. All the fingertips of the right hand are touching and pointing down. Exhale.

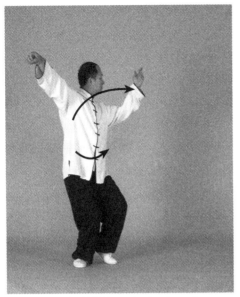

Figure 4-458: (W) Turn the body to face (W). At the same time move the left hand across the body, palm faces in. Inhale.

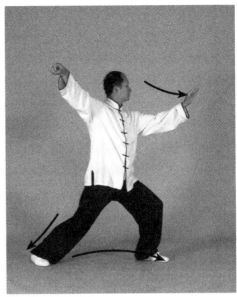

Figure 4-459: (W) Next, turn the palm out and fingers pointing forward. Step the left leg forward so the stance is mountain climbing stance (*deng shan bu*, 蹬山步), and push the left hand forward. Exhale.

103. The Snake Creeps Down (*She Shen Xia Shi*, 蛇身下势)

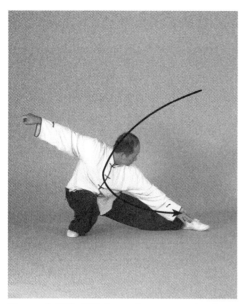

Figure 4-460: (W) Squat into tame the tiger stance (*fu hu bu*, 伏虎步) with weight on the right leg while swinging your left hand past your face and down to your left foot. Inhale.

104. Step Forward to the Seven Stars (Shang Bu Qi Xing, 上步七星)

The Chinese name of this form is "shang bu qi xing." Shang bu means step forward, and qi xing means seven stars. In China, the seven stars refer to the seven stars of the big dipper. In this form your body resembles the constellation, with your front leg the handle and your body and arms the bowl. Chinese people believe that the arrangement of the seven stars hides many fighting strategies. For example, qi xing zhen, (七星陣), which means seven star tactics, refers to ways of positioning and moving troops in battle. Qi xing bu means seven star steps and refers to ways of stepping and moving in combat. Qi xing is also used to refer to the cavities located on the chest. In this form you step forward to form the qi xing form and strike your opponent's qi xing area.

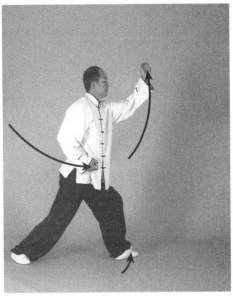 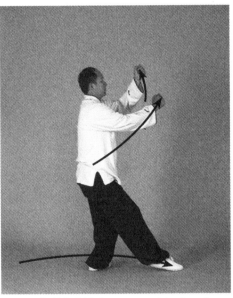

Figure 4-461: (W) Raise your body and lift the left fist up, while turning the left toes to the side. Start to exhale.

Figure 4-462: (W) Step your right foot forward on its toes into false stance (xuan ji bu or xu bu, 玄機步、虛步). Punch with your right fist under your left hand. Complete your exhalation.

Analysis

Your left hand leads the opponent's arm upward to expose his chest to your right punch and his groin to a kick from your right leg.

105. Step Back and Ride the Tiger (*Tui Bu Kua Hu*, 退步跨虎)

The Chinese name of this form is "tui bu kua hu." Tui bu means step back. Kua means to straddle, to encroach upon, or to pass over, and hu is tiger. Therefore, this form can be translated either "step back to ride the tiger" or "step back to pass over the tiger." The tiger is a very powerful and violent animal. If you desire to ride one, you had better hold on to the hair on his back tightly; otherwise you will fall and become his victim. If you want to pass over a sleeping tiger, you must also be careful not to touch the tiger and wake him. Generally speaking, this form implies that your hands hold onto the opponent, and your steps should be careful to set up the most advantageous position for yourself.

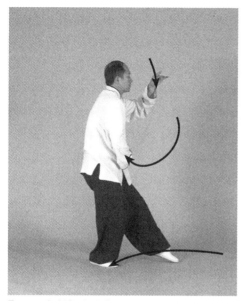

Figure 4-463: (W) Step back with your right leg once againt into false stance (*xuan ji bu or xu bu*, 玄機步、虛步) while scooping your right hand up, and cover down with your left arm. Inhale.

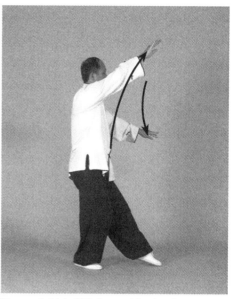

Figure 4-464: (W) Spread both of your arms upward and forward. Exhale.

Analysis

This form is commonly used when your opponent grabs your lapels with the intention of pulling you down or lifting you up. You must therefore first increase your stability by sitting back as if you were riding a tiger: firm and stable. In addition, you must grasp the opponent's arm tightly like you would hold on to the hair on the tiger's back. This will stop his attack. If, when your opponent grabs your chest, you sit back and also pull his arms toward you, you can pull him off balance or use your left leg to kick his groin.

106. Turn the Body and Sweep the Lotus with the Leg (Zhuan Shen Bai Lian, 轉身擺蓮)

The Chinese name of this form is "zhuan shen bai lian." Zhuan shen means to turn the body and bai lian is to sweep the lotus. There are three kicks in this form, one forward kick and two sweeping kicks. The feel of a sweeping kick is like a lotus leaf on a long stem, swinging from side to side in the wind.

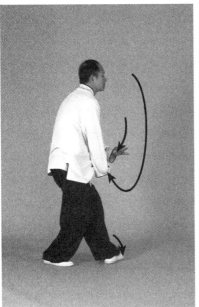

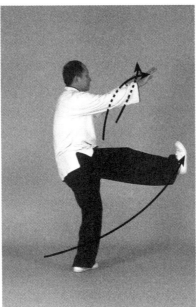

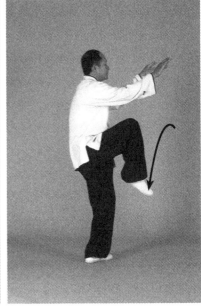

Figure 4-465: (W) Step the left leg down and turn the toes to the side while scooping both of your hands down to the abdominal area. Inhale.

Figures 4-466 and 4-467: (W) Spread both of your hands to the sides in front of your chest area, palms facing out, while kicking your right sole up to groin height and then bringing it back. Exhale.

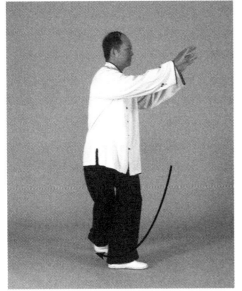

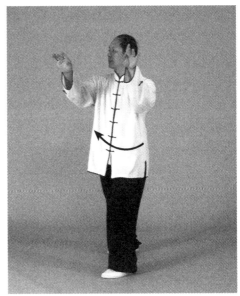

Figure 4-468: (W) Step your right leg behind you, to the left side of your left leg. Start to inhale.

Figures 4-469: (E) Turn your body 180 degrees on your heels to face (E). Complete your inhalation.

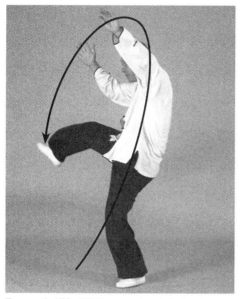 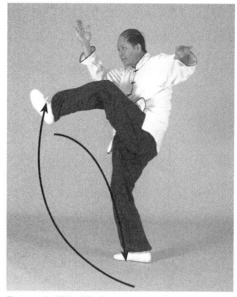

Figure 4-470: (E) Sweep the right leg in a clockwise circle. Slap both hands with your leg at the top of the circle. Exhale.

Figure 4-471: (E) Set the right leg down. Inhale. Immediately sweep the left leg out, up to touch right hand and then in; the heel is flat when the hand slaps it at the highest point. Exhale.

Analysis

There are three kicks involved in this form, a sole or toe kick and two high sweep kicks. When kicking high, it is very important to have a firm root, for without stability you are lost. When kicking high, you must kick very fast because when your raise your leg your lower body is exposed to attack, especially to sweeps and groin attacks.

107. Draw the Bow and Shoot the Tiger (Wan Gong She Hu, 彎弓射虎)

The Chinese name of this form is "wan gong she hu." Wan gong means to bend a bow, and she hu means to shoot a tiger. When a bow is bent, it stores energy. When the arrow is shot, it is fast and powerful. This tells you that you must first store jin in your posture, and when you strike, the strike must be fast. In this form, your right hand is shaped like a bow and your left arm is like an arrow.

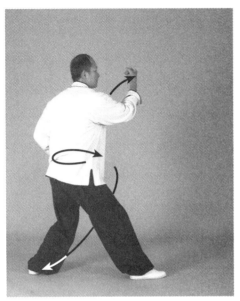

Figure 4-472: (W) Turn your body to face (W) and place your left foot to the rear; stand in four-six stance (si liu bu, 四六步); move the right fist up and your left fist to the waist. Inhale.

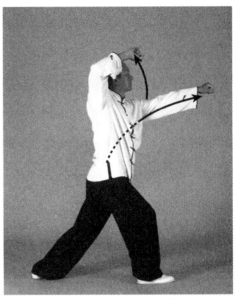

Figure 4-473: (W) Continue to block your right fist up while punching the left fist forward. The stance is mountain climbing stance (deng shan bu, 蹬山步). Exhale.

Analysis
Your right hand is used for deflecting and the left one for punching. Step backward as your arms move. This not only helps you yield and adjust distance, but also balances your speed and jin.

108. Twist the Body and Circle the Fist (*Pie Shen Chui*,　撇身捶)

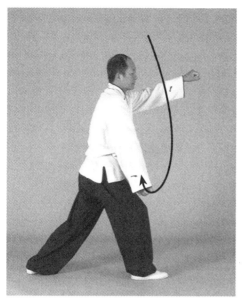

Figure 4-474: (W) Make a clockwise circle with the right arm in front of your body, while turning your body to the right into sitting on crossed legs stance (*zuo pan bu*, 坐盤步). Begin to inhale.

109. Step Forward, Deflect Downward, Parry, and Punch (*Jin Bu Ban Lan Chui*, 進步搬攔捶)

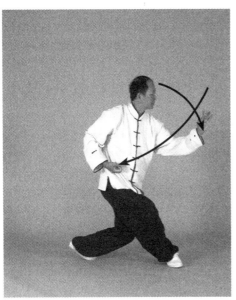

Figure 4-475: (W) Continue twisting to your right, and move your right hand to your waist while covering your left hand. Complete exhaling. The left arm swings across the body. Complete your inhalation.

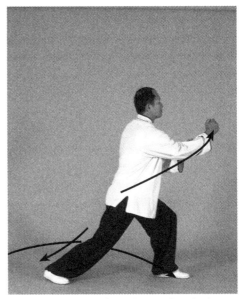

Figure 4-476: (W) Step forward with the left leg into mountain climbing stance (*deng shan bu*, 蹬山步) while punching your right fist forward and sliding your left hand to the inside of your right elbow area. When you step forward, inhale, and when you punch, exhale.

110. Seal Tightly (*Ru Feng Si Bi*, 如封似閉)

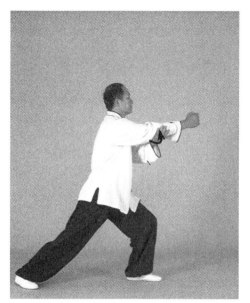

Figure 4-477: (W) Continue to slide your left hand under the right elbow, with the palm of your left hand facing in to your right arm. Start to inhale.

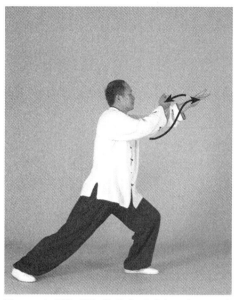

Figure 4-478: (W) Coil the left hand around the right forearm, move from the elbow to the wrist, and extend forward. When the left hand has reached its maximum extension, start to pull in the right fist. Continue to inhale.

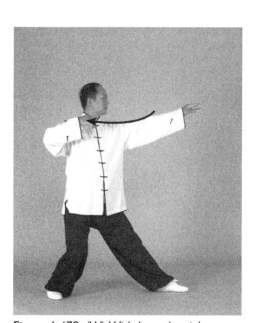

Figure 4-479: (W) Withdraw the right arm to chest area while sitting back in four-six stance (*si liu bu*, 四六步). Complete your inhalation.

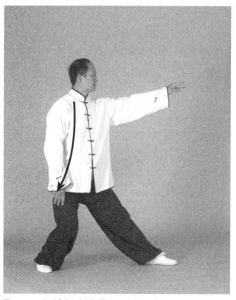

Figure 4-480: (W) Drop the right arm down. Exhale.

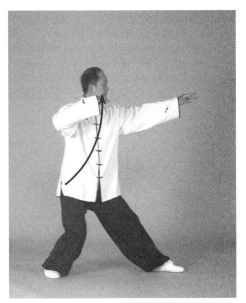

Figure 4-481: (W) Raise the right arm up so it is beside the ear. Inhale.

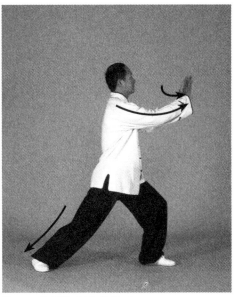

Figure 4-482: (W) Shift the stance to mountain climbing stance (*deng shan bu*, 蹬山步) and push the right palm forward. The left hand opens into a palm, pushing forward. Exhale.

111. Embrace the Tiger and Return to the Mountain (*Bao Hu Gui Shan,* 抱虎歸山)

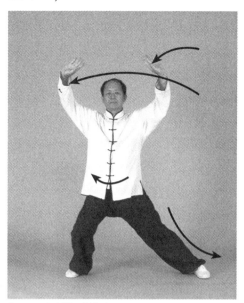

Figure 4-483: (N) Cross the hands and turn the body (N), and then open both of your arms. Lean to the right side. Inhale.

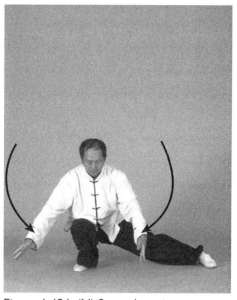

Figure 4-484: (N) Squat down into tame the tiger stance (*fu hu bu,* 伏虎步) while circling both arms out, down, and in. Weight is on the right leg. Begin to exhale.

112. Close Taiji (He Taiji, 合太極)

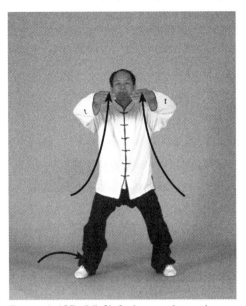

Figure 4-485: (N) Shift the weight to the left leg, raise the right knee, and step the right leg down in horse stance (ma bu, 馬步). Move both hands to the chest area. Arms are in a circle. Complete exhaling.

113. Return to the Original Stance (*Taiji Huan Yuan,* 太極還原)

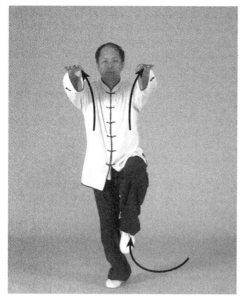

Figure 4-486 (N) Extend your arms, palms down, and raise the left knee. Begin to inhale.

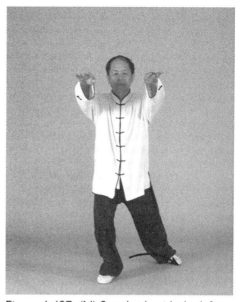

Figure 4-487: (N) Step back with the left leg. Continue your inhalation.

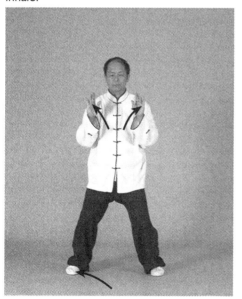

Figure 4-488: (N) Step back with the right leg while moving both of your hands to the upper chest. Finish inhalation.

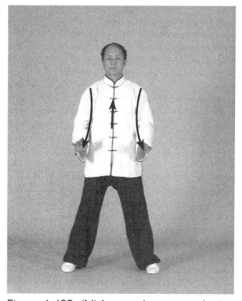

Figure 4-489: (N) Lower the arms and raise up the body so the original stance is assumed. Exhale.

End of the Third Part.

You should remember that this form is a traditional martial style of taijiquan. Every movement of each posture has its own martial purpose, essential artistic qualities, and a root for power manifestation. Just like a complex and difficult piece of music, it will take you a great investment of time and energy (i.e., gongfu) to practice, understand, and master. Only then will you fully feel and comprehend the essence of every movement. This devotion in turn will bring meaning to your practice.

In addition, you must also learn how to incorporate into your form the idea of using the mind to lead the qi to your imaginary target. In order to make the qi circulate strongly and smoothly, you must understand how to use your breathing properly. The final goal is to unify the external with the internal.

To get a more accurate idea of the correct movements in detail, it can be helpful to watch the companion videotape to this book. To understand the martial essence of each form, you should refer to the books: *Tai Chi Theory and Martial Power* and *Tai Chi Chuan Martial Applications*, published by YMAA.

Notes

1. 先求開展，后求緊湊，可臻于縝密矣。

2. *Tai Chi Theory and Martial Power,* Dr. Yang, Jwing-Ming, YMAA Publication Center, 1986, Appendix A, 3.

3. *Tai Chi Theory and Martial Power,* Dr. Yang, Jwing-Ming, YMAA Publication Center, 1986, Appendix A, 10.

4. 膝部似鬆非鬆。

5. 姿勢無過或不及，當求其中正。

6. 式式勢順，不拗不背，周身舒適。式式均勻。

7. *Tai Chi Theory and Martial Power,* Dr. Yang, Jwing-Ming, YMAA Publication Center, 1986, Appendix A, 1.

8. 無使有缺陷處,無使有凸凹處,無使有續斷處。

9. "Complex and Hidden Brain in the Gut Makes Cramps, Buttflies and Valium," by Sandra Blakeslee, *The New York Times*, Science, January 23, 1996.

10. 一舉動，周身俱要輕靈，尤須貫穿。

11. *Historical Record*, 史紀。"The History of the Confucius Family" 孔子世家。 楊家駱編著。 正中書局。Taipei, Taiwan, 1993.

12. 其根在腳，發于腿，主宰于腰，形于手指。由腳而腿而腰，總須完整一气。向前退后，乃能得機得勢。

CHAPTER 5

Conclusion

結論

Although this book has provided you with a theoretical foundation for your study of taijiquan, covering both internal qi cultivation and the physical postures, it still is only a basic reference of shallow depth. The purpose of this book is to be an introduction to taijiquan understanding and practice. If you are interested in furthering your study of taijiquan, you should refer to the following books, all published by YMAA Publication Center:

- *The Essence of Taiji Qigong*
- *Tai Chi Theory and Martial Power*
- *Tai Chi Chuan Martial Applications*
- *Taiji Chin Na*

You are also encouraged to study the following qigong books that could help you understand the internal side of taijiquan practice:

- *Qigong for Health and Martial Arts*
- *The Root of Chinese Qigong*
- *The Essence of Shaolin White Crane*

The art of taijiquan was created and has developed through a thousand years of accumulated knowledge, which in turn was gained through committed practice and honest evaluation of results. It is neither possible nor appropriate to reach to a more profound level in a short period of study. Remain humble and keep your mind open, and in time you will see this art revealed in all of its complexity and richness. Moreover, as the paths of science and spirituality begin to interweave, your appreciation of the profound simplicity that taijiquan reveals can have a deeper and more rewarding effect on your life.

APPENDIX A
Names of Traditional Yang Style Taijiquan Movements

	Page
1. **Beginning** (*Taiji Qi Shi*, 太極起勢)	192
2. **Grasp the Sparrow's Tail: Right** (*You Lan Que Wei*, 右攬雀尾)	194
3. **Grasp the Sparrow's Tail: Left** (*Zuo Lan Que Wei*, 左攬雀尾)	195
4. **Wardoff** (*Peng*, 掤)	196
5. **Rollback** (*Lu*, 攦)	197
6. **Press** (*Ji*, 擠)	199
7. **Push Forward** (*An*, 按)	200
8. **Single Whip** (*Dan Bian*, 單鞭)	201
9. **Lift Hands to the Up Posture** (*Ti Shou Shang Shi*, 提手上勢)	203
10. **The Crane Spreads Its Wings** (*Bai He Liang Chi*, 白鶴亮翅)	204
11. **Brush Knee and Step Forward: Left** (*Zuo Lou Xi Ao Bu*, 左摟膝拗步)	205
12. **Play the Guitar** (*Shou Hui Pi Pa*, 手揮琵琶)	207
13. **Twist Body, Brush Knee and Step Forward: Left** (*Zuo Lou Xi Ao Bu*, 左摟膝拗步)	208
14. **Twist Body, Brush Knee and Step Forward: Right** (*You Lou Xi Ao Bu*, 右摟膝拗步)	209
15. **Twist Body, Brush Knee and Step Forward: Left** (*Zuo Lou Xi Ao Bu*, 左摟膝拗步)	211
16. **Play the Guitar** (*Shou Hui Pi Pa*, 手揮琵琶)	212
17. **Twist Body, Brush Knee and Step Forward: Left** (*Zuo Lou Xi Ao Bu*, 左摟膝拗步)	213
18. **Twist Body and Circle the Fist** (*Pie Shen Chui*, 撇身捶)	214
19. **Step Forward, Deflect Downward, Parry and Punch** (*Jin Bu Ban Lan Chui*, 進步搬攔捶)	215
20. **Seal Tightly** (*Ru Feng Si Bi*, 如封似閉)	216
21. **Embrace the Tiger and Return to the Mountain** (*Bao Hu Gui Shan*, 抱虎歸山)	218
22. **Close Taiji** (*He Taiji*, 合太極)	219
Transition Form (*Guo Du Shi*, 過渡勢)	220

23. **Wardoff, Rollback, Press, and Push Forward** (*Peng Lu Ji An,* 掤攦擠按)   221

24. **Single Whip** (*Dan Bian,* 單鞭)   224

25. **Punch under the Elbow** (*Zhou Di Kan Chui,* 肘底看捶)   226

26. **Step Back and Repulse the Monkey: Left** (*Zuo Dao Nian Hou,* 左倒攆猴)   227

27. **Step Back and Repulse the Monkey: Right** (*You Dao Nian Hou,* 右倒攆猴)   228

28. **Step Back and Repulse the Monkey: Left** (*Zuo Dao Nian Hou,* 左倒攆猴)   229

29. **Diagonal Flying** (*Xie Fei Shi,* 斜飛勢)   230

30. **Lift Hands to the Up Posture** (*Ti Shou Shang Shi,* 提手上勢)   231

31. **The Crane Spreads Its Wings** (*Bai He Liang Chi,* 白鶴亮翅)   232

32. **Brush Knee and Step Forward: Left** (*Zuo Lou Xi Ao Bu,* 左摟膝拗步)   233

33. **Pick Up the Needle from the Sea Bottom** (*Hai Di Lao Zhen,* 海底撈針)   234

34. **Fan Back** (*Shan Tong Bei,* 扇通背)   235

35. **Turn, Twist Body, and Circle the Fist** (*Zhuan Shen Pie Shen Chui,* 轉身撇身捶)   236

36. **Step Forward, Deflect Downward, Parry and Punch** (*Jin Bu Ban Lan Chui,* 進步搬欄捶)   237

37. **Step Forward, Wardoff, Rollback, Press and Push Forward** (*Shang Bu Beng Lu Ji An,* 上步掤攦擠按)   238

38. **Single Whip** (*Dan Bian,* 單鞭)   241

39. **Wave Hands in the Clouds: Right** (*You Yun Shou,* 右雲手)   243

40. **Wave Hands in the Clouds: Left** (*Zuo Yun Shou,* 左雲手)   244

41. **Wave Hands in the Clouds: Right** (*You Yun Shou,* 右雲手)   245

42. **Single Whip** (*Dan Bian,* 單鞭)   246

43. **Stand High to Search Out the Horse** (*Gao Tan Ma,* 高探馬)   248

44. **Separate Right Foot** (*You Fen Jiao,* 右分腳)   249

45. **Separate Left Foot** (*Zuo Fen Jiao,* 左分腳)   250

46. **Turn and Kick with the Heel: 90 degrees** (*Zhuan Shen Deng Jiao,* 轉身蹬腳)   251

47. **Brush Knee and Step Forward: Left** (*Zuo Lou Xi Ao Bu,* 左摟膝拗步)   252

48. **Brush Knee and Step Forward: Right** (*You Lou Xi Ao Bu,* 右摟膝拗步)   253

49. **Step Forward and Strike Down with the Fist** (*Jin Bu Zai Chui,* 進步栽捶)   254

50. **Turn, Twist Body, and Circle the Fist** (*Zhuan Shen Pie Shen Chui,* 轉身撇身捶)   255

51. **Step Forward, Deflect Downward, Parry and Punch** (*Jin Bu Ban Lan Chui,* 進步搬欄捶)   256

52. **Kick Right** (*You Ti Jiao,* 右踢腳)   257

53. **Strike the Tiger: Right** (*You Da Hu,* 右打虎)   258

54. **Strike the Tiger: Left** (*Zuo Da Hu,* 左打虎)   259

55. **Kick Right** (*You Ti Jiao,* 右踢腳)   260

56. **Attack the Ears with the Fists** (*Shuang Feng Guan Er,* 雙風貫耳)   261

57. Kick Left (*Zuo Ti Jiao*, 左踢腳) 262

58. Turn and Kick with the Heel: 270 degrees (*Zhuan Shen Deng Jiao*, 轉身蹬腳) 263

59. Twist the Body and Circle the Fist (*Pie Shen Chui*, 撇身捶) 264

60. Step Forward, Deflect Downward, Parry, and Punch (*Jin Bu Ban Lan Chui*, 進步搬攔捶) 265

61. Seal Tightly (*Ru Feng Si Bi*, 如封似閉) 266

62. Embrace the Tiger and Return to the Mountain (*Bao Hu Gui Shan*, 抱虎歸山) 268

63. Close Taiji (*He Taiji*, 合太極) 269

Transition Form (*Guo Du Shi*, 過渡勢) 270

64. Wardoff, Rollback, Press, and Push Forward (*Peng Lu Ji An*, 掤攦擠按) 271

65. Single Whip (*Dan Bian*, 單鞭) 274

66. The Wild Horse Parts Its Mane: Right (*You Ye Ma Fen Zong*, 右野馬分鬃) 276

67. The Wild Horse Parts Its Mane: Left (*Zuo Ye Ma Fen Zong*, 左野馬分鬃) 277

68. The Wild Horse Parts Its Mane: Right (*You Ye Ma Fen Zong*, 右野馬分鬃) 278

69. Grasp the Sparrow's Tail: Left (*Zuo Lan Que Wei*, 左攬雀尾) 279

70. Wardoff, Rollback, Press, and Push Forward (*Peng Lu Ji An*, 掤攦擠按) 280

71. Single Whip (*Dan Bian*, 單鞭) 283

72. The Fair Lady Weaves with Shuttle: Left (*Zuo Yu Nu Chuan Suo*, 左玉女穿梭) 285

73. The Fair Lady Weaves with Shuttle: Right (*You Yu Nu Chuan Suo*, 右玉女穿梭) 286

74. The Fair Lady Weaves with Shuttle: Left (*Zuo Yu Nu Chuan Suo*, 左玉女穿梭) 287

75. The Fair Lady Weaves with Shuttle: Right (*You Yu Nu Chuan Suo*, 右玉女穿梭) 288

76. Grasp Sparrow's Tail: Left (*Zuo Lan Que Wei*, 左攬雀尾) 289

77. Wardoff, Rollback, Press, and Push Forward (*Peng Lu Ji An*, 掤攦擠按) 290

78. Single Whip (*Dan Bian*, 單鞭) 293

79. Wave Hands in the Clouds: Right (*You Yun Shou*, 右雲手) 295

80. Single Whip (*Dan Bian*, 單鞭) 296

81. The Snake Creeps Down (*She Shen Xia Shi*, 蛇身下勢) 298

82. The Golden Rooster Stands on One Leg: Right (*You Jin Ji Du Li*, 右金雞獨立) 299

83. Golden Rooster Stands on One Leg: Left (*Zuo Jin Ji Du Li*, 左金雞獨立) 300

84. Step Back and Repulse the Monkey: Left (*Zuo Dao Nian Hou*, 左倒撞猴) 301

85. Diagonal Flying (*Xie Fei Shi*, 斜飛勢) 302

86. Lift Hands to the Up Posture (*Ti Shou Shang Shi*, 提手上勢) 303

87. The White Crane Spreads Its Wings (*Bai He Liang Chi*, 白鶴亮翅) 304

88. Brush Knee and Step Forward: Left (*Zuo Lou Xi Ao Bu*, 左摟膝拗步)   305

89. Pick Up the Needle from the Sea Bottom (*Hai Di Lao Zhen*, 海底撈針)   306

90. Fan Back (*Shan Tong Bei*, 扇通背)   307

91. The White Snake Turns Its Body and Spits Poison (*Zhuan Shen Bai She Tu Xin*, 轉身白蛇吐信)   308

92. Step Forward, Deflect Downward, Parry, and Punch (*Jin Bu Ban Lan Chui*, 進步搬攔捶)   309

93. Step Forward, Wardoff, Rollback, Press, and Push Forward (*Shang Bu Peng Lu Ji An*, 上步掤攦擠按)   310

95. Wave Hands in the Clouds: Right (*You Yun Shou*, 右雲手)   315

96. Single Whip (*Dan Bian*, 單鞭)   316

97. Stand High to Search Out the Horse (*Gao Tan Ma*, 高探馬)   318

98. Cross Hands (*Shi Zi Shou*, 十字手)   319

99. Turn and Kick (*Zhuan Shen Shi Zi Tui*, 轉身十字腿)   320

100. Brush Knee and Punch Down (*Lou Xi Zhi Dang Chui*, 摟膝指襠捶)   321

101. Step Forward, Wardoff, Rollback, Press, and Push Forward (*Shang Bu Peng Lu Ji An*, 上步掤攦擠按)   322

102. Single Whip (*Dan Bian*, 單鞭)   325

103. The Snake Creeps Down (*She Shen Xia Shi*, 蛇身下勢)   327

104. Step Forward to the Seven Stars (*Shang Bu Qi Xing*, 上步七星)   328

105. Step Back and Ride the Tiger (*Tui Bu Kua Hu*, 退步跨虎)   329

106. Turn the Body and Sweep the Lotus with the Leg (*Zhuan Shen Bai Lian*, 轉身擺蓮)   330

107. Draw the Bow and Shoot the Tiger (*Wan Gong She Hu*, 彎弓射虎)   332

108. Twist the Body and Circle the Fist (*Pie Shen Chui*, 撇身捶)   333

109. Step Forward, Deflect Downward, Parry, and Punch (*Jin Bu Ban Lan Chui*, 進步搬攔捶)   334

110. Seal Tightly (*Ru Feng Si Bi*, 如封似閉)   335

111. Embrace the Tiger and Return to the Mountain (*Bao Hu Gui Shan*, 抱虎歸山)   337

112. Close Taiji (*He Taiji*, 合太極)   338

113. Return to the Original Stance (*Taiji Huan Yuan*, 太極還原)   339

Translation and Glossary of Chinese Terms

Ai 哀　Sorrow.

Ai 愛　Love, kindness.

An 按　One of the taijiquan basic thirteen postures. An means to push or press down. Often, it is also used as push forward or upward.

Ba Duan Jin 八段錦　Eight Pieces of Brocade. A wai dan qigong practice which is said to have been created by Marshal Yue Fei during the Southern Song dynasty (A.D. 1127-1279).

Ba Kua Chang (Baguazhang) 八卦掌　Means "eight trigram palms." The name of one of the Chinese internal martial styles.

Ba Mai 八脈　Referred to as the eight extraordinary vessels. These eight vessels are considered to be qi reservoirs, which regulate the qi status in the primary qi channels.

Ba Men 八門　Means "eight doors." Taijiquan is costructed out of thirteen basic postures, which includes eight basic body movment patterns and five stepping strategies. The right basic body movements are commonly compared to the eight trigrams in baguazhgang, and are called the "eight doors."

Ba Shi 八勢　Means "eight standing postures." These eight basic fundamental stances are commonly used in Northern styles of Chinese martial arts. They are also used in taijiquan.

Bagua 八卦　Literally, "eight divinations." Also called the eight trigrams. In Chinese philosophy, the eight basic variations; shown in the *Yi Jing* as groups of single and broken lines.

Baguazhang (Ba Kua Zhang) 八卦掌　Means "Eight Trigram Palms." The name of one of the Chinese internal martial styles.

Bai He 白鶴　Means "White Crane." One of the Chinese southern martial styles.

Bai, Yu-feng 白玉峰　A well known Chinese martial artist during the Song dynasty (Southern and Southern, A.D. 960-1278). Later, he and his son joined the Shaolin Temple. His monk's name was Qiu Yue Chan Shi.

Baihui (Gv-20) 百會　Literally, "hundred meetings." An important acupuncture cavity located on the top of the head. The baihui cavity belongs to the governing vessel.

Batuo 跋陀　An Indian Buddhist monk who came to China to preach Buddhism in A.D. 464.

Bei Kao 背靠　Using any part of the back to bump someone off balance is called bei kao.

Bruce Lee 李小龍　A well-known Chinese martial artist and movie star during the 1960s.

Cai 採　Plucking.

Canton (Guangdong) 廣東　A province in southern China.

Ce Kao 側靠　To bump someone off balance from the side.

Chan 纏 To wrap or to coil. A common Chinese martial arts technique.

Chan (Ren) 禪，忍 A Chinese school of Mahayana Buddhism which asserts that enlightenment can be attained through meditation, self-contemplation and intuition, rather than through study of scripture. Chan is called ren in Japan.

Chang 長 Long.

Chang Chuan (Changquan) 長拳 Means "long-range fist." Chang chuan includes all northern Chinese long-range martial styles.

Chang Jiang 長江 Literally, long river. Refers to the Yangtze River in southern China.

Chang, La-ta 張邋遢 Means "Sloppy Zhang." A nickname of Zhang, San-feng.

Changquan (Chang Chuan) 長拳 Means "long-range fist." Changquan includes all northern Chinese long-range martial styles.

Chen Jia Gou 陳家溝 Means "Chen's family ditch," and implies Chen's village. The place where Chen Style Taijiquan originated. Located in Huai Qing County, Henan Province, China.

Cheng, Gin-Gsao 曾金灶 Dr. Yang, Jwing-Ming's White Crane master.

Cheng, Man-Ching 鄭曼清 A well-known Chinese Taijiquan master in America during the 1960's.

Chi (Qi) 氣 The energy pervading the universe, including the energy circulating in the human body.

Chi Kung (Qigong) 氣功 The gongfu of qi, which means the study of qi.

Chiang, Kai-Shek 蔣介石 A well-known president in China.

Chin Na (Qin Na) 擒拿 Literally means "grab control." A component of Chinese martial arts which emphasizes grabbing techniques, to control your opponent's joints, in conjunction with attacking certain acupuncture cavities.

Chong Mai 衝脈 Thrusting vessel. One of the eight extraordinary qi vessels

Confucius 孔子 A Chinese scholar, during the period of 551-479 B.C., whose philosophy has significantly influenced Chinese culture.

Da 打 To strike. Normally, to attack with the palms, fists or arms.

Da Lu 大攄 Means "large rollback." One of the basic pushing hands practices in taijiquan.

Da Mo 達摩 The Indian Buddhist monk who is credited with creating the Yi Jin Jing and Xi Sui Jing while at the Shaolin monastery. His last name was Sardili and he was also known as Bodhidarma. He was once the prince of a small tribe in southern India.

Da Zhi 大智和尚 A Japanese Buddhist monk who lived in the Yuan dynasty, in the year A.D. 1312. After he studied Shaolin martial arts (barehands and staff) for nearly 13 years A.D. 1324, he returned to Japan and spread Shaolin Gongfu to Japanese martial arts society.

Da Zhou Tian 大周天 Literally, "grand cycle heaven." Usually translated grand circulation. After a nei dan qigong practitioner completes small circulation, he will circulate his qi through the entire body or exchange the qi with nature.

Dai Mai Hu Xi 帶脈呼吸 Belt vessel breathing. An advanced meditation breathing technique, which uses the mind to lead the qi to the qi belt vessel and expand the qi horizontally.

Dan Tian 丹田 "Elixir field." Located in the lower abdomen. It is considered the place which can store qi energy.

Dan Tian Qi 丹田氣 Usually, the qi which is converted from original essence and is stored in the lower dan tian. This qi is considered "water qi" and is able to calm down the body. Also called xian tian qi (pre-heaven qi).

Dao 道 The "way," by implication the "natural way."

Dao De Jing 道德經 *Morality Classic*. Written by Lao Zi.

Dao Jia 道家 The Dao family. Daoism. Created by Lao Zi during the Zhou dynasty (1122-934 B.C). In the Han dynasty c. A.D. 58, it was mixed with the Buddhism to become the Daoist religion (*Dao Jiao*).

Deng Feng Xian Zhi 登封縣志 Deng Feng County Recording. A formal historical recording in Deng Feng County, Henan, where the Shaolin Temple is located.

Deng Shan Bu 蹬山步 Means "mountain climbing stance." One of the eight basic fundamental stances.

Di 地 The earth. Earth, heaven (*tian*) and man (*ren*) are the three natural powers" (*san cai*).

Di Li Shi 地理師 Di li means "geomancy" and shi means "teacher." Therefore di li shi is a teacher or master who analyzes geographic locations according to the formulas in the *Yi Jing* (Book of Change) and the energy distributions in the earth. Also called Feng Shui Shi.

Dian 點 "To point" or "to press."

Dian Mai (Dim Mak) 點脈 Mai means "the blood vessel" (*xue mai*) or "the qi channel" (*qi mai*). Dian mai means "to press the blood vessel or qi channel."

Dian Qi 電氣 Dian means "electricity" and so dian qi means "electrical energy" (electricity). In China, a word is often placed before "qi" to identify the different kinds of energy.

Dian Xue 點穴 Dian means "to point and exert pressure" and xue means "the cavities." Dian xue refers to those qin na techniques which specialize in attacking acupuncture cavities to immobilize or kill an opponent.

Dian Xue massages 點穴按摩 One of Chinese massage techniques in which the acupuncture cavities are stimulated through pressing. Dian xue massage is also called acupressure and is the root of Japanese shiatsu.

Dim Mak (Dian Mai) 點脈 Cantonese of "dian mai."

Du Mai 督脈 Usually translated "governing vessel." One of the eight extraordinary vessels.

Emei 峨嵋 Name of a mountain in Sichuan Province, China.

Emei Da Peng Gong 峨嵋大鵬功 Da peng means roc, a legendary bird in ancient China. Emei Da Peng Gong is a qigong style developed under this name.

Fan Fu Hu Xi 反腹呼吸 Reverse abdominal breathing. Also commonly called "Daoist Breathing."

Fan Tong Hu Xi 返童呼吸 Back to childhood breathing. A breathing training in nei dan qigong through which the practitioner tries to regain control of the muscles in the lower abdomen. Also called "abdominal breathing."

Feng 封 "To seal" or "to cover."

Feng Shui Shi 風水師 Literally, "wind water teacher." Teacher or master of geomancy. Geomancy is the art or science of analyzing the natural energy relationships in a location, especially the interrelationships between "wind" and "water," hence the name. Also called di li shi.

Fu 夫 Fu has many meaning by itself. When it is placed together with gong, such as in "gong-fu," it means any effort which requires patience and time to accomplish.

Fu Hu Bu 伏虎步 Means "tame the tiger stance." One of the eight basic fundamental stances.

Fu Shi Hu Xi 腹式呼吸 Literally, "abdominal way of breathing." As you breathe, you use the muscles in the lower abdominal area to control the diaphragm. It is also called "back to (the) childhood breathing."

Fu Xi 伏羲   A legendary Chinese ruler around the period of 2852-2738 B.C, who is credited with the introduction of farming, fishing and animal husbandry. Fu Xi is also credited as the creator of taiji and bagua theory.

Fuyu 福裕   The name of a Shaolin head monk who is credited with building five additional Shaolin temples, excluding the Henan Shaolin temple, during the Chinese Huang Qing of Yuan dynasty A.D. 1212. These five were located at Jixian of Hebei province, He Lin of Wai Meng province, Changan of Shaanxi province, Taiyuan of Shanxi province, and Lo Yang of Henan province. Two of these "branch" temples were located in the south of China.

Fujian Province 福建   A province located in southeast China.

Ge 戈   Spear, lance or javelin; implies general weapons in this book.

Gong (Kung) 功   Energy or hard work.

Gong Jian Bu 弓箭步   Means "bow-arrow stance." One of the eight basic fundamental stances in Northern Chinese martial arts.

Gongfu (Kung Fu) 功夫   Means "energy-time." Anything which will take time and energy to learn or to accomplish is called gongfu.

Gu-Zheng 古箏   An ancient, string musical instrument.

Guang Cheng Zi 廣成子   An ancient Daoist qigong master.

Gui Qi 鬼氣   The qi residue of a dead person. It is believed by the Chinese Buddhists and Daoists that this qi reside is a so-called ghost.

Guohuen 國魂   Country soul or spirit.

Guoshu 國術   Abbreviation of "Zhongguo wushu," which means "Chinese martial techniques."

Ha 哈   A qigong sound which is commonly used to lead an over abundance of qi from inside the body out and therefore reduce over-accumulated qi.

Haidi 海底   Means "sea bottom." This is a name given by martial artists to the huiyin cavity (Co-1) in Chinese medicine. Perineum.

Han 漢   A dynasty in Chinese history (206 B.C.- A.D. 221).

Han, Ching-Tang 韓慶堂   A well known Chinese martial artist, especially in Taiwan in the last forty years. Master Han is also Dr. Yang, Jwing-Ming's Long Fist Grand Master.

He 和   Harmony or peace.

Hen 恨   Hate.

Hen 哼   A yin qigong sound which is the opposite of the 'ha' yang sound.

Henan 河南省   The province in China where the Shaolin Temple is located.

Hou Tian Fa 后天法 (後天法)   Means "Post-Heaven Techniques." An internal Qigong style dating from A.D. 550.

Hsing Yi Chuan (Xingyiquan) 形意拳   A style of internal Chinese martial arts.

Hua 化   "To neutralize."

Hua Quan 化拳   Means "Neutralizing Style." Taijiquan is also called Hua Quan, because it specializes in neutralizing the opponent's force into nothing.

Hua Tuo 華佗   A well known doctor in the Chinese Three Kingdoms Period (A.D. 221-265)

Huan 緩   Slow.

Huang Ting Ching 黃庭經   Means *Yellow Yard Classic*. The name of an ancient Qigong book.

Hubei province 湖北   A province in China.

Huo Qi 活氣   Vital qi. Also means the qi circulating in a living person.

Huo 火   Fire. One of the five elements.

Ji 擠   Means "to squeeze" or "to press."

Jia Dan Tian 假丹田   False dan tian. Daoists believe that the lower dan tian located on the front side of abdomen is not the real dan tian. The real dan tian corresponds to the physical center of gravity. The false dan tian is called qihai (qi ocean) in Chinese medicine.

Jian Kao 肩靠   Shoulder bump. Refers to the use of the shoulder to bump someone off balance.

Jin 金   Metal. One of the five elements.

Jin Bu 進步   Step forward. Taijiquan is constructed from thirteen basic postures, which includes basic moving patterns and strategic steppings. Jin bu is one of the five steppings.

Jin Gi Du Li 金雞獨立   Means "golden rooster standing on one leg stance." One of the basic fundamental stances in Northern Chinese martial arts.

Jin (Jing) 勁   Chinese martial power. A combination of "li" (muscular power) and "qi."

Jin Gong 勁功   Gongfu which specializes in the training of jin manifestation.

Jin Zhong Zhao 金鐘罩   Literally, "golden bell cover." A higher level of iron shirt training.

Jin, Shao-Feng 金紹峰   Dr. Yang, Jwing-Ming's White Crane grand master.

Jing (Jin) 勁   Chinese martial power. A combination of "li" (muscular power) and "qi."

Jing 精   Essence. The most refined part of anything.

Jing 靜   Calm.

Jing-Shen 精神   Literally, essential spirit. The meaning is the spirit of vitality.

Jueyuan 覺遠   The monk name of a Shaolin priest during the Chinese Song dynasty (A.D. 960-1278).

Jun-Bao 君寶   A nickname for Zhang, San-feng.

Jun Qing 君倩   A Daoist and Chinese doctor during the Chinese Jin dynasty (A.D. 265-420). Jun Qing is credited as the creator of the Five Animal Sports Qigong practice.

Kan 坎   One of the Eight Trigrams.

Kao 靠   Means "bump." One of the taijiquan thirteen postures.

Kao Tao 高濤   Master Yang, Jwing-Ming's first taijiquan master.

King Wen of Zhou 周文王   King Wen of Zhou. He was six feet tall, and it was he who interpreted the *Book of Changes (Yi Jing)*.

Kong Qi 空氣   Air.

Kung (Gong) 功   Means energy or hard work.

Kung Fu (Gongfu) 功夫   Means "energy-time." Anything which will take time and energy to learn or to accomplish is called kung fu.

Lan Zhou 蘭州   Name of a county in ancient times. Exact location unknown to the author.

Lao Zi 老子   The creator of Daoism, also called Li Er.

Laogong (P-8) 勞宮   Cavity name. On the pericardium channel in the center of the palm.

Le 樂   Joy or happiness.

Li 力   The power which is generated from muscular strength.

Li 離   One of the eight trigrams.

Li Er 李耳   Nickname of Lao Zi.

Li Sou 李叟   A well known Chinese martial artist during the Chinese Song dynasty (A.D. 960-1278).

Li, Mao-Ching 李茂清   Dr. Yang, Jwing-Ming's Long Fist master.

Li-Qi 力氣 When you use li (muscular power) you also need qi to support it. However, when this qi is led by a concentrated mind, the qi is able to manifest the muscular power to a higher level and is therefore called jin. Li-qi (or *qi-li*) is a general definition of jin and commonly implies manifested power.

Li, Qing-An 李清庵 An ancient Chinese Qigong master.

Li, Shi-Ming 李世民 The first Tang emperor.

Lian Qi 練氣 Lian means "to train, to strengthen and to refine." A Daoist training process through which your qi grows stronger and more abundant.

Liang 梁 A dynasty in Chinese history (A.D. 502-557).

Liang Wu 梁武 An emperor of the Chinese Liang dynasty.

Lie 挒 Split or rend. One of the thirteen basic postures in taijiquan.

Liu He Ba Fa 六合八法 Literally, "six combinations eight methods." One of the Chinese internal martial arts, its techniques are combined from taijiquan, xingyi and baguazhang. This internal martial art reportedly created by Chen Bo during the Song dynasty (A.D. 960-1279).

Lu 挭 Rollback. One of the thirteen basic postures in taijiquan.

Luo 絡 The small qi channels that branch out from the primary qi channels and are connected to the skin and to the bone marrow.

Ma Bu 馬步 Horse Stance. One of the basic stances in Chinese martial arts.

Mai 脈 Means "vessel" or "qi channel."

Mencius (372-289 B.C.) 孟子 A well-known scholar who followed the philosophy of Confucius during the Chinese Zhou dynasty (909-255 B.C.).

Mian 綿 Soft.

Mian Quan 綿拳 Means soft style. Taijiquan is also called mian quan because it is soft and relaxed.

Mu 木 Wood. One of the five elements.

Na 拿 Means "to hold" or "to grab." Also an abbreviation for Chin Na or Qin Na.

Nanking Central Guoshu Institute 南京中央國術館 A national martial arts institute organized by the Chinese government in 1926.

Nei Dan 內丹 Literally, internal elixir. A form of qigong in which qi (the elixir) is built up in the body and spread out to the limbs.

Nei Gong 內功 Internal gongfu. This implies those practices that involve internal qi training.

Nei Jia 內家 Internal family. Those styles that emphasize internal qi training.

Ni Fu Hu Xi 逆腹呼吸 Reversed Abdominal Breathing. Also called Fan Fu Hu Xi or Daoist breathing. Commonly practiced in Chinese martial arts and Daoist qigong.

Nei Shi Gongfu 內視功夫 Nei shi means "to look internally," so Nei Shi Gongfu refers to the art of looking inside yourself to read the state of your health and the condition of your qi.

Nu 怒 Anger

Peng 掤 Wardoff. One of the taijiquan basic thirteen postures.

Peng Kai 掤開 Push open. Peng means to arc your arms and use them to push or bounce something away.

Ping 平 Peace and harmony.

Putian 浦田 Name of a county in China's Fujian Province.

Qi (Chi) 氣 Chinese term for universal energy. A current popular model is that the qi circulating in the human body is bioelectric in nature.

Qian Kao 前靠 Forward bump. To bump someone off balance from his front.

Qi Hua Lun 氣化論 Qi variation thesis. An ancient treatise which discusses the variations of qi in the universe.

Qi Huo 起火 To start the fire. In qigong practice, when you start to build up qi at the lower dan tian.

Qi Qing Liu Yu 七情六欲 Seven emotions and six desires. The seven emotions are happiness, anger, sorrow, joy, love, hate and desire. The six desires are the six sensory pleasures associated with the eyes, nose, ears, tongue, body and mind.

Qi Shi 氣勢 Shi means the way something looks or feels. Therefore, the feeling of qi as it expresses itself.

Qi-Xue 氣血 Literally, "qi blood." According to Chinese medicine, qi and blood cannot be separated in our body and so the two words are commonly used together.

Qigong (Chi Kung) 氣功 The gongfu of qi, which means the study of qi.

Qihai (Co-6) 氣海 Means "qi ocean." An acupuncture cavity belonging to the conception vessel.

Qin (Chin) 擒 Means "to catch" or "to seize."

Qin Na (Chin Na) 擒拿 Literally means "grab control." A component of Chinese martial arts which emphasizes grabbing techniques to control your opponent's joints, in conjunction with attacking certain acupuncture cavities.

Qing dynasty 清朝 A dynasty in Chinese history; The last Chinese dynasty (A.D. 1644-1912).

Qiu Yue Chan Shi 秋月禪師 A Shaolin monk during the Chinese Song dynasty (A.D. 960-1278). His layman name was Bai, Yu-feng.

Quan-Yi 全一 A nickname of Zhang, San-feng.

Re Qi 熱氣 Re means warmth or heat. Generally, re qi is used to represent heat. It is used sometimes to imply that a person or animal is still alive since the body is warm.

Ren 人 Man or mankind.

Ren 仁 Humanity, kindness or benevolence.

Ren (Chan) 忍 Means "to endure." A Chan Buddhist meditation passed down by Da Mo.

Ren Mai 任脈 Conception Vessel. One of the eight extraordinary vessels.

Ren Qi 人氣 Human qi.

Ren Shi 人事 Literally, human relations. Human events, activities and relationships.

Ru Jia 儒家 Literally, "Confucian family." Scholars following Confucian thoughts; Confucianists.

Ruan Bian 軟鞭 A soft whip commonly made from leather or animal tendons. The bian is a whip which can be made from leather, tendons, rattan, or even wood.

Ruan Ying Bian 軟硬鞭 A soft-hard whip commonly made from rattan.

San Bao 三寶 Three treasures. Essence (*jing*), energy (*qi*) and spirit (*shen*). Also called san yuan (three origins).

San Cai 三才 Three powers. Heaven, earth and man.

San Cai Shi 三才勢 Three power posture. A standing meditation posture in taijiquan practice.

San Da (San Shou) 散打、散手 Literally, "random striking" or "random hands." Implies techniques executed randomly. This means free sparring.

San Gong 散功   Literally, "energy dispersion." A state of premature degeneration of the muscles where the qi cannot effectively energize them. It can be caused by earlier overtraining.

San Shi Qi Shi 三十七勢   Thirty-seven postures. Taijiquan is also called thirty-seven postures because, from the thirteen basic moving patterns, it derives into thirty-seven postures.

San Shou (San Da) 散手、散打   Literally, "random hands or random striking." Implies techniques executed randomly. This means free sparring.

San Yuan 三元   Three origins. Also called "san bao" (three treasures). Human essence (*jing*), energy (*qi*) and spirit (*shen*).

Sardili 沙地利   The last name of Da Mo. Also known as Bodhidarma.

Seng Bing 僧兵   Monk soldiers. The monks who also trained martial arts to protect the property of the temple.

Shang Dan Tian 上丹田   Upper dan tian. Located at the third eye, it is the residence of the shen (*spirit*).

Shang Kao 上靠   Upward bump. To bump someone off balance through an upward bumping force.

Shao Yuan 邵元和尚   A Japanese Buddhist monk who went to Shaolin Temple in A.D. 1335. During this stay, he mastered calligraphy, painting, chan theory (i.e., *ren*) and Shaolin Gongfu. He returned to Japan in A.D. 1347 and was considered a "country spirit" (*guohuen*) by the Japanese people. This confirms that Shaolin martial techniques were imported into Japan for at least seven hundred years.

Shaolin 少林   "Young woods." Name of the Shaolin Temple.

Shaolin Temple 少林寺   A monastery located in Henan Province, China. The Shaolin Temple is well known because of its martial arts training.

Shen 神   Spirit. According to Chinese qigong, the qhen resides at the upper dan tian (the third eye).

Shen 深   Deep.

Shi Er Jing 十二經   The twelve primary qi channels in Chinese medicine.

Shi Er Zhuang 十二庄   Twelve postures. The name of a qigong training style.

Shi San Shi 十三勢   Thirteen postures. Taijiquan is also called "thirteen postures" because it is constructed from thirteen basic moving patterns.

Shi Xiang Zu 師襄子   Name of Confucius' music teacher.

Shi, You-San 石友三   A military warlord during the Chinese civil war in the 1920's. He was known as the one who burned the Shaolin Temple in 1928.

Shuai 摔   Means "to throw." An abbreviation of "shuai jiao" (wrestling).

Shuai Jiao 摔交   Chinese wrestling. Part of Chinese martial arts.

Shui 水   Water. One of the five elements

Shun Fu Hu Xi 順腹呼吸   Smooth Abdominal Breathing. Also called Normal Abdominal Breathing. Also called Buddhist Breathing.

Si Ji Gong 四季功   Four Seasons Gong. A type of qigong practice which helps make the body's seasonal qi transition more smooth.

Si Liu Bu 四六步   Four-six stance. One of the eight basic fundamental stances.

Si Qi 死氣   Dead Qi. The qi remaining in a dead body. Sometimes called "ghost qi" (*gui qi*).

Si Xin Hu Xi 四心呼吸   A qigong nei dan practice in which a practitioner uses his mind with the coordination of the breathing to lead the qi to the centers of the palms and feet.

Song 宋   A dynasty in Chinese history (A.D. 960-1278).

Southern Song dynasty 南宋 After the Song was conquered by the Jin race from Mongolia, the Song people moved to the south and established another country, called Southern Song (A.D. 1127-1278).

Suan Ming Shi 算命師 Literally, "calculate life teacher." A fortune teller who is able to calculate your future and destiny.

Sui dynasty 隋 A dynasty in China during the period of (A.D. 589-618).

Sui Qi 髓氣 "Marrow qi". The qi circulating in the bone marrow.

Sun, Lu-Tang (1861-1932) 孫祿堂 A well known martial artist in the early 1920's. He mastered many styles, such as baguazhang, xingyiquan, and taijiquan. He is also the creator of Sun Style Taijiquan.

Sun, Yat-Sen 孫中山 Father of China.

Tai Chi Chuan (Taijiquan) 太極拳 A Chinese internal martial style that based on the theory of taiji (grand ultimate).

Tai Xi 胎息 Embryo Breathing. One of the final goals in regulating the breath, Embryo Breathing enables you to generate a "baby shen" at the huang ting (yellow yard).

Taiji 太極 Means "grand ultimate." It is this force which generates two poles, yin and yang.

Taiji Qigong 太極氣功 A qigong training specially designed for taijiquan practice.

Taijiquan (Tai Chi Chuan) 太極拳 A Chinese internal martial style which is based on the theory of taiji (grand ultimate).

Taipei 台北 The capital city of Taiwan located in the north.

Taiwan 台灣 An island to the southeast of mainland China. Also known as "Formosa."

Taiwan University 台灣大學 A well known university located in northern Taiwan.

Taizuquan 太祖拳 A style of Chinese external martial arts.

Tamkang 淡江 Name of a University in Taiwan.

Tamkang College Guoshu Club 淡江國術社 A Chinese martial arts club founded by Dr. Yang when he was studying in Tamkang College.

Tang 趟 A martial sequence. Normally, a sequence is constructed from many techniques, and become a routine practice form. Also commonly called "taolu."

Tang dynasty 唐 A dynasty in Chinese history during the period A.D. 713-907.

Taolu 套路 A martial sequence. Normally, a sequence is constructed from many techniques and become a routine practice form. Also commonly called "tan."

Ti 踢 Means "to kick."

Ti Sui Xi 体髓息 Skin Marrow Breathing.

Ti Xi 体息 Body breathing or skin breathing. In qigong, the exchanging of qi with the surrounding environment through the skin.

Tian 天 Heaven or sky. In ancient China, people believed that Heaven was the most powerful natural energy in this universe.

Tian Mountain 天山 Literally, "sky mountain." The name of a mountain located in Xinjiang Province, China.

Tian Qi 天氣 Heaven qi. It is now commonly used to mean the weather, since weather is governed by heaven qi.

Tian Ren He Yi 天人合一 Literally, "heaven and man unified as one." A high level of qigong practice in which a qigong practitioner, through meditation, is able to communicate his qi with heaven's qi.

Tian Shi 天時 Heavenly timing. The repeated natural cycles generated by the heavens such as: seasons, months, days and hours.

Tianron (SI-17) 天容 An acupuncture cavity belonging to the small intestine primary qi channel.

Tiao Qi 調氣 To regulate the qi.

Tiao Shen 調身 To regulate the body.

Tiao Shen 調神 To regulate the spirit.

Tiao Xi 調息 To regulate the breathing.

Tiao Xin 調心 To regulate the emotional mind.

Tie Bu Shan 鐵布衫 Iron shirt. Gongfu training which toughens the body externally and internally.

Tie Sha Zhang 鐵砂掌 Literally, "iron sand palm." A special martial arts conditioning for the palms.

Tu 土 Earth. One of the five elements.

Tui Bu 退步 "Step backward." One of the taijiquan thirteen postures. Taijiquan is constructed from eight basic moving patterns (eight doors) and five strategic steppings (five steppings). Tui bu is one of the five steppings.

Tui Kao 腿靠 Leg bump. To use the thigh to bump someone off balance.

Tui Na 推拿 Means "to push and grab." A category of Chinese massages for healing and injury treatment.

Tun Kao 臀靠 Hip bump. To use the hip to bump someone off balance

Tuo Tian Shi 托天勢 Holding up the heaven posture. A common qigong posture which is used to stretch the torso and raise up the spirit of vitality

Wa Shou 瓦手 Tile hand. The hand form of taijiquan is also called tile hand, because it resembles the shape of a Chinese roof tile.

Wai Dan Chi Kung (Wai Dan Qigong) 外丹氣功 External elixir qigong. In wai dan qigong, a practitioner will generate qi to the limbs and then allow the qi to flow inward to nourish the internal organs.

Wai Dan 外丹 External elixir. External qigong exercises in which a practitioner will build up the qi in his limbs and then lead it into the center of the body for nourishment.

Wai Jia 外家 External family. Those martial schools which practice the external styles of Chinese martial arts.

Wai Jin 外勁 External power. The type of jin where the muscles predominate and only local qi is used to support the muscles.

Wang, Zong-Yue 王宗岳 A well known taijiquan master in the 1920's.

Wei Qi 衛氣 Protective qi or guardian qi. The qi at the surface of the body which generates a shield to protect the body from negative external influences such as colds.

Wen Wang Cao 文王操 A piece of music composed by king Wen of Zhou.

Wilson Chen 陳威伸 Dr. Yang, Jwing-Ming's friend.

Wu 武 Means "martial."

Wu Bu 五步 Five steppings. Taijiquan is constructed from eight basic moving patterns and five steppings.

Wu Qin Shi 五禽戲 Five Animal Sports. A set of medical qigong practice created by Jun Qing during Chinese Jin dynasty (A.D. 265-420).

Wu Tiao 五調   Five regulations. This includes: regulating the body, breathing, mind, qi, and spirit.

Wu Xin 五心   Five centers. The face, the laogong cavities in both palms, and the yongquan cavities on the bottoms of both feet.

Wu Xin Hu Xi 五心呼吸   One of the qigong nei dan practices in which a practitioner uses his mind in coordination with breathing to lead the qi to the center of the palms, feet and head.

Wu Zhen Ren 伍真人   An ancient Daoist qigong master.

Wudang Mountain 武當山   A mountain located in Fubei Province in China.

Wu, Jian-Quan (1870-1942) 吳鑒泉   A famous taijiquan master in the 1930's. He is credited as the creator of Wu Style Taijiquan.

Wuji Qigong 無極氣功   A style of taiji qigong practice.

Wuji 無極   Means "no extremity."

Wushu 武術   Literally, "martial techniques."

Wuxing 五行   Five elements

Wuyi 武藝   Literally, "martial arts."

Xi 細   Slender.

Xi 喜   Joy, delight, and happiness.

Xi Kao 膝靠   "Knee bump." To use the knee to bump someone off balance.

Xi Sui Gong 洗髓功   Gongfu for marrow and brain washing qigong practice.

Xi Sui Jing 洗髓經   Literally, *Washing Marrow/Brain Classic*, usually *translated Marrow/Brain Washing Classic*. A qigong training which specializes in leading qi to the marrow to cleanse it or to the brain to nourish the spirit for enlightenment. It is believed that xi sui jing training is the key to longevity and achieving spiritual enlightenment.

Xia Dan Tian 下丹田   Lower dan tian. Located in the lower abdomen, it is believed to be the residence of water qi (original qi).

Xia Kao 下靠   "Downward bump." To bump someone off balance through a downward bumping action.

Xian Jin 顯勁   The jins which are manifested externally and can be seen.

Xian Tian Qi 先天氣   Pre-birth qi or pre-heaven qi. Also called dan tian qi. The qi which is converted from original essence and is stored in the lower tian. Considered to be "water qi," it is able to calm the body.

Xiao Jiu Tian 小九天   Small Nine Heaven. A qigong style created around A.D. 550.

Xiao Lu 小擺   "Small rollback." A taijiquan pushing hands technique.

Xiao Zhou Tian 小周天   Literally, small heavenly cycle. Also called small circulation. In qigong, when you can use your mind to lead qi through the conception and governing vessels, you have completed "xiao zhou tian."

Xiao 孝   Filial piety.

Xin 心   Means "heart." Xin means the mind generated from emotional disturbance.

Xin 信   Trust.

Xingyi 形意   An abbreviation of Xingyiquan.

Xingyiquan (Hsing Yi Chuan) 形意拳   One of the best known Chinese internal martial styles created by Marshal Yue Fei during the Chinese Song dynasty (1103-1142 A.D.).

Xinjiang Province 新疆   A Chinese province located in western China.

Xinzhu Xian 新竹縣   Birthplace of Dr. Yang, Jwing-Ming in Taiwan.

Xiong Kao 胸靠 "Chest bump." To use the chest to bump someone off balance.

Xiu Qi 修氣 Cultivate the qi. Cultivate implies to protect, maintain and refine. A Buddhist Qigong training.

Xu Bu 虛步 "False stance." One of the eight basic fundamental stances. Also called xuan ji bu.

Xuan Ji Bu 玄機步 Tricky stance." One of the eight basic fundamental stances. Also called xu bu.

Yan 言 Talking or speaking.

Yang 陽 Too sufficient. One of the two poles. The other is yin.

Yang Quan 楊拳 Yang Style Taijiquan is also called Yang Quan.

Yang Shou 陽手 "Yang hand." Any time the palm is facing outward in taijiquan.

Yang, Chen-fu (1883-1836) 楊澄甫 A well known Yang Style Taijiquan master in the 1930's. He was part of the third generation of Yang Style Taijiquan practitioners.

Yang, Lu-chan (1799-1872) 楊露禪 Also name Fu-kuai. The creator of Yang Style Taijiquan.

Yang, Jwing-Ming 楊俊敏 Author of this book.

Yang, You-Ji 養由基 A famous archer during the Chinese Spring and Autumn period (722-481 B.C).

Yao Duan 拗斷 To break off by twisting.

Yao Zhe 拗折 To bend by twisting.

Yi 意 Wisdom mind. The mind generated from wise judgment.

Yi 義 Justice or righteousness.

Yi Jin Jing 易筋經 Literally, *Changing Muscle/Tendon Classic*, usually called *The Muscle/Tendon Changing Classic*. Credited to Da Mo around 550 A.D., this book discusses wai dan qigong training for strengthening the physical body.

Yi Jing 易經 *Book of Changes*. A book of divination written during the Zhou dynasty (1122-255 B.C).

Yi Shou Dan Tian 意守丹田 Keep your yi on your lower dan tian. In qigong training, you keep your mind at the lower dan tian in order to build up qi. When you are circulating your qi, you always lead your qi back to your lower dan tian before you stop.

Yi Yi Yin Qi 以意引氣 Use your yi (wisdom mind) to lead your qi. A qigong technique. Yi cannot be pushed, but it can be led. This is best done with the yi.

Yin 陰 Deficient. One of the two poles. The other is yang.

Yin Shou 陰手 "Yin hand." Any time the palm is facing inward in taijiquan. Also implied are the techniques which are hidden and not obvious to the opponent.

Ying Bian 硬鞭 A hard whip, usually made from a hard wood.

Ying Gong 硬功 Hard gongfu. Any Chinese martial training which emphasizes physical strength and power.

Yongquan (K-1) 湧泉 Bubbling well. Name of an acupuncture cavity belonging to the kidney primary qi channel.

You 悠 Long, far, meditative, continuous, slow and soft.

You Pan 右盼 "Look to the right." One of the taijiquan thirteen postures.

Yu 欲 Desire.

Yuan dynasty 元代 A Chinese dynasty during the period of (A.D. 1206-1368).

Yuan Jing 元精 Original essence. The fundamental, original substance inherited from your parents, it is converted into original qi.

Yuan Qi 元氣 Original qi. The qi created from the original essence inherited from your parents.

Yue Fei 岳飛 A Chinese hero in the Southern Song dynasty (A.D. 1127-1279). Said to have created Ba Duan Jin, xingyiquan and Yue's Ying Zhua.

Yun 勻 Uniform or even.

Zhang Dao-Ling 張道陵 A Daoist who combined scholarly Daoism with Buddhist philosophies and created Religious Daoism (*Dao Jiao*) during the Chinese Eastern Han dynasty (25-221 A.D.).

Zhang, San-Feng 張三豐 Chang, San-Feng is credited as the creator of taijiquan during the Song dynasty in China (960-1127 A.D.).

Zhang, Xiang-San 張詳三 A well known Chinese martial artist in Taiwan.

Zhen Dan Tian 真丹田 The real dan tian, which is located at the physical center of gravity.

Zheng Hu Xi 正呼吸 Formal Breathing. More commonly called Buddhist Breathing.

Zheng Fu Hu Xi 正腹呼吸 Normal Abdominal Breathing. Also called Shun Fu Hu Xi, which means "Smooth Abdominal Breathing."

Zheng Qi 正氣 Righteous qi. When a person is righteous, it is said that he has righteous qi which evil qi cannot overcome.

Zhi 止 Stop.

Zhong 忠 Loyalty.

Zhong Dan Tian 中丹田 Middle dan tian. Located in the area of the solar plexus, it is the residence of fire qi.

Zhong Ding 中定 "Firm the center." One of the taijiquan thirteen postures.

Zhong Guo Wushu 中國武術 Chinese Wushu.

Zhong Guo 中國 Literally, "central country." This name was given by the neighboring countries of China. China was considered the cultural and spiritual center from the point of view of the Asian countries in ancient times.

Zhou 肘 "Elbow." To use the elbow to execute defensive or offensive techniques in taijiquan.

Zhou 周 Roundness or completeness.

Zhuang Zhou 莊周 A contemporary of Mencius who advocated Daoism.

Zhuang Zi 莊子 Zhuang Zhou. A contemporary of Mencius who advocated Daoism. Zhuang Zi also means the works of Zhuang Zhou.

Zuo Dun 坐蹲 "Squat stance." One of the eight fundamental stances in Northern Chinese martial arts training.

Zuo Gu 左顧 "See the left." One of the taijiquan thirteen postures.

Zuo Pan Bu 坐盤步 "Sitting on crossed legs stance." One of the eight basic fundamental stance in Northern Chinese martial arts training.

ZuoWan 坐腕 "Settling the wrist." When taijiquan uses the palm to strike, right before contact, the wrist is settled to firm the posture and alignment of the palm.

Taijiquan Classical Yang Style DVD

This appendix offers a simple navigation guide to using the companion DVD and this book. Using both book and DVD for learning is an excellent way to deepen your taijiquan knowledge.

Techniques (DVD Edition)	This Book Section	Page
• Taijiquan Lecture	1.3 - 1.9	30-50
• Taijiquan 13 Postures	3.1	107
Eight Doors	3.2	110
Five Steppings	3.4	127
• Fundamental Eight Stances	4.4	140
• Taiji Qigong	4.5	145
Stretching and Warming Up	4.5	151-156
Primary Qigong Set	4.5	161-174
Rocking Qigong Set	4.5	175-178
Stepping Qigong Set	4.5	179-186
• Yang Style Taijiquan Sequence		
Piece by Piece Taijiquan Sequence		
Part 1	4.6	192-220
Part 2	4.6	221-270
Part 3	4.6	271-339
Continuous Tajijquan Sequence		
In Depth Analysis		
Part 1		
Part 2		
Part 3		
Slideshow of All Pieces		
Fa Jing Demonstration	4.2	135
Help/Instructions		

DVD Extras

Yin/Yang Symbol—When you see the symbol throughout the DVD, press ENTER key on your remote to access In-Depth Analysis for that piece. Use Skip Forward and Back buttons to move to the next or previous pieces.

Index

abdomen 64
Acupuncture 60
an 40, 41, 108, 116, 117, 118, 177, 200
Arcing the Arms 148
Attack the Ears with the Fists 261
Ba Duan Jin 80, 154
bagua 110
Baguazhang xi, 82, 349, 375, 376
Bai He 160, 173, 204, 232, 304
balance 91
battery, electrical 64
Batuo 6
Beginning Taiji 192
bioelectricity 55, 59, 60, 64, 146
blood 72
Book of Changes 56
Bow-Arrow Stance 141
Boxer Rebellion 9
breathing 92, 188
Bruce Lee xi, 10, 11, 13
Brush Knee and Punch Down 321
Brush Knee and Step Forward: Left 205,
    208, 211, 213, 233, 252, 305
Brush Knee and Step Forward: Right 209,
    253
Brush Knee and Twist Step 185
Buddhism 6, 7, 78, 83
cai 40, 119, 184
Canton 7, 82
carbon 70
center 132
Central Kingdom 4
Chang Dao Zhen Yan 92
Chang Jiang 13
Chang, Kai-shek 9, 10
Changquan 41
Chang, San-feng 108, 109
Chen, Chang-xing 33
Cheng, Man-ching 11–12
Chen Jia Gou 32, 33
Chen style taijiquan 35
chest 139
chi. *See* qi
Chiang, Kai-shek 9, 10
chi kung. *See* qigong
Chinese xi
Chinese Athletic Committee 9

Chinese Civil War 9
chin na 135
Close Taiji 219, 269, 338, 345, 347, 348
common knowledge 2, 3
Confucianism 21, 79
Confucius 77, 95, 190
Crane Spreads Its Wings 204, 232, 304
Cross Hands 319
Cultural Revolution 9, 12
Dai Mai Hu Xi 147
da lu 130
Da Mo xi, 6, 7, 16, 17, 54, 73, 81, 86
Dan Bian 201, 224, 241, 246, 274, 293,
    296, 313, 316, 325, 347
dan tian 65, 66, 68, 69, 94, 162
Dao 3, 21, 29, 35, 36, 45, 57, 92, 93, 107
Dao De Jing 78, 107, 109
Daoism 21, 78, 79, 107
Dao Jia 78
Da Zhi 8
Da Zhou Tian 38, 75, 147
Deflect Downward 215, 237, 256, 265,
    309, 334
Deng Feng County Recording 6
Deng Feng Xian Zhi 6
Deng Shan Bu 141
Diagonal Flying 181, 230, 302
Dian Mai 351
Di Li Shi 351
Draw the Bow and Shoot the Tiger 332
Eagle Attacks Its Prey 171
eight doors 107, 110, 111, 113, 115, 117,
    119, 121, 123, 125
eight postures 40
eight stances 140
eight trigrams 39, 56, 108, 110
elbows 138, 151
electromagnetic energy 55
Embrace the Tiger and Return to the Moun-
    tain 218, 268, 337
Embracing Arms 176
Embracing the Moon on the Chest 148
Emei 82, 150
Emei Da Peng Gong 150
emotions 83
Essence of the Five Fists 8
Europe 13

Expand the Chest to Cleanse the Body 163
external elixir 76
external movements 189
external styles 15
Fair Lady Weaves with Shuttle: Left 285, 287
Fair Lady Weaves with Shuttle: Right 286, 288
False Dan Tian 65
False Stance 143
Fan Back 235, 307
Fan Tong Hu Xi 351
feet 139–140
Feng Shui Shi 351
five directions 41
five elements 109
five steppings 127
food 63, 71
Four Gate Breathing 45
Four-Six Stance 142
Fu Hu Bu 143
Fujian Province 23
fundamental eight stances 140–143
Fu Xi 108
Fuyu 15
Golden Rooster Stands on One Leg: Left 300
Golden Rooster Stands on One Leg: Right 299
Golden Rooster Stands on One Leg Stance 144
gongfu xi, 3, 82
Gong Jian Bu 141
Gong Shou 148
Grand Circulation 38, 75, 147
Grasp the Sparrow's Tail: Left 195, 279, 289
Grasp the Sparrow's Tail: Right 194
Guoshu 1, 9, 34
ha 33
Han 6, 8, 74, 77, 78, 79
hands 137
Hao style taijiquan 35
hard styles 18, 20
head 138
hen 33, 46, 352
Henan 6, 15, 32, 33
herbs 80
hips 139
Hong Kong 10, 12, 13

Horse Stance 141
Hua 33
Hua Quan 33, 352
Hua Tuo 80
Hubei province 1
Hui Zhong Bao Yue 148
Hu Xi 45, 147
imagined opponent 191
India 6, 78
Indo-China 10, 12, 13
Indonesia 10
internal elixir 76
internal feeling 189
internal styles 15
Japan 6, 8, 10, 59, 74
ji 41, 114
Jiang, Fa 32
Ji Ben Ba Shi 140
jin 17, 18, 40, 42
Jin Bu 127, 215, 237, 254, 256, 265, 309, 334
Jin Gi Du Li 144
Jueyuan 7
Jun Qing 80
kan 84, 86, 87
kan and li 86
kao 124, 126
kicking 20, 133
Kick Left 262
Kick Right 257, 260
King Wen of Zhou 108, 190
knees 139
Korea 10, 21, 27
kung fu 3, 13
Lan Zhou 7
Lao Zi 78, 107
Large Bear Swims in the Water 169
large rollback 130, 131
Left and Right to Open the Mountain 170
Left and Right to Push the Mountains 165
legs 139
li 17, 84
Liang dynasty 7, 16, 31, 81
Liang Wu 7
lie 40, 121
Li Er 107
Lift Hands to the Up Posture 203, 231, 303
Lion Rotates the Ball 172
Li Sou 7, 8

Li style taijiquan 32, 35
Liu He Ba Fa xi, 18, 20, 82
loosening up the Joints 151
lu 40, 112, 197, 221
Lu-chan 33
Ma Bu 141
Malaysia 10
Manchus 8, 21
marrow 73
Marrow Washing qigong 59
martial arts
    and western society xi, 1, 11
    history of 3, 4, 5, 6
    outside China 10
    styles 1, 4, 13–19
Martial Arts Investigation Team 10
martial arts styles 1
martial qigong 81, 82–84
medical qigong 79, 104
meditation 29, 145, 146, 147
Mencius 77, 354
Mian Quan 33
Ming dynasty 31
Ming Lang Ying Qi Xiu Lei Gao 31
Mingmen (Gv-4) 65
Ming Shi Fang Ji Zhuan 31
Ming Tai Zu 31
Mongols 21
monks, Buddhist 7, 23, 24–25
Mountain Climbing Stance 141
movement 189
Muscle/Tendon Changing Qigong 81
Nanking Central Guoshu Institute 1, 9, 34
Nan Lei Ji Wang Zheng Nan Mu Zhi Ming
    31
nei dan 47, 76, 77
northern styles 13
nu 285
Opium War 8
Parry 215, 237, 256, 265, 309, 334
Peng 40, 110, 178, 196, 221, 271, 280,
    290, 310, 322
Philippines 10
Pick Up the Needle from the Sea Bottom
    234, 306
Pie Shen Chui 183, 214, 236, 255, 264,
    333
Play the Guitar 207, 212
postures 34, 136

Pour the Qi into the Baihui 164
Press 116, 177, 199, 221, 238, 271, 280,
    290, 310, 322
Primary Set (taiji qigong) 161
Punch 215, 226, 237, 256, 265, 309, 321,
    328, 334
punching 133
Punch under the Elbow 226
Push Forward 200, 221, 238, 271, 280,
    290, 310, 322
pushing hands 48
Putian 23
qi
    and hormones 63
    and spirit 103
    balance 55
    channels 61
    circulation xii, 47, 148
    cultivation 103
    cycles 58
    defined 53–54, 54, 97
    generation 47
    leading 94, 102
    modern definition 58
    regulating 37, 101
    regulation 97
    reservoirs 61
    types 54, 56
    with yin and yang 85
qigong
    and bioelectricity 59, 62
    and scholars 77
    Bone Marrow Washing 73
    defined xi, 54, 56–59, 57
    history 53
    Marrow/Brain Washing 83
    martial 81
    medical 79
    modern definition 61
    Muscle/Tendon Changing 81
    religious 83
    training 64, 75, 84, 87, 88, 98, 145
    types of 73, 74, 75, 77, 77–83, 79, 81
    with yin and yang 75, 87
Qihai (Co-6) 65
Qi Hua Lun 56
Qi is Sunk to the Dan Tian 162
Qin dynasty 74
Qing dynasty 8, 9

qin na (chin na) 20, 133
Qiu Yue Chan Shi 8, 349, 355
real dan tian 65
regulating the body 36, 44, 89, 99
regulating the breathing 36, 45, 99
regulating the emotional mind 45
regulating the mind 37, 93, 95, 100
regulating the qi 37, 97, 101
regulating the spirit 38, 97, 103
relaxation 46, 90
religious qigong 83
Ren Qi 355
Re Qi 355
respiration 70
Return to the Original Stance 339
Rocking Set (taiji qigong) 175
Rollback 197, 221, 238, 271, 280, 290,
    310, 322
rooting 45, 54, 84, 86, 90
Ru Jia 78
Saber 42
scholar qigong 77
Seal Tightly 216, 266, 335
Separate Left Foot 250
Separate Right Foot 249
Settle the Wrists and Push the Palms 167
Shaolin Historical Records 8
Shaolin Temple 6, 7, 8, 9, 10, 15, 17, 24,
    41, 81
Shaolin Temple Record 8
Shao Yuan 8
Shi Xiang Zu 190
shoulders 138
Si Liu Bu 142
Single Whip 201, 224, 241, 246, 274, 283,
    293, 296, 313, 316, 325
Sitting on Crossed Legs Stance 142
Si Xin Hu Xi 45, 147
Small Circulation 38, 75, 145, 147
Small Circulation meditation 75
small rollback 130
Snake Creeps Down 298, 327, 347, 348
soft-hard styles 18, 20
soft styles 18, 20
Song dynasty 7, 17, 21, 31, 32, 80
southern styles 13
spear xiii, 43
Squat Stance 144
staff 43, 51

Stand High to Search Out the Horse 248,
    318
Step Back and Repulse the Monkey: Left
    227, 229, 301
Step Back and Repulse the Monkey: Right
    228
Step Back and Ride the Tiger 329
Step Forward 215, 237, 238, 256, 265, 309,
    310, 322, 334
Step Forward and Strike Down with the Fist
    254, 321
Step Forward to the Seven Stars 328
Stepping Leg 184
still sitting meditation 146
still standing meditation 147
stretching 151, 153
Strike the Tiger: Left 259
Strike the Tiger: Right 258
striking 20
Sui dynasty 7
Sun Style 32, 35
Sun style taijiquan 35
sword 42, 51
taiji fighting set 49
taiji qigong 140, 145, 160
Taiji Qi Shi 192
taijiquan
    and health 2
    history 1, 2, 30, 31, 36
    practice 29, 43–45, 45, 46, 134–136, 135,
        187
    sequence 47, 134
    styles 30, 32, 33, 35
Taiwan 10, 12, 13, 80, 96
Taiwan University 96, 373
Tai Xi 146
Tame the Tiger stance 143
Tamkang College Guoshu Club 373
Tang dynasty 7
Theory of Qi's Variation 56
thighs 139
thirteen postures 41, 107, 137
Thrust the Chest and Arc the Chest 159
ti 203
Tian Mountain 25
tiao qi 37, 97
tiao shen 36, 38, 44, 89, 97
tiao xi 36, 45, 91
tiao xin 37, 93

ti xi 147
torso, stretching 154
traditional Chinese medicine 79
Transition Form 220, 270
tu 308
Tui Bu 129, 329
Turn and Kick 251, 263, 320
Turn the Body and Sweep the Lotus with the Leg 330
Turn, Twist Body, and Circle the Fist 236, 255
Twist Body and Circle the Fist 183, 214
Twist Body, Brush Knee and Step Forward: Left 208, 211, 213
Twist Body, Brush Knee and Step Forward: Right 209
Twist the Body and Circle the Fist 264, 333
wai dan 47, 76, 77
waist 139
Wang Zong 32
Wardoff 40, 178, 196, 221, 238, 271, 280, 290, 310, 322
warming up 151, 156, 188
Wave Hands in the Clouds 179
Wave Hands in the Clouds: Left 244
Wave Hands in the Clouds: Right 243, 245, 295, 315
Waving the Spine and Massaging the Internal Organs 158
weapons 3, 41–42
Wen Wang Cao 190
whipping speed 19
White Crane Spreads Its Wings 173, 304
White Crane Waves Its Wings 160
White Snake Turns Its Body and Spits Poison 308, 348
Wild Horse Parts Its Mane: Left 277
Wild Horse Parts Its Mane: Right 276, 278
wing chun 11
World War II 9, 10
wrestling 20, 133
wrists 137, 151
Wudang Mountain 1
wuji 82
wushu 13, 51, 104, 359, 361
Wu style taijiquan 32, 33, 35
Wuu style taijiquan 35
wuyi 3
Wu Zhen Ren 93

Xiao Zhou Tian 38, 75, 147
xin 87
xingyi 359
xingyiquan xi, 21, 22, 82
Xinjiang Province 25
Xi Sui Gong 75
Xi Sui Jing 7, 17
Xuan Ji Bu 143
Xu Bu 143
yang 84
Yang, Cheng-fu 34
Yang family lineage 33, 34
Yang Jian 33
Yang Qi 33
Yang Quan 33
Yang style taijiquan 35
Yangtze River 13, 14
Yang Yu 33
yelling 189
Yellow River 4, 15
yi 87, 95, 102, 140
Yi Jing 30, 31, 56, 57, 107, 108, 109
Yi Jin Jing 7, 17
yin 40, 62, 84, 146
yin and yang 1, 4, 30, 31, 36, 38, 39, 40, 62, 76, 82, 84, 85, 86, 87, 88, 96, 107, 108, 109, 145, 148, 187, 192
yinjiao (Co-7) 65
You Pan 131
yu 285
Yue Fei 21, 80, 81
Yun Shou 179, 243, 244, 245, 295, 315
Zhang, San-feng xi, 26, 31, 32, 40
Zhao Bao style taijiquan 35
zhi 321
zhong 4, 132, 148
Zhong Ding 132
Zhong Guo 4
zhou 122, 147
Zhuang Zhou 78
Zhuang Zi 78
Zuo Dun 144
Zuo Gu 129
Zuo Pan Bu 142

About the Author

Dr. Yang, Jwing-Ming, Ph.D. 楊俊敏博士

Dr. Yang, Jwing-Ming was born on August 11, 1946 in Xinzhu Xian, Taiwan, Republic of China (新竹縣,台灣,中華民國). He started his wushu (武術) and kung fu (*gongfu,* 功夫) training when he was fifteen years old in Shaolin White Crane (少林白鶴) under Master Cheng, Gin-gsao (曾金灶, 1911-1976). As a child, Master Cheng learned Taizuquan (太祖拳) from his grandfather. When he was fifteen years old, he started learning White Crane Style from Master Jin, Shao-feng (金紹峰) and followed him for 23 years until Master Jin's death.

After thirteen years of study, from 1961 to 1974, under Master Cheng, Dr. Yang became an expert in the White Crane Style of Chinese martial arts, including the bare hands and various weapons such as saber, staff, spear, trident, two short rods, and many others. Under Master Cheng, he also studied White Crane Qigong (氣功), qin na (or *chin na,* 擒拿), he (推拿), dian xue (點穴按摩) massage, and herbal treatment.

At the age of sixteen, Dr. Yang began the study of Yang Style Taijiquan (楊氏太極拳) under Master Gao, Tao (高濤). He later continued his study of taijiquan under several other masters and senior practitioners, such as Master Li, Mao-ching (李茂清) and Mr. Wilson Chen (陳威伸) in Taipei (台北). Master Li learned taijiquan from the well-known Master Han, Ching-tang (韓慶堂), and Mr. Chen learned from Master Zhang, Xiang-san (張祥三). Under these masters, Dr. Yang mastered the taiji bare-hand sequence, the two-man fighting sequence, pushing hands, taiji sword, taiji saber, and taiji qigong.

When Dr. Yang was eighteen years old, he entered Tamkang College (淡江學院) in Taipei Xian to study physics. During this time, he began studying traditional Shaolin Long Fist (少林長拳) under Master Li, Mao-ching in the Tamkang College Guoshu Club (淡江國術社) from 1964 to 1968 and eventually became an assistant instructor to Master Li. From Master Li, he learned northern-style wushu, including bare-hand and kicking techniques, and numerous weapons. In 1971, he completed his Master of Science degree in physics at National Taiwan University (台灣大學) before serving in the Chinese Air Force from 1971 to 1972. He taught physics at the Junior Academy of the Chinese Air Force (空軍幼校) while also teaching wushu. Honorably discharged in 1972, he returned to Tamkang College to teach physics and resume his study under Master Li, Mao-ching.

Dr. Yang moved to the United States in 1974 to study mechanical engineering at Purdue University. At the request of a few colleagues, he began to teach gongfu, founding the Purdue University Chinese Gongfu Research Club in 1975. He also taught college-credit courses in taijiquan. In May 1978, he was awarded a Ph.D. in mechanical engineering from Purdue University.

In 1980, Dr. Yang moved to Houston to work for Texas Instruments and also founded Yang's Shaolin Kung Fu Academy, now under the direction of his disciple Jeffery Bolt. In 1982, he moved to Boston and founded Yang's Martial Arts Academy.

In 1984, he gave up his engineering career to devote his time to research, writing, and teaching of Chinese martial arts. In 1986, he moved YMAA to the Jamaica Plain area of Boston and established this location as Yang's Martial Arts Association (YMAA) headquarters. YMAA became a division of Yang's Oriental Arts Association, Inc. (YOAA, Inc.) in 1989.

Dr. Yang has been involved in Chinese wushu since 1961, studying Shaolin White Crane, Shaolin (*Bai He*) Long Fist, and Taijiquan (*Chanqquan*) under several different masters. He has taught for more than forty years: seven years in Taiwan, five years at Purdue University, two years in Houston, twenty-six years in Boston, and five years at his YMAA California Retreat Center. He has taught seminars all around the world, sharing his knowledge of Chinese martial arts and qigong: in Argentina, Austria, Barbados, Botswana, Belgium, Bermuda, Canada, China, Chile, England, Egypt, France, Germany, Holland, Hungary, Iran, Ireland, Italy, Latvia, Mexico, Poland, Portugal, Saudi Arabia, Spain, South Africa, Switzerland, and Venezuela.

YMAA has grown into an international organization that includes 60 schools spread across 19 countries: Argentina, Belgium, Canada, Chile, France, Holland, Hungary, Iran, Ireland, Italy, Poland, Portugal, Qatar, Spain, South Africa, Sweden, Switzerland, the United Kingdom, and the United States. YMAA publications, books, and videos have been translated into French, Italian, Spanish, Polish, Czech, Bulgarian, Russian, Hungarian, and Farsi.

In 2005, Dr. Yang established the YMAA California Retreat Center (楊氏武藝協會特訓中心), a dedicated training ground for a small committed group of selected students. Located in the mountainous regions of northern California, the center was formed to host a 10-year training program, directed and taught by Dr. Yang himself, beginning in September 2008. It is Dr. Yang's wish that through this effort, he will be able to preserve traditional Chinese martial arts to the same standards and quality of ancient times. He remains the chief supervisor of YMAA International and in January 2008, his youngest son Nicholas has succeeded him as president of YMAA.

Dr. Yang has published numerous other volumes on the martial arts and qigong:
1. *Shaolin Chin Na,* Unique Publications, Inc., 1980
2. *Shaolin Long Fist Kung Fu,* Unique Publications, Inc., 1981
3. *Yang Style Tai Chi Chuan,* Unique Publications, Inc., 1981
4. *Introduction to Ancient Chinese Weapons,* Unique Publications, Inc., 1985
    A Martial Arists Guide to Ancient Chinese Weapons, revised edition, YMAA Publication Center, 1999
5. *Chi Kung for Health and Martial Arts,* YMAA Publication Center, 1985
    Qigong—Health and Martial Arts, revised edition, YMAA Publication Center, 1998
6. *Northern Shaolin Sword,* YMAA Publication Center, 1985
7. *Advanced Yang Style Tai Chi Chuan Vol. 1—Tai Chi Theory and Martial Power,* YMAA Publication Center, 1986

Tai Chi Theory and Martial Power, revised edition, YMAA Publication Center, 1996

8. *Advanced Yang Style Tai Chi Chuan Vol. 2—Tai Chi Chuan Martial Applications,* YMAA Publication Center, 1986
Tai Chi Chuan Martial Applications, revised edition, YMAA Publication Center, 1996

9. *Analysis of Shaolin Chin Na,* YMAA Publication Center, 1987, 2004

10. *The Eight Pieces of Brocade—Ba Duan Jin,* YMAA Publication Center, 1988
Eight Simple Qigong Exercises for Health, revised edition, YMAA Publication Center, 1997

11. *The Root of Chinese Qigong—The Secrets of Qigong Training,* YMAA Publication Center, 1989, 1997

12. *Muscle/Tendon Changing and Marrow/Brain Washing Chi Kung—The Secret of Youth,* YMAA Publication Center, 1989
Qigong the Secret of Youth, Da Mo's Muscle Tendon Changing and Marrow Brain Washing Qigong, revised edition, YMAA Publication Center, 2000

13. *Hsing Yi Chuan—Theory and Applications,* YMAA Publication Center, 1990
Xingyiquan—Theory and Applications, revised edition, YMAA Publication Center, 2003

14. *The Essence of Tai Chi Chi Kung—Health and Martial Arts,* YMAA Publication Center, 1990
The Essence of Taiji Qigong—Health and Martial Arts, revised edition, YMAA Publication Center, 1998

15. *Qigong for Arthritis,* YMAA Publication Center, 1991
Arthritis Relief, revised edition, YMAA Publication Center, 2005

16. *Chinese Qigong Massage—General Massage,* YMAA Publication Center, 1992
Qigong Massage—Fundamental Techniques for Health and Relaxation, revised edition, YMAA Publication Center, 2005

17. *How to Defend Yourself,* YMAA Publication Center, 1992

18. *Baguazhang—Emei Baguazhang,* YMAA Publication Center, 1994
Baguazhang—Theory and Applications, revised edition, YMAA Publication Center, 2008

19. *Comprehensive Applications of Shaolin Chin Na—The Practical Defense of Chinese Seizing Arts,* YMAA Publication Center, 1995

20. *Taiji Chin Na—The Seizing Art of Taijiquan,* YMAA Publication Center, 1995

21. *The Essence of Shaolin White Crane,* YMAA Publication Center, 1996

22. *Back Pain—Chinese Qigong for Healing and Prevention,* YMAA Publication Center, 1997
Back Pain Relief—Chinese Qigong for Healing and Prevention, revised edition, YMAA Publication Center, 2004

23. *Taijiquan Classical Yang Style—The Complete Form and Qigong,* YMAA Publication Center, 1999
Tai Chi Chuan—Classical Yang Style, revised edition, YMAA Publication Center, 2010

24. *Taijiquan Theory of Dr. Yang, Jwing-Ming—The Root of Taijiquan,* YMAA Publication Center, 2003

25. *Qigong Meditation—Embryonic Breathing,* YMAA Publication Center, 2003

26. *Qigong Meditation—Small Circulation,* YMAA Publication Center, 2006

27. *Tai Chi Ball Qigong—Health and Martial Arts,* YMAA Publication Center, 2010

Dr. Yang has also published the following DVDs:

1. *Chin Na In Depth Courses 1–4,* YMAA Publication Center, 2003

2. *Chin Na In Depth Courses 5–8,* YMAA Publication Center, 2003

3. *Chin Na In Depth Courses 9–12,* YMAA Publication Center, 2003

4. *Eight Simple Qigong Exercises for Health—The Eight Pieces of Brocade,* YMAA Publication Center, 2003

5. *Shaolin White Crane Gong Fu Basic Training Courses 1&2,* YMAA Publication Center, 2003

6. *Shaolin White Crane Hard and Soft Qigong,* YMAA Publication Center, 2003

7. *Taijiquan, Classical Yang Style (Long Form Taijiquan),* YMAA Publication Center, 2003

8. *Analysis of Shaolin Chin Na,* YMAA Publication Center, 2004

9. *Shaolin Kung Fu Fundamental Training,* YMAA Publication Center, 2004

10. *Baguazhang (Eight Trigrams Palm Kung Fu),* YMAA Publication Center, 2005

11. *Essence of Taiji Qigong,* YMAA Publication Center, 2005

12. *Qigong Massage,* YMAA Publication Center, 2005

13. *Shaolin Long Fist Kung Fu Basic Sequences,* YMAA Publication Center, 2005

14. *Taiji Pushing Hands Courses 1&2,* YMAA Publication Center, 2005

15. *Taiji Sword, Classical Yang Style,* YMAA Publication Center, 2005

16. *Taiji Ball Qigong Courses 1&2,* YMAA Publication Center, 2006

17. *Taiji Fighting Set—88 Posture, 2-Person Matching Set,* YMAA Publication Center, 2006

18. *Taiji Pushing Hands Courses 3&4,* YMAA Publication Center, 2006

19. *Understanding Qigong DVD 1—What is Qigong? Understanding the Human Qi Circulatory System,* YMAA Publication Center, 2006

20. *Understanding Qigong DVD 2—Keypoints of Qigong & Qigong Breathing,* YMAA Publication Center, 2006

21. *Shaolin Saber Basic Sequences,* YMAA Publication Center, 2007

22. *Shaolin Staff Basic Sequences,* YMAA Publication Center, 2007

23. *Simple Qigong Exercises for Arthritis Relief,* YMAA Publication Center, 2007

24. *Simple Qigong Exercises for Back Pain Relief,* YMAA Publication Center, 2007

25. *Taiji & Shaolin Staff Fundamental Training,* YMAA Publication Center, 2007

26. *Taiji Ball Qigong Courses 3&4,* YMAA Publication Center, 2007

27. *Understanding Qigong DVD 3—Embryonic Breathing,* YMAA Publication Center, 2007

28. *Understanding Qigong DVD 4—Four Seasons Qigong,* YMAA Publication Center, 2007

29. *Understanding Qigong DVD 5—Small Circulation,* YMAA Publication Center, 2007

30. *Understanding Qigong DVD 6—Martial Arts Qigong Breathing,* YMAA Publication Center, 2007

31. *Five Animal Sports Qigong,* YMAA Publication Center, 2008

32. *Saber Fundamental Training,* YMAA Publication Center, 2008

33. *Shaolin White Crane Gong Fu Basic Training Courses 3&4,* YMAA Publication Center, 2008

34. *Taiji 37 Postures Martial Applications,* YMAA Publication Center, 2008

35. *Taiji Saber, Classical Yang Style,* YMAA Publication Center, 2008

36. *Taiji Wrestling—Advanced Takedown Techniques,* YMAA Publication Center, 2008

37. *Taiji Yin/Yang Sticking Hands,* YMAA Publication Center, 2008

38. *Xingyiquan (Hsing I Chuan),* YMAA Publication Center, 2008

39. *Northern Shaolin Sword,* YMAA Publication Center, 2009

40. *Sword Fundamental Training,* YMAA Publication Center, 2009

41. *Taiji Chin Na in Depth,* YMAA Publication Center, 2009

42. *YMAA 25-Year Anniversary,* YMAA Publication Center, 2009

43. *Shuai Jiao—Kung Fu Wrestling,* YMAA Publication Center, 2010

BOOKS FROM YMAA

6 HEALING MOVEMENTS
101 REFLECTIONS ON TAI CHI CHUAN
108 INSIGHTS INTO TAI CHI CHUAN
ADVANCING IN TAE KWON DO
ANALYSIS OF SHAOLIN CHIN NA 2ND ED
ANCIENT CHINESE WEAPONS
ART OF HOJO UNDO
ARTHRITIS RELIEF, 3RD ED.
BACK PAIN RELIEF, 2ND ED.
BAGUAZHANG, 2ND ED.
CARDIO KICKBOXING ELITE
CHIN NA IN GROUND FIGHTING
CHINESE FAST WRESTLING
CHINESE FITNESS
CHINESE TUI NA MASSAGE
CHOJUN
COMPREHENSIVE APPLICATIONS OF SHAOLIN CHIN NA
CROCODILE AND THE CRANE: A NOVEL
CUTTING SEASON: A XENON PEARL MARTIAL ARTS THRILLER
DESHI: A CONNOR BURKE MARTIAL ARTS THRILLER
DIRTY GROUND
DR. WU'S HEAD MASSAGE
DUKKHA REVERB
DUKKHA, THE SUFFERING: AN EYE FOR AN EYE
DUKKHA UNLOADED
ENZAN: THE FAR MOUNTAIN, A CONNOR BURKE MARTIAL ARTS THRILLER
ESSENCE OF SHAOLIN WHITE CRANE
EXPLORING TAI CHI
FACING VIOLENCE
FIGHTING ARTS
FORCE DECISIONS: A CITIZEN'S GUIDE
FOX BORROWS THE TIGER'S AWE
INSIDE TAI CHI
KAGE: THE SHADOW, A CONNOR BURKE MARTIAL ARTS THRILLER
KATA AND THE TRANSMISSION OF KNOWLEDGE
KRAV MAGA: WEAPON DEFENSES
LITTLE BLACK BOOK OF VIOLENCE
LIUHEBAFA FIVE CHARACTER SECRETS
MARTIAL ARTS ATHLETE
MARTIAL ARTS INSTRUCTION
MARTIAL WAY AND ITS VIRTUES
MASK OF THE KING
MEDITATIONS ON VIOLENCE
MIND/BODY FITNESS
MUGAI RYU
NATURAL HEALING WITH QIGONG
NORTHERN SHAOLIN SWORD, 2ND ED.
OKINAWA'S COMPLETE KARATE SYSTEM: ISSHIN RYU
POWER BODY
PRINCIPLES OF TRADITIONAL CHINESE MEDICINE
QIGONG FOR HEALTH & MARTIAL ARTS, 2ND ED.
QIGONG FOR LIVING
QIGONG FOR TREATING COMMON AILMENTS

QIGONG MASSAGE
QIGONG MEDITATION: EMBRYONIC BREATHING
QIGONG MEDITATION: SMALL CIRCULATION
QIGONG, THE SECRET OF YOUTH: DA MO'S CLASSICS
QUIET TEACHER: A XENON PEARL MARTIAL ARTS THRILLER
RAVEN'S WARRIOR
ROOT OF CHINESE QIGONG, 2ND ED.
SCALING FORCE
SENSEI: A CONNOR BURKE MARTIAL ARTS THRILLER
SHIHAN TE: THE BUNKAI OF KATA
SHIN GI TAI: KARATE TRAINING FOR BODY, MIND, AND SPIRIT
SIMPLE CHINESE MEDICINE
SIMPLE QIGONG EXERCISES FOR HEALTH, 3RD ED.
SIMPLIFIED TAI CHI CHUAN, 3RD ED.
SUDDEN DAWN: THE EPIC JOURNEY OF BODHIDHARMA
SUNRISE TAI CHI
SUNSET TAI CHI
SURVIVING ARMED ASSAULTS
TAE KWON DO: THE KOREAN MARTIAL ART
TAEKWONDO BLACK BELT POOMSAE
TAEKWONDO: A PATH TO EXCELLENCE
TAEKWONDO: ANCIENT WISDOM FOR THE MODERN WARRIOR
TAEKWONDO: DEFENSES AGAINST WEAPONS
TAEKWONDO: SPIRIT AND PRACTICE
TAO OF BIOENERGETICS
TAI CHI BALL QIGONG: FOR HEALTH AND MARTIAL ARTS
TAI CHI BOOK
TAI CHI CHUAN CLASSICAL YANG STYLE (REVISED EDITION)
TAI CHI CHUAN MARTIAL APPLICATIONS, 2ND ED.
TAI CHI CONNECTIONS
TAI CHI DYNAMICS
TAI CHI QIGONG, 3RD ED.
TAI CHI SECRETS OF THE ANCIENT MASTERS
TAI CHI SECRETS OF THE WU & LI STYLES
TAI CHI SECRETS OF THE WU STYLE
TAI CHI SECRETS OF THE YANG STYLE
TAI CHI THEORY & MARTIAL POWER, 2ND ED.
TAI CHI WALKING
TAIJI CHIN NA
TAIJI SWORD: CLASSICAL YANG STYLE
TAIJIQUAN THEORY OF DR. YANG, JWING-MING
TENGU: THE MOUNTAIN GOBLIN, A CONNOR BURKE MARTIAL ARTS THRILLER
TRADITIONAL CHINESE HEALTH SECRETS
TRADITIONAL TAEKWONDO
WAY OF KATA
WAY OF KENDO AND KENJITSU
WAY OF SANCHIN KATA
WAY TO BLACK BELT
WESTERN HERBS FOR MARTIAL ARTISTS
WILD GOOSE QIGONG
WISDOM'S WAY
WOMAN'S QIGONG GUIDE
XINGYIQUAN, 2ND ED.

more products available from . . .

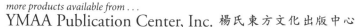

YMAA Publication Center, Inc. 楊氏東方文化出版中心

1-800-669-8892 • info@ymaa.com • www.ymaa.com

DVDS FROM YMAA

ADVANCED PRACTICAL CHIN NA IN-DEPTH

ANALYSIS OF SHAOLIN CHIN NA

BAGUAZHANG: EMEI BAGUAZHANG

CHEN STYLE TAIJIQUAN

CHIN NA IN-DEPTH COURSES 1–4

CHIN NA IN-DEPTH COURSES 5–8

CHIN NA IN-DEPTH COURSES 9–12

FACING VIOLENCE: 7 THINGS A MARTIAL ARTIST MUST KNOW

FIVE ANIMAL SPORTS

JOINT LOCKS

KNIFE DEFENSE: TRADITIONAL TECHNIQUES AGAINST A DAGGER

KUNG FU BODY CONDITIONING 1

KUNG FU BODY CONDITIONING 2

KUNG FU FOR KIDS

KUNG FU FOR TEENS

LOGIC OF VIOLENCE

NORTHERN SHAOLIN SWORD : SAN CAI JIAN, KUN WU JIAN, QI MEN JIAN

QIGONG MASSAGE

QIGONG FOR HEALING

QIGONG FOR LONGEVITY

QIGONG FOR WOMEN

SABER FUNDAMENTAL TRAINING

SANCHIN KATA: TRADITIONAL TRAINING FOR KARATE POWER

SHAOLIN KUNG FU FUNDAMENTAL TRAINING: COURSES 1 & 2

SHAOLIN LONG FIST KUNG FU: BASIC SEQUENCES

SHAOLIN LONG FIST KUNG FU: INTERMEDIATE SEQUENCES

SHAOLIN LONG FIST KUNG FU: ADVANCED SEQUENCES 1

SHAOLIN LONG FIST KUNG FU: ADVANCED SEQUENCES 2

SHAOLIN SABER: BASIC SEQUENCES

SHAOLIN STAFF: BASIC SEQUENCES

SHAOLIN WHITE CRANE GONG FU BASIC TRAINING: COURSES 1 & 2

SHAOLIN WHITE CRANE GONG FU BASIC TRAINING: COURSES 3 & 4

SHUAI JIAO: KUNG FU WRESTLING

SIMPLE QIGONG EXERCISES FOR ARTHRITIS RELIEF

SIMPLE QIGONG EXERCISES FOR BACK PAIN RELIEF

SIMPLIFIED TAI CHI CHUAN: 24 & 48 POSTURES

SUNRISE TAI CHI

SUNSET TAI CHI

SWORD: FUNDAMENTAL TRAINING

TAEKWONDO KORYO POOMSAE

TAI CHI BALL QIGONG: COURSES 1 & 2

TAI CHI BALL QIGONG: COURSES 3 & 4

TAI CHI CHUAN CLASSICAL YANG STYLE

TAI CHI CONNECTIONS

TAI CHI ENERGY PATTERNS

TAI CHI FIGHTING SET

TAI CHI PUSHING HANDS: COURSES 1 & 2

TAI CHI PUSHING HANDS: COURSES 3 & 4

TAI CHI SWORD: CLASSICAL YANG STYLE

TAI CHI SYMBOL: YIN YANG STICKING HANDS

TAIJI & SHAOLIN STAFF: FUNDAMENTAL TRAINING

TAIJI CHIN NA IN-DEPTH

TAIJI 37 POSTURES MARTIAL APPLICATIONS

TAIJI SABER CLASSICAL YANG STYLE

TAIJI WRESTLING

UNDERSTANDING QIGONG 1: WHAT IS QI? • HUMAN QI CIRCULATORY SYSTEM

UNDERSTANDING QIGONG 2: KEY POINTS • QIGONG BREATHING

UNDERSTANDING QIGONG 3: EMBRYONIC BREATHING

UNDERSTANDING QIGONG 4: FOUR SEASONS QIGONG

UNDERSTANDING QIGONG 5: SMALL CIRCULATION

UNDERSTANDING QIGONG 6: MARTIAL QIGONG BREATHING

WHITE CRANE HARD & SOFT QIGONG

WUDANG KUNG FU: FUNDAMENTAL TRAINING

WUDANG SWORD

WUDANG TAIJIQUAN

XINGYIQUAN

YANG TAI CHI FOR BEGINNERS

YMAA 25-YEAR ANNIVERSARY DVD

more products available from . . .

YMAA Publication Center, Inc. 楊氏東方文化出版中心

1-800-669-8892 • info@ymaa.com • www.ymaa.com